Clinical Gastroenterology in the Elderly

Gastroenterology and Hepatology

Executive Editor

J. Thomas LaMont, M.D.

Chief, Division of Gastroenterology
Beth Israel Hospital
Boston, Massachusetts
and
Irving W. Rabb Professor of Medicine
Harvard Medical School
Boston, Massachusetts

Clinical Gastroenterology in the Elderly

edited by

Alvin M. Gelb

Beth Israel Medical Center, New York
and Albert Einstein College of Medicine
Bronx, New York

Marcel Dekker, Inc.   New York•Basel•Hong Kong

Library of Congress Cataloging-in-Publication Data

Clinical gastroenterology in the elderly / edited by Alvin M. Gelb.
   p. cm.-- (Gastroenterology and hepatology ; 2)
   Includes index.
   ISBN 0-8247-9398-6 (hardcover : alk. paper)
   1. Geriatric gastroenterology. I. Gelb, Alvin M.
  II. Series: Gastroenterology and hepatology (New York, N.Y.) ; 2.
  [DNLM: 1. Digestive System Diseases--in old age. 2. Digestive
System Diseases--therapy. WI 140 C6405 1996]
  RC802.4.A34C55 1996
  618.97'633--dc20
  DNLM/DLC
  for Library of Congress
                                               96-23406
                                                CIP

The publisher offers discounts on this book when ordered in bulk quantities. For more information, write to Special Sales/Professional Marketing at the address below.

This book is printed on acid-free paper.

MARCEL DEKKER, INC.
270 Madison Avenue, New York, New York 10016

Current printing (last digit):
10 9 8 7 6 5 4 3 2 1

Printed in the United States of America

To my daughter, Janet, of blessed memory
and for my sons, who follow in my footsteps

Do not cast me off in my old age;
When my strength fails do not forsake me!

Psalm 71, verse 9

Preface

Why study the elderly? One simple reason is that they make up a large part of our patient population. There are all kinds of statistics indicating that people are living longer, especially those over the age of 80. One does not need statistical evidence, however, to know this. If you walk down almost any street in an urban center, you cannot help seeing the numbers of elderly people. If you go to cities where retirees congregate, you cannot help but be overwhelmed by the population density. Physicians are encountering the elderly in their practice much more than in past years. It is not rare to have several patients in their 80s and 90s in an office or hospital at one time.

What is it we are attempting in this book and whom are we trying to reach? A prime target audience is gerontologists, who in their day-to-day practice frequently encounter gastroenterological problems. Perhaps a fifth of medical problems are of this nature. Many of these problems can be handled by the gerontologist, and do not need to be referred to a gastroenterologist.

We are also attempting to lay down some general principles for gastroenterologists on how to shift their focus when dealing with the elderly. Only a few years ago, gastroenterologists received little or no training in geriatrics. And we are trying to reach generalists, to provide them with specific principles of gastroenterology. It is to the busy practitioner or house staff officer in need of a quick—but focused—reference source that this book is aimed.

Although there are books on geriatrics with chapters on gastroenterology, and even books devoted exclusively to geriatric gastroenterology, an up-to-date reference source, such as this book, is necessary because progress in this field is occurring very rapidly—almost as rapidly as the number of geriatric patients is increasing. These same patients are increasingly availing themselves of medical care. Today, we are caring for older patients in unforeseen ways: doctors who do not specialize in geriatrics but treat a wider spectrum of patients are being forced to think more and more about the care of the very old. We hope this book will be useful to them.

Does the study of geriatrics have validity apart from the study of general medicine? Or, put another way, are the elderly special or are they the tail end of a curve? I am reminded of a debate that took place in the 19th century regarding pediatrics. The question then was, is pediatrics a specialty, or are babies and children just little adults? A hundred years later, that debate seems ludicrous. Everyone agrees that pediatrics is a legitimate specialty. The debate concerning geriatrics as a special study may very well seem equally ludicrous a hundred years from now. I am also reminded of the folk saying, "Once an adult, twice a child." If the beginning of life deserves special attention, perhaps the end of life merits special attention as well.

People who divide youth, middle age, and old age into early and late stages also have a point. In this book, we are not very concerned with the active, vigorous people who are in the "youth" of old age; it is the "old" old on whom we concentrate, since they have special problems peculiar to the last decades of life. It is impossible to state an exact age at which there is a transition to "old" old. We will know someone who is "young" at 90 or "old" at 60.

What distinguishes geriatric gastroenterology from more general gastroenterology? The answer falls along several lines. There is the differing incidence of certain diseases in the elderly. More than that, however, is the comorbidity factor. In the elderly, there is often not one disease but many other diseases that have to be considered in the therapeutic decisions and prognosis. Even if comorbidity does not enter the picture, there is diminished reserve as people age. There is also diminished therapeutic benefit to be gained as life expectancy decreases. To put it succinctly, the risk/benefit ratio is increased as people age, and influences therapeutic decisions.

Finally, in this preface I want to thank the many people, in addition to the authors, who helped in the creation of this book. They are those who made suggestions, edited, or typed. Their efforts are appreciated.

Alvin M. Gelb

Contents

Contributors

Howard L. Beaton, M.D. Chief of Surgery, New York Downtown Hospital, New York, New York

Karl T. Bednarek, M.D. Associate Attending, Department of Medicine, Beth Israel Medical Center, New York, New York

Mark Chu, D.O. Department of Medicine, Beth Israel Medical Center, New York, New York

David J. Clain, M.D., F.A.C.P., F.R.C.P. Associate Professor of Medicine, Albert Einstein College of Medicine, Bronx, and Head, Department of Liver Diseases, Beth Israel Medical Center, New York, New York

Seth A. Cohen, M.D. Attending Physician, Department of Medicine, Beth Israel Medical Center, New York, New York

Bradley A. Connor, M.D. Clinical Instructor and Assistant Attending Physician, Division of Digestive Diseases, Department of Medicine, The New York Hospital–Cornell Medical Center, New York, New York

Henry Ferstenberg, M.D. Associate Clinical Professor, Albert Einstein College of Medicine, Bronx, and Department of Surgery, Beth Israel Medical Center, New York, New York

Jeffrey S. Gamss, M.D. Gastroenterologist, Beth Israel Medical Center, New York, New York

Alvin M. Gelb, M.D. Chief, Division of Gastroenterology, Department of Medicine, and Attending Physician, Beth Israel Medical Center, New York, and Professor of Medicine, Albert Einstein College of Medicine, Bronx, New York

Hillel S. Hammerman, M.D.   Associate Director, Division of Gastroenterology, North Division, Beth Israel Medical Center, New York, New York

Daniel Helburn, M.D.   Gastroenterologist, Hamden Internal Medicine, Hamden, Connecticut

Franklin E. Kasmin, M.D., F.A.C.P.   Attending Gastroenterologist, Beth Israel Medical Center, New York, New York

Arthur E. Lindner, M.D.   Associate Professor, Department of Medicine, New York University School of Medicine, New York, New York

Carole A. Michelsen, M.D.   Director of Geriatric Medicine, Department of Medicine, Beth Israel Medical Center, New York, New York

Michael Ruoff, M.D.   Clinical Professor, Department of Medicine, New York University School of Medicine, New York, New York

Ellen J. Scherl, M.D.   Associate Attending, Division of Gastroenterology, Department of Medicine, Beth Israel Medical Center, and Assistant Attending, Department of Gastroenterology, Mount Sinai Hospital, New York, New York

Beth Schorr-Lesnick, M.D., F.A.C.P., F.A.C.G.   Assistant Professor of Medicine, Albert Einstein College of Medicine, Bronx, and Assistant Attending, Department of Medicine, Beth Israel Medical Center, New York, New York

Jerome H. Siegel, M.D., F.A.C.P., F.A.C.G.   Chief, Division of Endoscopy, North Division, Beth Israel Medical Center, New York, and Associate Clinical Professor of Medicine, Albert Einstein College of Medicine, Bronx, New York

Wataru Tamura, M.D.   Chief Resident in Medicine, Beth Israel Medical Center, New York, New York

Robert A. Weiss, M.D.   Associate Attending, Division of Gastroenterology, Department of Medicine, Beth Israel Medical Center, New York, New York

Clinical Gastroenterology in the Elderly

The Aged in General—Demographics, Physiology, Immunology, and Pharmacology

Alvin M. Gelb
Beth Israel Medical Center, New York, and Albert Einstein College of
Medicine, Bronx, New York

I. INTRODUCTION AND DEMOGRAPHICS

Physicians have been criticized for what they do, and for what they do not do, for the elderly. In *Modern Maturity,* the magazine of the American Association of Retired Persons, an article from *U.S. News and World Report* is summarized (1). The report states that the article is on the "medical mistreatment of the elderly," a widely held belief, especially among the elderly. Among the points made is that "medical neglect of the aged begins before illness strikes" and that "few screening guidelines refer specifically to people over 65." It advises the elderly to speak up, to question assertions based solely on age, and to get the family involved. That this perception of neglect of the elderly is widespread is real. Even if untrue, it is something with which the healing professions have to deal. It is obvious to physicians that even at the same chronological age, elderly persons may be at very different physiological age and comorbidity may be very different. Making screening guidelines to cover all, or even the majority, of elderly people is difficult if not impossible. It may be necessary to make separate guidelines for separate decades of life, factoring in comorbidity.

Certain guidelines that apply in a general way to all people, may apply also to the elderly. At all ages people should eat a nutritious diet and refrain from smoking. Exercise is advised for all, but it is generally recognized that the elderly may be limited by the physiology of aging and whatever illnesses they suffer. In a general way and from the physician's viewpoint, the elderly are a group that have a diminished reserve and a diminished life expectancy even without comorbidity.

Whatever the reason, the fact is that the healing professions are increasingly concerned with the health and maintenance problems of the elderly. Both in medical schools and in hospitals, there are new geriatric services which are growing quite rapidly. The National Institutes of Health in the United States is becoming much more focused on the problems of the elderly. More attention is being paid in the medical literature. Both articles and textbooks are more concerned with diseases of the aged. This book, even this entire series of books, is evidence of that attention.

It is worthwhile to consider some of the factors driving this increased interest in the elderly. First of all, there are the demographics (2–4). The elderly, who made up 4.5% of the population in the United States in 1990, are projected to constitute 13.1% by the year 2005. This growth is seen worldwide: 250 million people over 65 are being projected for the year 2025. At least in developed countries, the genesis of some of our current problems lies in the success of medical efforts, especially public health, which has significantly reduced early mortality, resulting in an increased lifespan. Appreciation of the need for hygienic measures to control infectious diseases, along with vaccines and antibiotics, had led to many more people surviving long enough to be considered elderly. Even among the elderly, life expectancy is increasing. In the United States, life expectancy increased about 1.4% from 1970 to 1990. There may be, however, a limit to this increase in survival. It has been suggested that there may be a compression so that morbidity and mortality will come closer together at the end of life.

The aging of the population and the possible compression of mortality and morbidity is resulting in a second factor which must be considered, the allocation of resources. At least in the United States at this time, where there is a large deficit, there is much debate about the healthcare portion of the budget. What to do for the elderly, and how to do it, is a large part of the debate. The 13% of our population over 65 receive about 33% of our healthcare budget. A *New York Times* article of June 18, 1993, states that even with contemplated reductions, Medicare costs would increase from a 1992 level of $129 billion, to $220 billion in 1998 (5). Without reductions, the cost in 1998 would be $258 billion a year.

Another factor discussed in the article in the *New York Times* concerning the Medicare debate is the increasing concern of the media with health problems in today's society. Articles appear on the front page of the newspaper chronicling the latest medical developments. There are columnists assigned both to give the latest medical news and to discuss it for the layperson. Not only in the newspapers is health being considered, but various organizations, including hospitals, are publishing brochures for the lay public and holding seminars. Pharmaceutical companies and hospitals advertise in newspapers, in magazines, and on billboards. The role of television in promoting health consciousness cannot be underestimated. "Health fairs" are being sponsored by all sorts of organizations.

This healthcare concern of the population is occurring at the same time as another phenomenon. People are increasingly organizing into special-interest groups and are becoming more aggressive in lobbying for their concerns. The elderly are no exception to this. They are making known their concerns in both writing and speaking.

To be considered is how all these trends impact on the individual physician in the practice of medicine: what to do when the daily newspaper or television carries the latest medical development before he even receives the medical journal in which the development is published, let alone has time to read it. He gets calls from patients concerning things he knows little or nothing about. The media need to present material as established fact, rather than with uncertainty that is characteristic of medicine as to the potential for something new to be real or to be eventually supplemented by another development.

Despite these things, the elderly are calling on the practitioner more and more, appearing more frequently in the waiting rooms. Not only are there more of them but they are more health conscious. It is not a rarity for a physician to see in a single day several patients in their 80s and some in their 90s. There is even a rare patient over 100. The physician must consider, in addition to the presenting problem, the aging process itself and how it affects presentation. Also to be considered are the difficulty in doing diagnostic tests, other diseases that may be present, and the response to multiple drugs. The elderly may give poor histories because of mental defect, which also may lead to nutritional problems. The gastroenterologist must be involved in the problems of aging, since about 20% of illnesses are gastrointestinal, and mortality from GI problems is of significant proportions. One cannot help but notice that the aged are being discussed at medical conferences more often in recent times.

II. PHYSIOLOGY

Gerontology is at an early state in its development. There is a great deal of variation in the observations made in different types of cells and species. Differences in methods contribute to this variation, which is often contradictory.

There are many theories of aging, some of which relate to our genes being programmed at birth (6). Modifier genes, which suppress degenerative changes, which at some point become ineffective, are one theory of aging. There may be differences in repetition of DNA, or there may be differences in the ability of DNA to repair itself. Gene redundancy may vary. Another theory is that aging may be due to accumulation of defects in macromolecules. Chromosomal aberrations, perhaps due to ionizing radiation or heat, have been considered. Changes in DNA are thought to be related to age changes. DNA is damaged by physical, chemical, and biological factors. The role of aging on RNA synthesis or on alterations in the nucleus is unknown.

Nongenetic theories have also been considered. Hormonal factors and autoimmunity have been discussed. Free radicals and cross-linkage may also play a part. Energy restriction and supplementation of borderline deficiencies of vitamins and minerals may have a role in achieving longevity, either directly or through other mechanisms.

Discussion of aging, a failure to maintain hemostasis, must involve connective tissue, the chemistry of which is complex beyond the scope of this book. Some of the things that affect connective tissue are important to consider (7). These include collagen cross-linking, gene splicing degenerative enzymes, cytokines, and the effect of radiation disease. The loss of elasticity with aging is obvious. There is an increase in the ratio of fat to lean body mass.

III. IMMUNOLOGY

There is much evidence that aging affects the immune system. In the past two decades there has been an explosion of our knowledge about this system, and there have been many experiments on young versus old animals (8, 9). If one believes that tumor formation is a failure of immunosurveillance, that in itself is evidence for immunosenescence. Vaccination is less successful in older people. The effect of aging on the thymus, which affects T-lymphocytes, is clear. It is the T-cells that are most affected by aging. Bone marrow function and B-cell formation are relatively preserved. Changes in thymic hormones are critical. Inhibition of calcium influx in the aging T-cell may result in inactivation of the T-cell, which in turn may inhibit cytokine secretion. Those T-cells that do become activated may be limited in their ability to continue the cell cycle. It is known that DNA repair mechanisms are diminished. The ratio of T-cell subsets generally remains the same.

The cytokine most extensively studied is interleukin-2 (IL-2), whose synthesis markedly decreases with aging. Those cells that do produce IL-2 continue their same level of production, but the number of such cells is reduced.

An increase in suppressor mechanisms may contribute to aging of the immune system. Antibodies to antibodies also have a role. The role of nutritional factors in maintaining the immune system is not clear. Nor is it clear what is due to disease and what is normal aging.

The prevention of senescence in the immune system becomes important. The roles of potentially reversible causes such as malnutrition, disease, and medications have to be considered, along with the use of vaccines in the elderly. In the future we may see the development of pharmaceutical approaches to age-related changes in the immune system.

IV. PHARMACOLOGY

About a quarter of all prescribed medications are used by people older than 65. It is estimated by the year 2030, it will be 40% (9). There are both a lack of information about these drugs and a lack of knowledge among physicians. How the medication is distributed in the body depends on absorption, distribution, and elimination by liver and kidneys (10, 11). The changes in these parameters with aging is, in turn, dependent on altered anatomy and physiology. Increase in fat and decrease in lean mass in older people affect drug distribution. Fat-soluble medicines distribute more widely, and water-soluble ones less widely, in the aged. Protein binding may be altered, and there may be reduced hepatic metabolism. Reduced renal elimination of drugs is probably due to reduced renal function in the aged.

Not only are there effects on metabolism, but there may also be changes in responsiveness of different organs. The chemistry of this is complex. Adverse reactions may occur, the incidence increasing with age. In those over 65 years, it probably occurs in 10–20% of people.

The problems caused by polypharmacy, which is widespread in the aged, are important. The more drugs taken, the greater the risk of an adverse reaction. Old people take on the average somewhere between three and eight medications. The nature and severity of comorbidity must also be considered. The mental status of the elderly is important in that it may affect their ability to take medication as ordered—their ability to follow instructions. The physician has to be aware not only of the pharmacology of the medicine, but of the nature and capabilities of the person for whom the medicine is prescribed. If possible, older persons should know the common adverse reactions of prescribed medications.

REFERENCES

1. Podolsky D, Silberner J. The doctor is out. Modern Maturity 1993; 36(1):91.
2. Katz S. Gastrointestinal disease of the elderly; introduction to the series. Prac Gastroenterol 1993; 17(5):9.

3. Grundy E. The epidemiology of aging. In: Brocklehurst JC, Tallis RC, Fillit HM, eds. Textbook of Geriatric Medicine and Gerontology, 4th ed. Edinburgh: Churchill Livingstone, 1992:3–20.
4. Holt PR. General perspectives on the aged gut. Clin Geriatr Med 1991; 7(2):185–189.
5. Pear R. Cutting health dollars to heal deficit. New York Times 1993; Jun 18:A21(col 4–6).
6. Davies I. Theories and general principles of aging. In: Brocklehurst JC, Tallis RC, Fillit. Textbook of Geriatric Medicine and Gerontology, 4th ed. New York: Churchill Livingstone, 1992:26–60.
7. Kefalides NA, Alper R. Aging and connective tissues. In: Brocklehurst JC, Tallis RC, Fillit. Textbook of Geriatric Medicine and Gerontology, 4th ed. New York: Churchill Livingstone, 1992:61–70.
8. Weigle WO. Effects of aging on the immune system. Hosp Pract 1989; 24(12):112–119.
9. Wexler ME. Aging and the immune system. Infect Dis Clin Pract 1994; 3(6):464–467.
10. Woodhouse KW, Wynne HA. The pharmacology of aging. In: Brocklehurst JC, Tallis RC, Fillit. Textbook of Geriatric Medicine and Gerontology, 4th ed. New York: Churchill Livingstone, 1992:1129–1142.
11. Mayersohn M. Special pharmacokinetic considerations in the elderly. In: Evans WE, Schentag JJ, Jusko WJ, eds. Applied Pharmacokinetics: Principles of Therapeutic Drug Monitoring. 2d ed. Spokane, WA: Applied Therapeutics, 1986:220–293.

2

Assessment of the Elderly Patient

Alvin M. Gelb
Beth Israel Medical Center, New York, and Albert Einstein College of Medicine, Bronx, New York

I. ATTITUDES AND EXPECTATIONS

In any discussion of the encounter between a patient and the physician, the attitudes and expectations of both parties must be considered. The need for this discussion is particularly true in geriatrics.

First to be considered is the attitude of the doctor, who is usually considerably younger than the patient (1). Attitude is influenced by the general culture we live in; quite simply, we live in a culture that worships youth and abhors aging. Millions of dollars are spent both in advertising and in merchandising to promote the cult of youth, and the public spends more millions in its pursuit. It is naïve to think that doctors can escape this cultural barrage. The systematic study of the old and their diseases is relatively new, and only now are medical students and residents being exposed to geriatrics in a formal manner in order to counter some of the cultural stereotypes.

Another factor in the attitude of younger physicians is what psychiatrics call denial. In confronting the aged patient, perhaps one who is dying, doctors are faced with the reality that they also will age and die. This reality colors their attitude. Sometimes they deal with this by distancing themselves from emotional involvement with the patient. It is even possible that some of the conflict between the young physician and his own parents may resonate in the encounter with the geriatric patient. It has been my observation that young physicians in training contemplate major illness in a geriatric patient as occurring almost in a different species. Major illness, however, especially fatal illness in a patient close in age to the young doctor, often has major emotional impact. They identify with the young patient in a way they do not with the older patient.

The last thing to be considered from the point of view of the physician is that caring for a geriatric patient adds to the work load of an already busy doctor. The patient is slow in every phase of the encounter, walking slowly into the examining room, slowly undressing and dressing, often needing aid along the way. The patient is often confused, making it difficult to obtain an accurate history. The diagnosis and treatment may not be straightforward, since there may be multiple diseases and treatments to consider. A treatment that may be appropriate for one condition may not be appropriate for another and has to be modified. Polypharmacy must be considered; instructions may not be remembered, and often have to be repeated. There is often confusion necessitating follow-up phone calls. Additional time is often necessary, and the physician's schedule may be greatly upset.

Second, the attitudes and expectations of geriatric patients must be explored. Expectations may be quite unrealistic (2, 3). They remember when they were young, when all systems worked well, and when they had no symptoms. They may not realize that much of what they now experience is part of normal aging, about which the physician can do little. The patient is aware of failing memory, muscular and arthritic complaints, and other functional problems. Only temporary relief can be given; sometimes no relief. On occasion, in an attempt to alleviate symptoms, more serious disease is caused. The legendary quest for the fountain of youth continues. There is a bit of humor that says if an elderly person awakes without pains, he should check the obituary page of the local newspaper before arising, to see if he is listed. As with all humor, there is a grain of truth.

Another problem to be considered is the fact that some older patients consult physicians frequently. By seeing the patient so often the doctor may be lulled into assuming the current problem is of the same self-limiting nature as were the previous problems. The current problem may not be seen for what it is because "wolf" has been cried too often.

There is a concise pamphlet entitled "Working With Your Older Patient: A Clinician's Handbook" distributed by the National Institutes of Health. In it many excellent points are made. The elderly population is very diverse. Some are frail; some healthy. Some desire a paternalistic approach, while others will challenge the physician. Cultural or ethnic heritage varies, as does level of education. Significant symptoms are often dismissed as "part of aging." Expectations may vary. Some want to be kept comfortable no matter what, while others want to prolong life at any cost. Religious beliefs enter into this, as well as into other aspects.

Older people often have sensory defects such as hearing and visual deficits. Sometimes their sensorium is clouded. The clinician must go slowly, and allow time for response. Past history, medications, family history, and social history are more important in the elderly than in younger patients. The elderly often have to be encouraged to discuss sensitive issues. These sensitive areas may include sexuality, incontinence, elder abuse, depression, long-term care, terminal care, and death.

Both the patient and the caregiver should be educated and encouraged to ask questions, but do not overload them with too much and too technical information. Keep treatment, especially medications, as simple as possible. Providing written instructions may help. The importance of the role that the family and other caregivers play cannot be overemphasized.

II. PRESENTATION OF DISEASE

Before proceeding to the details in the diagnostic process, it should be appreciated that elderly patients, more so than younger patients, have atypical symptoms, signs, and test results (4). In fact, symptoms, signs, or tests may be normal even in the face of major, life-threatening disease. The absence or mildness of symptoms may lead to significant delay in seeking medical help and may lead to delay on the part of the physician in appreciating the seriousness of what is happening.

Why symptoms, signs, and test results may not reflect the severity of the disease that is occurring is not clear. A possible reason for some of this may be that mental faculties may not be as clear as formerly, and there may be a degree of confusion. That objective findings are altered may be due to such things as changes in the immune system, which can alter the response to disease. Our understanding of how and why the elderly experience disease and the influence of comorbidity is very limited.

III. HISTORY

Obtaining the history can be difficult (5). There may be confusion and/or memory deficits, or there may be other sensory deficits. As already alluded to, important symptoms may be atypical or absent. The patient may be bothered more by something that has little importance to the physician, who may thus neglect a symptom of a disease with major ramifications. A careful review of symptoms is necessary. Vague words are often used regarding the nature and duration of symptoms. The patient may not stay focused on the problem being considered, bringing forth much extraneous material.

Medications are a problem because of memory defects. The patient may not know what is being taken. The medications themselves may cause or add to confusion. The patient may be hesitant about asking questions or asking that the directions be repeated or written. He may try to fake the fact that he is confused.

Problems with social situation, alcoholism, financial matters, or other stresses that may affect symptoms are often not disclosed. Some patients may talk too much and may camouflage essential material in a querulous manner. Others may talk too little, not giving sufficient clues to the nature of the problem. A significant factor is the frequent presence of depression, which may not be recognized but may color the history. Problems arise with both the overreporting and underreporting of symptoms. The patient may feel if he does not complain enough or is not sufficiently dramatic he will not get the doctor's attention. On the other hand, he may feel that if he complains too much, the doctor will be annoyed.

IV. PHYSICAL EXAMINATION

It is a cliché that a complete examination must be done, but in fact attention must be directed more extensively to certain items than is necessary in younger people (5). Nutrition and hydration must be carefully considered. Does the patient have sufficient teeth, either natural or artificial, to accomplish adequate nutrition? Is the patient drinking enough, or is there evidence of dehydration? The carotid arteries should be checked for bruits. The spine should be checked for range of motion, since arthritis is so common. Cancer being so frequent in the elderly, breasts and rectum must be examined carefully. Circulatory problems should be considered, especially in the vessels of the leg. Consideration should be given to glaucoma and dysequilibrium, both of which are common.

V. LABORATORY AND SPECIAL PROCEDURES

Routine laboratory tests often show a minor degree of abnormality. Reserve in many organs has been used up, and there is less margin. The tests that measure the status of the heart, liver, and kidneys may be slightly abnormal, even though there is no significant disease. Conversely, as has been previously stated, tests may be normal or minimally abnormal even in the face of serious disease. In the history, physical exam, and laboratory, attention should be directed not only to the dominant disease, but to the comorbidity and to diminished reserve, remembering that in the elderly the risk/benefit rate is increased.

VI. SPECIALIZED TESTS

Specialized tests may be more of a problem with the elderly, both in the preparation for the tests and in their performance and interpretation. Many tests are invasive, carrying with them significant risk. There is sometimes ambivalence on the part of the physician. He asks himself whether the test is really necessary, whether it is worth putting the elderly patient through so much discomfort, whether the elderly patient can manage the preparation. The cardiopulmonary risk must also be considered.

Barium studies by the radiologist in elderly patients have been studied (6, 7). Reports in the literature indicate that about 60–70% of barium meal examinations are of either good or excellent quality. There was no relationship between age and mobility, and the ability to obtain an adequate exam. At least in preparation for a barium enema, patients over 75 years of age are no more likely than those aged 55 to 74 to have problems with preparation (8). My personal experience is that preparation for barium enema is taxing on elderly patients, especially those who have no one to help them. Hospitalizing the patient may help, but in the current regulatory climate this may be difficult or impossible. In the performance of the test, experience is that the difficulty of the barium study is related to the patient's mental status–his ability to cooperate and follow directions. Sometimes, with barium enema studies, a balloon has to be used to allow the patient to retain the barium well enough for an adequate study.

Gastrointestinal endoscopy in the very elderly, especially those who have or have had cardiopulmonary disease, is a problem (9, 10). The difficulty of preparation, especially for colonoscopy, must be considered. The dosage of sedative medication must frequently be reduced. There may be periods when oxygen saturation is below normal. Cardiac irregularities, both rhythm and ECG changes, have been observed in patients who are being monitored. It is stated that elderly patients should have nasal oxygen and cardiopulmonary monitoring during endoscopy. It is not clear that those measures alter morbidity or mortality. The experience of most endoscopists is that more time, effort, and care must be spent on the very elderly patient. Where it has been studied in a systematic fashion, endoscopy is safe, well tolerated, and helpful even in patients aged 80 or more.

Computerized tomography requires the patient to remain motionless for an extended period of time, which may be difficult for an elderly person and cause a problem in obtaining a reliable study.

The problem of decreased mental faculties, a problem in many aged patients, enters into consideration in all specialized tests several different ways. There is often a problem in obtaining informed consent for the procedure to be done. The instructions to the patient may not be understood, and the patient may thus arrive for the exam not adequately prepared. The physician may not even be aware that the elderly patient does not understand instructions. The confused patient may be so passive that the doctor assumes he is being heard and understood, even when he is not.

The last thing to be considered is the fundamental attitude of the doctor toward disease, especially in the very elderly. Are the results, even if positive, worthwhile, leading to a course of action that will add significantly to useful, comfortable life? On the other hand, is this test an academic exercise done merely to satisfy the intellectual curiosity of the doctor, of no benefit to the patient, possibly prolonging an existence no longer desired? Both physicians and society are wrestling with many basic ethical questions such as these, for which there are no simple answers.

REFERENCES

1. Butler RN. The doctor and the aged patient. In: Reichel W, ed. The Geriatric Patient. New York: HP Publishing, 1978:199–206.
2. Besdine RW. Clinical evaluation of the elderly patient. In: Hazzard WR, Andres R, Bierman EL, Blass JP, eds. Principles of Geriatric Medicine and Gerontology. 2d ed. New York: McGraw-Hill, 1990:175–183.
3. Cassel CK, Walsh JR, Shepard M, Riesenberg D. Clinical evaluation of the patient. In: Cassell CK, Riesenberg DE, Sorenson LB, Walsh JR, eds. Geriatric Medicine. 2d ed. New York: Springer-Verlag, 1990:102–110.
4. France MJ, Vuletic JC, Koelmeyer TD. Does advancing age modify the presentation of disease? Am J Forensic Med Pathol 1992; 13(2):120–123.
5. Steinberg FU. Evaluation and treatment of the geriatric patient. In: Steinberg FU, ed. Care of the Geriatric Patient: In the Tradition of EV Cowdry. St. Louis: Mosby, 1983:39–46.
6. Sangster G, Williams CE, Garvey CJ Jr, Baldwin RN. Disability and the diagnostic quality of barium meals in elderly patients. Age Ageing 1992; 21(2):135–138.
7. Hawkins SP, Rowlands PC, Shorvon PJ. Barium meals in the elderly: a quality reassurance. Br J Radiol 1991; 64(758):113–115.
8. Grad RM, Clarfield AM, Rosenbloom M, Perrone M. Adequacy of preparations for barium enema among elderly outpatients. Can Med Assoc J 1991; 144(10):1257–1261.
9. Lieberman DA, Wuerker CK, Katon RM. Cardiopulmonary risk of esophago-gastroduodenoscopy. Gastroenterology 1985; 88(2):468–472.
10. Cooper BT, Neumann CS. Upper gastrointestinal endoscopy in patients aged 80 years or more. Age Ageing 1986; 15(6):343–349.

3

Esophageal Disease

Robert A. Weiss
Beth Israel Medical Center, New York, New York

I. INTRODUCTION

While diseases of the esophagus are common in patients of all ages, some are unique to the elderly (1). Examples include Zenker's diverticulum, dysphagia caused by cervical osteophytes; dysphagia aortica; and presbyesophagus. Other diseases may begin when the patient is young but not present clinically until many years later, as in the case of Barrett's esophagus and esophageal adenocarcinoma, whose frequencies increase with chronic gastroesophageal reflux disease of long duration. Still others, such as dysmotilities, become more frequent with advancing age. Finally, the effects of medications and coexisting medical conditions must be considered (2) (Table 1).

The most common subjective complaint in a patient with esophageal disease is dysphagia. It can be classified based on the location of the swallowing difficulty. *Oropharyngeal dysphagia* consists of difficulty propelling the bolus from the oral cavity into the cervical esophagus; *transport dysphagia* involves problems in the passage of the bolus through the body of the esophagus; and *esophagogastric dysphagia* denotes problems with the movement of the bolus from the distal esophagus into the proximal stomach.

II. OROPHARYNGEAL DYSPHAGIA

Normal oropharyngeal deglutition is accomplished by both voluntary and reflexive control and requires adequate protection of the airway. During the act of swallowing the pharynx is converted from a respiratory conduit

Table 1 Diseases and Conditions
Associated with Old Age

Diseases unique to the elderly
  Zenker's diverticulum
  Cervical osteophytes
  Dysphagia aortica
Onset at younger age; delayed presentation
  Barrett's esophagus
  Adenocarcinoma
Increased frequency with advancing age
  Dysmotility
  "Pill" esophagitis
  Underlying diseases

to a food pathway thereby preventing nasal regurgitation or passage of the ingested bolus into the airway. It is essential that no food residue remain in the hypopharynx following a swallow. This is accomplished by approximation of the muscular soft palate to the posterior wall of the pharynx to protect against nasal regurgitation as well as elevation of the larynx and hyoid bone both to close off the airway and to pull open the upper esophageal sphincter (3). Contraction of the pharyngeal constrictors clears the remaining residue from the hypopharynx.

Trupe et al. (4) have reported incidences of swallowing abnormalities involving the mouth, pharynx, and upper esophageal sphincter ranging from 30% to 50% in elderly nursing home patients. In contrast, the incidence of dysphagia ranges from 10% to 15% in hospitalized patients of all ages.

Patients with oropharyngeal dysphagia will report food lodging in the throat, difficulty initiating the act of swallowing, aspiration or regurgitation of liquid food through the nose, and coughing during swallowing. The latter occurs due to incomplete closure of the glottis, resulting in the passage of food into the respiratory tract (5).

There is a great deal of evidence that aging alone does not cause significant impairment in swallowing. Most physiologic swallowing mechanisms remain intact in the elderly. There may be some slowing of oropharyngeal motility and an increase in the duration of the oropharyngeal swallow. In general, in the elderly patient oropharyngeal dysphagia is usually the result of a specific illness or pathologic condition. These include neurologic, neuromuscular, systemic, immunologic, and psychiatric entities (6) (Table 2).

Diseases involving the swallowing center in the brainstem or the cranial nerves that regulate swallowing (V, VII, IX, X, and XII) can result in

Table 2 Oropharyngeal Dysphagia

Central nervous system
  Stroke
  Parkinsonism
  Multiple Sclerosis
  Wilson's disease
Neuromuscular disorders
  Peripheral neuropathy
  Myasthenia gravis
  Polymyositis/dermatomyositis
  Metabolic (thyroid; diabetes)
Structural lesions
  Tumors
  Strictures
  Webs
  Cervical osteophytes
  Zenker's diverticulum
UES dysfunction
  Hypertensive UES
  Hypotensive UES
  Cricopharyngeal achalasia

oropharyngeal dysphagia. Examples include major strokes (7) and pseudo-bulbar palsy. In *Parkinson's disease* there may be tremors of the tongue and hesitancy in initiating swallows. In addition there may be failure of relaxation of the upper esophageal sphincter (UES) as well of incoordination of UES relaxation with pharyngeal contraction (8). Other CNS diseases in which oropharyngeal dysphagia may occur include multiple sclerosis, amyotrophic lateral sclerosis, and Wilson's disease.

Dysphagia may also be associated with a variety of diseases affecting the peripheral nervous system or the muscles involving the tongue, hypopharynx, and UES. In myasthenia gravis, muscle weakness occurs with repetitive contractions. Dysphagia occurs in approximately two-thirds of affected patients, most often men above the age of 70. There may be associated ptosis and diplopia (9). Other diseases include diabetes mellitus with neuropathy (10), skeletal muscle disorders such as polymyositis and dermatomyositis (11, 12), and metabolic myopathies as seen with thyrotoxicosis (13) and hyperthyroidism.

Oropharyngeal dysphagia may also result from local structural lesions causing obstruction. Intrinsic lesions include carcinoma, strictures, and webs. Included is the Plummer-Vinson syndrome, consisting of sideropenic dysphagia and postcricoid webs, most often seen in middle-aged females. Other clinical findings include glossitis, cheilosis, achlorhydria, splenomegaly, and koilonychia. There is an association with hypopharyngeal carcinoma that may present after several years (14). Extrinsic compression of the upper esophagus is seen with inflammatory conditions such as abscesses, cervical lymphadenopathy, prior neck surgery (particularly thyroid or parathyroid), and enlargement of surrounding structures. This may occur with thyromegaly and, less commonly, with the presence of cervical osteophytes (15).

A cause of dysphagia and other symptoms is Zenker's diverticulum, which is an outpouching of the posterior pharyngeal wall just proximal to the UES. It may be due to an area of congenital weakness of the muscle fibers in the back of the pharynx as well as cricopharyngeal dysfunction leading to high pharyngeal pressures (16). There may also be an association of incomplete UES relaxation with pharyngeal contraction (17).

About 85% of cases occur in people above the age of 50. Symptoms are initially those of oropharyngeal dysphagia. If the diverticulum is large enough to retain food, patients may complain of a feeling of fullness and gurgling in the neck, coughing, and aspiration. Postprandial and nocturnal regurgitation of undigested food may occur. Less commonly, obstructive symptoms may result from compression of the esophagus by a large diverticulum. Treatment is usually surgical, and involves diverticulectomy with or without myotomy (18, 19). There are also reports of endoscopic diverticulotomy for Zenker's diverticulum. This procedure may afford patients a shorter hospital stay with equal efficacy compared with traditional surgical procedures (20).

There are a variety of functional abnormalities of the UES in the elderly that may result in oropharyngeal dysphagia. A *hypertensive UES* causes a sensation of spasm or globus. With a *hypotensive UES* there is regurgitation from the esophagus into the pharynx (21). *Cricopharyngeal achalasia* refers to incomplete relaxation of the UES. There may also be associated premature sphincter closure or a delay in relaxation of the sphincter (22).

In the diagnostic evaluation of patients with oropharyngeal dysphagia, particular attention to the neurologic exam is crucial, as is careful palpation of the head and neck for a neoplasm. The diagnostic study of choice is a barium X-ray of the pharynx and UES with rapid-sequence videofluoroscopy (23). Manometric studies may be indicated.

The treatment of oropharyngeal dysphagia depends on the underlying disease process. With neurologic, muscular, systemic, or metabolic disorders, therapy is targeted at the underlying disorder. Tumors of the head and neck are treated by surgical resection where possible; in other cases radiation and/or chemotherapy are used. With disorders of cricopharyngeal function, there may be a role for surgical myotomy (24), provided there is no evidence for gastroesophageal reflux (25).

III. ESOPHAGEAL DYSPHAGIA

The etiology of esophageal dysphagia may be either *neuromuscular,* manifest as a functional motility disorder, or *mechanical,* as seen with obstructing lesions from a variety of intrinsic or extrinsic causes (Table 3). Clues to the diagnosis may be provided by the history. Important distinguishing features are whether dysphagia occurs with solids as opposed to liquids, progressive vs. intermittent symptoms, and the presence or absence of pyrosis. Functional motility disorders generally result in dysphagia for both liquids and solids, while obstructing lesions tend to be progressive and initially cause dysphagia only for solid foods (26).

In the elderly population, the functional motility disorders include achalasia, diffuse esophageal spasm, and scleroderma. Mechanical etiologies resulting in obstruction include neoplasms, rings or webs, strictures, vascular anomalies, and esophageal injury due to certain medications.

Achalasia consists of the triad of increased lower esophageal sphincter (LES) resting or baseline pressure, failure of the LES to completely relax in response to a swallow, and aperistalsis in the body of the esophagus. Clinically there are slowly progressive dysphagia for both solids and liquids, gradual weight loss, and generally no complaint of chest pain. Undigested food and secretions may remain in the esophagus and result in coughing and aspiration, particularly at night, when the patient is recumbent. As the onset of achalasia is insidious, the diagnosis may be delayed for several

Table 3 Esophageal Dysphagia

Motility disorders
  Achalasia
  Diffuse esophageal spasm
  Scleroderma
Presbyesophagus
Structural disorders
  Tumors
  Strictures
  Rings/webs
  Vascular anomalies
  "Pill" esophagitis

---

years. The pathophysiology of achalasia relates to defective ganglionic cells in the myenteric (Auerbach's) plexus in the wall of the esophagus.

In patients with achalasia, a plain film of the chest may show a dilated esophagus with retained food and secretions producing an air-fluid level. The normal gastric air bubble is absent in about one-half of cases (27). The esophagram shows a dilated, frequently tortuous esophagus with a so-called bird's beak tapering at the esophagogastric junction. This corresponds to the zone of increased pressure in the LES. In achalasia of long duration, the esophagus may assume a sigmoid appearance due to the marked dilatation and tortuosity.

Not only does achalasia carry an increased risk of malignancy. It should be noted that similar abnormal motility may be secondary to underlying malignancies that may infiltrate the submucosa of the distal esophagus. Tumors include distal esophageal and proximal gastric carcinomas as well as lung cancer (particularly oat cell carcinoma), pancreatic cancer, hepatocellular carcinoma (28), sarcomas, mesotheliomas (29), and lymphomas.

Idiopathic achalasia usually has its onset in the 20-to-40-year age group and is uncommon above the age of 50. Thus, in the elderly, the diagnosis of achalasia should prompt a search for a possible underlying malignancy. In patients over the age of 50 who also have dysphagia of under 1 year's duration and weight loss of more than 15 lb, malignancy should be strongly suspected (30). There is an important role for endoscopy with brushings and biopsy. In primary achalasia the endoscope usually passes through the high-pressure area with slight pressure. If, however, there is difficulty in advancing the endoscope into the stomach, the presence of an underlying tumor should be considered. If endoscopic ultrasonography (EUS) is available, it may be useful in the detection of submucosal tumors at the esophagogastric junction (31).

Diffuse esophageal spasm (DES) consists of dysphagia to both solids and liquids, chest pain, and distinctive findings on manometry (32). The pain may resemble that of angina pectoris and in the elderly may be a source of diagnostic uncertainty (33). Barium films of the esophagus may be normal or may reveal a variety of patterns that are variously referred to as tertiary contractions and corkscrew esophagus. Esophageal manometry shows high-amplitude contractions of prolonged duration, frequently repetitive and simultaneous. Of clinical relevance is the fact that these contractions are nonperistaltic. A variant of DES is known as the *nutcracker esophagus,* in which the contractions are of extremely high (>180 mm Hg) amplitude (34).

The most important thing the physician must do is to exclude coronary artery disease as the source of the chest pain. Of patients with chest pain whose coronary arteries are evaluated angiographically, approximately 33%

will be found to have esophageal motility disorders (35), of which DES is most common (36). Since gastroesophageal reflux may provoke esophageal spasm, it is important to evaluate esophageal pH prior to planning therapy.

Therapy consists of nitrates (37) or calcium channel blockers (38) to relax the smooth muscle of the esophagus. If present, gastroesophageal reflux must be aggressively treated. Most importantly, many patients will improve once coronary artery disease has been ruled out with the reassurance that their condition is not life-threatening (39).

The esophagus is involved in over 80% of patients with *scleroderma* (40), especially those with Raynaud's phenomenon. These patients present with progressive dysphagia to solids and liquids, similar to the picture seen with achalasia. There is also, however, a high frequency of pyrosis due to the associated gastroesophageal reflux disorder. This is explained by the manometric findings of decreased LES pressure and diminished peristalsis in the lower (smooth-muscle) portion of the esophagus. Therapy is directed at the gastroesophageal reflux.

A possible entity of considerable interest in the elderly is *presbyesophagus.* It is defined as an age-related change in esophageal motility and function (41). A 1964 study by Soergel et al. (42) examined patients in the ninth decade of life and noted the presence of frequent nonperistaltic, tertiary contractions along with delayed esophageal emptying, a decrease in LES relaxation, and upward displacement of the LES into an intrathoracic position. Other studies have demonstrated a relative weakness in the amplitude of peristaltic contractions (43) and slower velocity of contractions in the upper esophagus (44).

Autopsy studies of the esophagus in elderly patients without clinically apparent esophageal disease have demonstrated morphologic changes that show a decrease in the number of myenteric ganglion cells in Auerbach's plexus. Thickening of the smooth-muscle layer was also seen. A heavy lymphocytic infiltrate was also noted in the myenteric plexus (45).

Presbyesophagus is probably of little clinical significance. It may reflect the increased frequency of other underlying medical conditions that occur in the elderly, such as stroke and diabetes, rather than a primary decrease in esophageal function. Changes in esophageal motility that may be relevant in younger patients may actually be considered normal in the elderly (46).

IV. ESOPHAGOGASTRIC DYSPHAGIA

Esophagogastric dysphagia occurs when there is difficulty in transferring a food bolus from the distal esophagus into the stomach. It can arise from a variety of causes.

Lower esophageal rings or webs can present with intermittent dysphagia to solids, usually nonprogressive in nature. These rings, also known as Schatzki rings, are thin, membranous projections of mucosa located in the vicinity of the squamocolumnar junction (47).

The onset of dysphagia is usually abrupt, and symptoms are those of esophageal obstruction. The initial episode often occurs while the patient is eating steak or bread and has been termed the "steakhouse syndrome" for this reason. Symptoms usually occur when the diameter of the esophageal lumen is narrowed to 12 mm or less (48). The diagnosis can be made by barium esophagography or esophagoscopy (Fig. 1). Treatment usually consists of rupture of the ring, either by bougienage or pneumatic dilatation.

Diaphragmatic or *hiatal hernias* can occur at all ages, but their frequency increases with advancing age (49). In patients above the age of 70 they may be present in 70% of cases (50). This increased incidence with advancing age may be related to age-related changes in the musculature of the hiatus as well as a decrease in the elasticity of the connective tissues of the diaphragm.

The most common type of hiatal hernia is the direct, or sliding, hernia, which accounts for about 90% of cases. The significance, however, of a hiatal

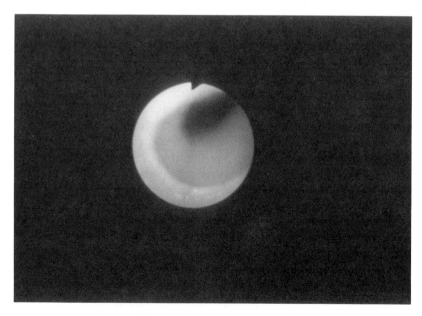

Figure 1   Endoscopic view of a Schatzki ring.

hernia as a causative factor for gastroesophageal reflux is controversial (51). Of greater significance are the strength of the lower esophageal sphincter and its function in providing a barrier against reflux. The role of the crura of the diaphragm in preventing reflux has only recently come under consideration.

Gastroesophageal reflux does *not* occur with significantly increased frequency in the elderly (52). It is important, however, to consider whether there are significant age-related changes in the physiologic mechanisms that act to prevent reflux and whether the symptoms and complications of gastroesophageal reflux disease (GERD) are different in the elderly population.

Several mechanisms are involved in preventing reflux. The most important one is the lower esophageal sphincter (LES). In the healthy elderly population no major differences in the manometrics of LES contraction are consistently noted except for a reduction in the amplitude of contractions following a swallow (53). This does not, however, necessarily correlate with the frequency of reflux in the elderly. What role the crura of the diaphragm play is unclear.

Other important factors to consider include the resistance of the esophageal mucosa to the refluxed material, esophageal clearance (54), gastric emptying, and the nature of the refluxate itself (55). There is decrease in the volume of saliva production and in the concentration of salivary bicarbonate in the elderly. One study has demonstrated a decrease in salivary bicarbonate in response to the instillation of acid into the esophagus; the measurement of acid clearance from the esophagus, however, was not addressed in this study (56).

In the elderly, gastric acid secretion may be decreased and there is an increased incidence of achlorhydria (57). Thus the refluxate is often less acidic, and as a result the severity of heartburn may be less than in the young. In contrast, the elderly consume more medications that may predispose to GERD by lowering the LES pressure. These include cardiac medications such as nitrates, calcium channel blockers, and lidocaine; theophylline; anticholinergic agents; antidepressants; and benzodiazepines.

The usual symptoms of GERD are pyrosis, regurgitation, and occasionally aspiration with wheezing. Other pathological processes that can result in a similar clinical picture include injury to the esophagus by caustic agents such as acids or alkali, radiation esophagitis, cholecystitis, and infectious processes such as candidiasis or herpetic esophagitis. Many patients with GERD complain of dysphagia. This may be the result of a motility disorder (58) or, in 10% of cases, stenosis or stricture of the esophagus (59). Dysphagia associated with a stricture is usually felt at the level of the distal esophagus (Fig. 2). If there is associated spasm, the symptoms may be localized at a different level. Symptoms tend to be intermittent and slowly progressive. In cases of stricture, carcinoma must be ruled out by endoscopic biopsy.

In general, despite the fact that GERD in the elderly tends to present with milder symptoms of heartburn and regurgitation than in the young, because of the longstanding duration of disease as well as age-related physiological changes, the elderly are more prone to the severe complications of GERD including severe esophagitis (Fig. 3), strictures, and Barrett's esophagus (60).

A complication of GERD, *Barrett's esophagus* is a disorder in which the normal squamous epithelium of the lower esophagus is replaced by columnar epithelium. Prolonged gastroesophageal reflux causes damage to the stratified squamous mucosa and results in a metaplastic reaction manifest by an overgrowth of gastric columnar cells (61). This lesion may also be seen after esophagogastrectomy, total gastrectomy, and esophagojejunal anastomosis.

Most cases of Barrett's esophagus occur over the age of 50. The most common complaints are the same as those of reflux. Radiologically there may be a hiatus hernia, esophageal stricture, ulceration, or mucosal nodular-

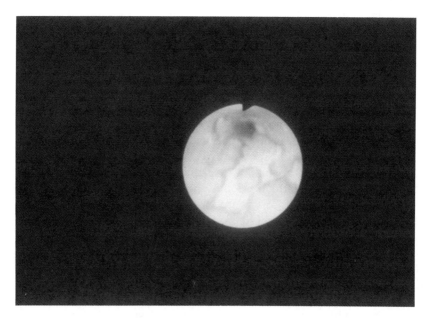

Figure 2 Peptic esophageal stricture.

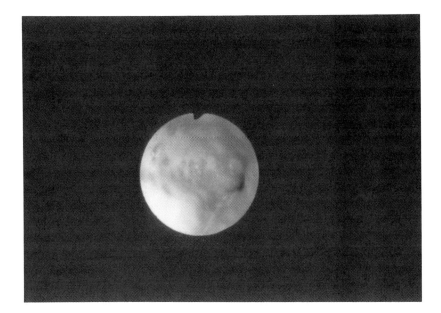

Figure 3 Severe erosive esophagitis.

ity. Hiatus hernia is seen in about 85% of cases of Barrett's esophagus and is usually associated with reflux (62).

The most serious long-term complication of Barrett's esophagus is the development of adenocarcinoma of the distal esophagus. This is usually preceded by dysplasia of the metaplastic epithelium (63). In established cases of Barrett's esophagus, esophagoscopy with biopsy and cytologic brushings must be done; how often is unclear.

The persistence of Barrett's epithelium despite intensive antireflux therapy must be considered a premalignant lesion. The presence of high-grade dysplasia or carcinoma in situ is an indication for resection of the involved area of the esophagus. While antireflux surgery such as fundoplication may relieve the symptoms of reflux, it does not result in complete regression of the metaplastic columnar epithelium, nor does it prevent the progression to adenocarcinoma.

The treatment of GERD in the elderly is similar to that in the younger population. The various treatment modalities will be reviewed with special emphasis on problems that can arise in the elderly as a result of therapy.

Phase I therapy consists of modifications in lifestyle such as the avoidance of eating for at least 3 hours prior to bedtime, and avoiding the recumbent position postprandially. Other measures include weight loss where appropriate, and elevation of the head of the bed (64). The use of a wedge to elevate the entire head of the bed may be particularly useful (65). Elevation of the head of the bed has a snergistic effect when combined with H_2 receptor antagonists (Fig. 4). Dietary measures include decreasing fat intake and avoiding irritants such as citrus juices, caffeine, and alcohol. Tobacco should be avoided as it lowers LES pressure.

Certain medications that are commonly consumed by the elderly may worsen GERD by lowering LES pressure. These include theophylline, anticholinergic agents, beta-adrenergic agonists, alpha-adrenergic antagonists, calcium channel blockers, and benzodiazepines (66).

Antacids are effective as part of phase I therapy but must be used with caution in the elderly. Particular attention should be paid to hypercalcemia, diarrhea, or constipation. Sodium overload is of concern, especially in patients with congestive heart failure. Antacids may also interfere with the absorption of other drugs.

Phase II therapy consists of systemic medication. The most widely used are the H_2 blockers (67). Since in the elderly there is a higher incidence of altered mental status, these medications may aggravate this (68). Also, the bioavailability of medications metabolized by the cytochrome P450 system may be altered. Examples include warfarin, theophylline, and benzodiazepines. Sucralfate has some efficacy in the treatment of reflux (69). Its major advantage in the elderly is its lack of systemic absorption and thus low potential for toxic side effects. It may cause constipation due to its

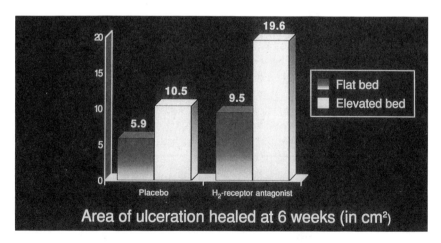

Figure 4 Effect of elevation of the head of bed on GERD. (*Source:* Ref 64.)

aluminum content and may interfere with the absorption of concurrently administered medications. Omeprazole is the most potent suppressor of gastric acid secretion. Its once-a-day dosing regimen is helpful in the elderly in facilitating compliance. High healing rates of esophagitis have been demonstrated in numerous studies (70). Omeprazole binds to the hepatic cytochrome P450 system and may affect the metabolism of other medications. Recently it has been approved for long-term, or maintenance, therapy for gastroesophageal reflux with erosive esophagitis.

If suppression of acid secretion does not succeed in improvement, the addition of a prokinetic agent may be of value. A prokinetic agent more widely used is the dopamine antagonist metoclopramide. It works by increasing LES pressure and speeding gastric emptying (71). There is a high incidence of side effects including drowsiness, muscle tremors or spasms, extrapyramidal reactions, and tardive dyskinesia. The newest available prokinetic agent is cisapride, a peripheral dopamine antagonist. It works by increasing LES tone, improving esophageal peristalsis, and promoting gastric emptying. This drug may be particularly useful in the elderly because of its lack of central nervous system side effects (72).

Antireflux surgery is indicated for symptoms refractory to medical management and for complications such as bleeding, stricture, esophageal ulceration, Barrett's esophagus, and chronic aspiration of refluxed material into the bronchial tree (73,74). In the elderly, the risk/benefit ratio of major surgery must be carefully assessed, especially in the presence of underlying medical conditions.

In summary, GERD is a common disorder that affects all age groups. Its presentation may be diverse, and multiple therapeutic options are available. All patients with GERD should modify their diet and lifestyles as described above. Therapeutic options range from antacids to H_2 blockers, proton pump inhibitors, and prokinetic agents. In refractory cases surgery may be indicated (75) (Table 4).

Another entity that deserves particular consideration in the elderly is medication-induced esophageal injury, or *pill esophagitis* (76). Elderly patients usually consume more medications than do younger patients. Other factors that increase the risk of injury to the esophagus by medications (77) include decreased production of saliva, the recumbent position, and the greater frequency of anatomic or motility disorders of the esophagus (78). The three anatomic locations where pill impaction is more likely to occur (79) are the level of the aortic arch, the region adjacent to the left atrium (80), and just above the lower esophageal sphincter (81).

Medications that are prone by their chemical nature to produce injury to the esophagus (Table 5) include doxycycline, potassium chloride, quinidine, and ferrous sulfate (82). Esophagitis may also develop in up to 20%

Table 4 Treatment of Gastroesophageal
Reflux Disease

Phase I therapy
  Weight loss
  Dietary
  Positional
  Antacids
Phase II therapy
  H_2 blockers
  Sucralfate
  Omeprazole
  Prokinetic agents
Surgery

---

of patients on long-term nonsteroidal antiinflammatory agents (83). The most frequently reported symptoms are retrosternal chest pain and odynophagia. If the injury is severe enough to produce a stricture, there may be dysphagia. Barium swallow and/or esophagoscopy may reveal mucosal edema, exudate, nodularity, discrete ulcerations, and strictures (84).

Treatment consists of the discontinuation of the offending agent(s), administration of medication in the upright position with adequate amounts of water, and avoiding recumbency after the ingestion of pills. Ulcerations can be treated with sucralfate or acid reduction therapy. If indicated, strictures should be dilated.

Infections of the esophagus are another important cause of inflammatory lesions that may produce difficulty swallowing. While the various organisms responsible are most commonly seen in patients with the acquired immunodeficiency syndrome (AIDS), there are underlying medical conditions in elderly patients that may predispose to colonization and infection. These

Table 5 Drugs That Can Exacerbate GERD

Progesterone	Theophylline*
Anticholinergics	Dopamine
Alpha-adrenergic antagonists	Beta-adrenergic agonists
Diazepam	Prostaglandins
Narcotics	Calcium channel blockers

Adapted from: Gastroesophageal Reflux Disease: Pathology, Diagnosis, Therapy. Mount Kisco, NY. Futura Publishing Co Inc: 1985:212.
* Animal studies only.

include malignancies, diabetes mellitus, malnutrition, surgery, and the use of certain medications—in particular, broad-spectrum antibiotics, cortico-steroids, and immunosuppressive and cytotoxic agents.

The most common etiology agent of esophageal infection is *Candida albicans* (85). Predisposing factors include a high-carbohydrate diet, diminished esophageal peristalsis, and an increased density of fungal populations in the elderly in general. Symptoms include dysphagia, odynophagia, and a retrosternal burning sensation as food passes down the inflamed esophagus. There may or may not be associated oral thrush. The diagnosis is supported by a barium esophagram showing plaques which result in a granular or nodular appearance to the esophageal mucosa. However, esophageal candidiasis may also be present even with a normal barium study. The most reliable method of diagnosing *Candida* esophagitis is esophagoscopy with biopsies and cytologic brushings (86). The endoscopic appearance of the mucosa includes raised white plaques, friability, and frank ulceration (87) (Fig. 5). Mild cases usually respond to nystatin troches or ketoconazole (88). In more severe cases or with failure to respond to oral agents, systemic therapy with amphotericin B may be required. Fluconazole, a newer oral antifungal agent, has been shown to be efficacious in *Candida* esophagitis.

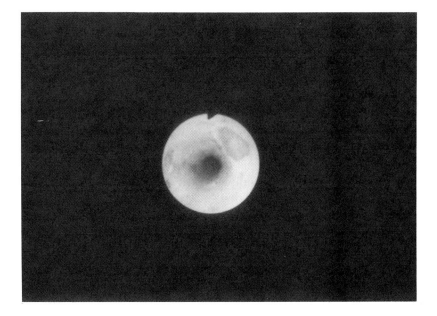

Figure 5   Endoscopic view of *Candida* esophagitis.

Cytomegalovirus and herpes simplex virus infection of the esophagus are seen in patients with underlying debilitating diseases and with a compromised immune system (89). The symptoms are odynophagia and retrosternal chest pain. The diagnosis is suggested by barium studies which characteristically show flat, punched-out ulcers with a clean base. The most reliable method of diagnosis is endoscopy with biopsy, brush cytology, and viral culture. The endoscopic appearances may include vesicular lesions, erosive changes, and ulceration (90). It is important to note that viral infection of the esophagus may coexist with esophageal candidiasis. Treatment is usually directed at the underlying disorder. For infection with herpes simplex virus, acyclovir is given orally. Cytomegalovirus infection requires treatment with an intravenous agent. Ganciclovir (DHPG) and foscarnet are both effective, but they have a high incidence of systemic toxicity.

Acute esophagitis may result as a complication of intrathoracic radiation. Symptoms include substernal burning, dysphagia, and odynophagia. In severe cases, strictures or tracheoesophageal fistulae may develop. The onset of symptoms is usually within the first 3 weeks of commencing radiation therapy, and symptoms may persist for several weeks after completion of treatment (91). Radiation esophagitis is dose-related. There are no specific radiologic or endoscopic features that are specific for this disorder. Mucosal biopsies are usually done at endoscopy. There may be thickening of the squamous epithelial layer, prominence of subepithelial collagen, and small-vessel telangiectasia (92).

Several interesting vascular anomalies can present in the elderly and have dysphagia as their manifestation. *Dysphagia lusoria* occurs when an aberrant right subclavian artery compresses the upper portion of the esophagus. Anatomically this results when the artery arises as the fourth branch of the aortic arch and then courses around the left and posterior aspect of the esophagus and trachea. This anomaly usually presents in childhood with dysphagia and dyspnea. It may remain clinically silent, however, until many years later and then present for the first time due to vascular degenerative changes associated with aging (93). The diagnosis of dysphagia lusoria is suggested by barium esophagography which shows a characteristic indentation of the esophagus at the T3 or T4 vertebral level. Angiography confirms the diagnosis and outlines the vascular anatomy. Treatment is surgical and consists of resection with reconstruction of the aberrant vessel or interposition of a graft.

Dysphagia aortica is less common than dysphagia lusoria. It results from a thoracic aortic aneurysm impinging on the proximal esophagus (which is relatively mobile) and compression of the distal esophagus (which is relatively fixed) between the sclerotic aorta posteriorly and the heart or esophageal hiatus anteriorly (94). Most patients are above the age of 70 and present with dysphagia to solids. Dysphagia aortica also results from elongation and tortuosity of the descending thoracic aorta as part of the normal aging process (95). Most patients with dysphagia aortica will do well with simple dietary changes such as avoiding bulky and solid foods. If symptoms of esophageal obstruction are severe, surgery may be needed, at which time the distal esophagus is mobilized at the hiatus (96).

Esophageal cancer is a major entity of clinical importance in the elderly. The usual age range at presentation is 50–70, and the disease is more frequent in men (97). There are several well-recognized risk factors, including alcohol, tobacco, nitrates, nitrosamines, and thermal irritation. Other clinical conditions that predispose to the development of esophageal carcinoma include achalasia, previous ingestion of caustic agents, the Plummer-Vinson syndrome, achalasia, and a history of gastric surgery.

The vast majority (95%) of esophageal carcinomas are of the squamous cell type. The most frequent site of involvement is the middle third, followed by the bottom third and then the top third. Adenocarcinoma of the esophagus can be due to longstanding Barrett's esophagus or may represent a cancer of gastric origin (cardiac or fundic region) which has extended proximally.

Most patients present with dysphagia which tends to be progressive, initially causing difficulty in swallowing solids. When more advanced, the patient may have trouble swallowing liquids including saliva. Dysphagia is a sign of advanced disease because the esophagus is easily distensible and dilates prior to the onset of symptoms. Late symptoms include halitosis due to the retention of undigested food, weight loss, hoarseness (signifying impingement on the recurrent laryngeal nerve), aspiration into the bronchial tree, tracheoesophageal fistula, and bleeding.

The diagnosis of esophageal carcinoma is made by barium X-ray studies and/or esophagoscopy. Tumors may appear polypoid, ulcerating, or infiltrating. Stricturing may be present. At endoscopy, biopsies as well as cytologic brushings should be obtained. Brushings are particularly relevant in cases of esophageal strictures through which the endoscope cannot be passed. Sometimes dilation is needed to facilitate the examination, and this is best done under fluoroscopic guidance.

The primary modalities of therapy for cancer of the esophagus are surgical resection (98) and radiation therapy (99). Unfortunately the diagnosis of esophageal carcinoma is usually made when the disease is already at an advanced stage. The reasons for this include the extensive network of submucosal lymphatics and the absence of a serosa, thus allowing for early localized spread of the disease as well as difficulty in surgically resecting the tumor. Computerized tomography is done preoperatively to determine resectability. Recently, endoscopic ultrasonography (EUS) has also been used to assess the extent of local spread and determine resectability (100).

Less than half of cases are found to be candidates for surgical resection at the time of presentation. Among those resected, postoperative mortality is about 25%, and the 5-year survival rate is under 10% (101). Surgical mortality rates increase with advancing age, usually due to associated underlying medical conditions including cardiac and pulmonary diseases.

In a series published by Nakayama, surgery for potential cure was possible in only 40% of cases. The remaining 60% had a palliative procedure performed. The indications for palliation include large, nonresectable tumors, local or distant metastases, and presence of underlying medical illnesses that increase the risk of surgery (102).

Several methods of palliation are available, and all have the goal of improving symptoms of dysphagia and obstruction and managing salivary secretions. These include insertion of an esophageal prosthesis (103), laser ablation of the tumor (104), and photodynamic therapy. Alternatively, a percutaneous gastrostomy can be placed endoscopically to provide nutritional support (105).

In the debilitated elderly patient, radiotherapy may be an alternative for patients with squamous cell carcinoma as this tumor is radiosensitive (106).

REFERENCES

1. Castell DO. Gastrointestinal disorders in the elderly. Gastroenterol Clin North Am 1990; 19:235–254.
2. Friedman LS, ed. Gastrointestinal disorders in the elderly. Gastroenterol Clin North Am 1990; 19:xi.
3. Jacob P, Kahrilas PJ, Logeman JA, Shah V, Ha T. Upper esophageal sphincter opening and modulation during swallowing. Gastroenterology 1989; 97: 1469–1478
4. Trupe EH, Siebens H, Siebens A. Prevalence of feeding and swallowing disorders in a nursing home. Arch Phys Med Rehabil 1984; 65:651–652.
5. Belsey R. Pulmonary complaints of esophageal diseases. Br J Dis Chest 1960; 54:342–348.
6. Sonies BC. Oropharyngeal dysphagia in the elderly. Clin Geriatr Med 1992; 8:569–577.
7. Gordon C, Hewer R, Wade D. Dysphagia in acute stroke. Br Med J 1987; 295:411–414.
8. Logemann JA, Blonsky ER, Boshes B. Dysphagia in parkinsonism. JAMA 1975; 231:69.
9. Osserman KE. Myasthenia Gravis. New York: Grune & Stratton, 1958.
10. Hollis JB, Castell DO, Braddom RL. Esophageal function in diabetes mellitus and its relation to peripheral neuropathy. Gastroenterology 1977; 73:1098–1102.

11. Jacob H et al. The esophageal motility disorder of polymyositis. Arch Intern Med 1983; 143:2262.

12. Grunebaum M, Salinger H, Radiologic findings in polymyositis-dermatomyositis involving the pharynx and upper esophagus. Clin Radiol 1971; 22:97.

13. Christensen J. Esophageal manometry in myxedema. Gastroenterology 1967; 52:1130 (abstract).

14. Jones RF M. The Patterson-Brown-Kelly syndrome–its relationship to iron deficiency and post cricoid carcinoma. Part I. J Laryngol Otol 1961; 75:529–543.

15. Lambert JR, Tepperman PS, Jimenez J, Newman A. Cervical spine disease and dysphagia: four new cases and a review of the literature. Am J Gastroenterol 1981; 76:35–40.

16. Cook IJ, Blumbergs P, Cash K, et al. Structural abnormalities of the cricopharyngeus muscle in patients with pharyngeal (Zenker's) diverticulum. J Gastroenterol Hepatol 1992; 7:556–562.

17. Cook IJ, Gabb M, Panagopoulos V, et al. Pharyngeal (Zenker's) diverticulum is a disorder of upper esophageal sphincter opening. Gastroenterology 1992; 103:1229–1235.

18. Lerut T, van Raemdonck D, Guelinckx P, et al. Zenker's diverticulum: Is a myotomy of the cricopharyngeus useful? How long should it be? Hepato-Gastroenterol 1992; 39:127–131.

19. Barthlen W, Feussner H, Hannig C, Holscher AH, Siewert JR. Surgical therapy of Zenker's diverticulum: low risk and high efficiency. Dysphagia 1990; 5:13.

20. Wayman DM, Byl FM, Adour KK. Endoscopic diverticulotomy for the treatment of Zenker's diverticulum. Otolaryngol Head Neck Surg 1991; 104:448–452.

21. Fulp S et al. Aging-related alterations in human upper esophageal sphincter function. Am J Gastroenterol 1990; 85:1569.

22. Palmer ED. Disorders of the cricopharyngeus muscle: a review. Gastroenterology 1976; 71:510–519.

23. Dodds WJ, Logemann JA, Stewart ET. Radiologic assessment of abnormal oral and pharyngeal phases of swallowing. AJR 1990; 154:965.

24. Bonavina L, Khan NA, DeMeester TR. Pharyngeoesophageal dysfunctions: the role of cricopharyngeal myotomy. Arch Surg 1985; 120:541.

25. Henderson RD, Maryratt G. Cricopharyngeal myotomy as a method of treating cricopharyngeal dysphagia secondary to gastroesophageal reflux. J Thorac Cardiovasc Surg 1977; 74:721–725.

26. Cattau EL, Castell DO. Symptoms of esophageal dysfunction. Adv Intern Med 1982; 27:151–181.

27. Castell DO. Gastrointestinal disorders in the elderly. Gastroenterol Clin North Am 1990; 19:227.

28. Tucker HJ, Snape WJ, Cohen S. Achalasia secondary to carcinoma: manometric and clinical features. Ann Intern Med 1978; 89:315.

29. Subramanyam K. Achalasia secondary to malignant mesothelioma of the pleura. J Clin Gastroenterol 1990; 12:183.

30. Tucker HJ, Snape WJ, Cohen S. Achalasia secondary to carcinoma: manometric and clinical features. Ann Intern Med 1978; 89:315.
31. Dancygier H, Classen M. Endoscopic ultrasonography in esophageal diseases. Gastrointest Endosc 1989; 35:220.
32. Roth HP, Fleshler B. Diffuse esophageal spasm. Ann Intern Med 1964; 61:914–923.
33. Kline M, Chesne R, Sturdevant RAI, McCallum RW. Esophageal disease in patients with angina-like chest pain. Am J Gastroenterol 1981; 75:116–123.
34. Brand DL, Martin D, Pope CE II. Esophageal manometrics in patients with angina-like chest pain. Dig Dis 1977; 22:300–304.
35. Ferguson SC, Kodges K, Hersh T, Jinich H. Esophageal manometry in patients with chest pain and normal coronary arteriogram. Am J Gastroenterol 1981; 75:124–127.
36. Fleshler B. Diffuse esophageal spasm. Gastroenterology 1967; 52:559–564.
37. Swamy N. Esophageal spasm: clinical and manometric response to nitroglycerin and long-acting nitrates. Gastroenterology 1977; 72:23–27.
38. Bortolotti M, Labo G. Clinical and manometric effects of nifedipine in patients with esophageal achalasia. Gastroenterology 1981; 80:39–44.
39. Richter JE. Gastroesophageal reflux disease in the elderly. Geriatr Med Today 1989; 8:27.
40. Zamost B et al. Esophagitis in scleroderma. Gastroenterology 1987; 92:421.
41. Fulp S et al. Ageing-related alterations in human upper esophageal sphincter function. Am J Gastroenterol 1990; 85:1569.
42. Soergel KH, Zboralski F, Amberg JR. Presbyesophagus: esophageal motility in nonagenarians. J Clin Invest 1964; 43:1472–1479.
43. Richter JE et al. Esophageal manometry in 95 healthy adult volunteers: variability of pressures with age and frequency of "abnormal" contractions. Dig Dis Sci 1987; 32:583.
44. Hollis JB, Castell DO. Esophageal function in elderly men: a new look at presbyesophagus. Ann Intern Med 1974; 80:371–374.
45. Eckardt V, LeCompte PM. Esophageal ganglia and smooth muscle in the elderly. Dig Dis 1978; 23:443–448.
46. Khan TA, Shragge BW, Chrispin JS, Lind JF. Esophageal motility in the elderly. Am J Dig Dis 1977; 22:1049–1054.
47. Schatzki R, Gary JE. Dysphagia due to a diaphragm-like localized narrowing in the lower esophagus ("lower esophageal ring"). AJR 1953; 70:911–922.
48. Goyal RK, Glancy JJ, Spiro HM. Lower esophageal ring. N Engl J Med 1970; 282:1298–1305.
49. Stilson W et al. Hiatal hernia and gastroesophageal reflux. Radiology 1969; 93:1323.
50. Pridie RB. Incidence and coincidence of hiatus hernia. Gut 1966; 7:188–189.
51. Cohen S, Harris L. Does hiatus hernia affect competence of the gastroesophageal sphincter? N Engl J Med 1971; 284:1053–1056.
52. Spence RAJ et al. Does age influence normal gastroesophageal reflux? Gut 1985; 26:799.
53. Soergel KH, Zboralski F, Amberg JR. Presbyesophagus: esophageal motility in nonagenarians. J Clin Invest 1964; 43:1472–1479.

54. Mittal R, Lange R, McCallum R. Identification and mechanism of delayed esophageal acid clearance in subjects with hiatus hernia. Gastroenterology 1987; 92:130.

55. Richter JE, Castell DO. Gastroesophageal reflux: pathogenesis, diagnosis and therapy. Ann Intern Med 1982; 97:93–103.

56. Sonnenberg A et al. Salivary secretion in reflux esophagitis. Gastroenterology 1982; 83:889.

57. Kekki M et al. Age and sex-related behavior of gastric acid secretion at the population level. Scand J Gastroenterol 1982; 17:737.

58. Olsen AM, Schlegel JF. Motility disturbances caused by esophagitis. J Thorac Cardiovasc Surg 1965; 50:607–612.

59. Skinner DB. Symptoms. In: Skinner DB, Belsey RHR, Hendrix TR, Zuidema GD, eds. Gastroesophageal Reflux and Hiatal Hernia. Boston: Little, Brown, 1972:37.

60. Richter JE. Gastroesophageal reflux disease in the elderly. Geriatr Med Today 1989; 8:27.

61. Allison PR, Johnstone AS. The oesophagus lined with gastric mucous membrane. Thorax 1953; 8:87–101.

62. Robbins AH, Vincent ME, Saini M, Schimmel EM. Revised radiologic concepts of the Barrett esophagus. Gastrointest Radiol 1978; 3:377–381.

63. McDonald GB, Brand DL, Thorning DR. Multiple adenomatous neoplasms arising in columnar-lined (Barrett's) esophagus. Gastroenterology 1977; 72:1317–1321.

64. Johnson L, DeMeester T. Evaluation of elevation of the head of the bed, bethanechol, and antacid foam tablets on gastroesophageal reflux. Dig Dis Sci 1981; 26:673.

65. Hamilton J et al. Sleeping on a wedge diminishes exposure of the esophagus to refluxed acid. Dig Dis Sci 1988; 33:581.

66. Castell DO. The lower esophageal sphincter: physiologic and clinical aspects. Ann Intern Med 1975; 83:390–401.

67. Colin-Jones DG. Histamine-2 receptor antagonists in gastroesophageal reflux. Gut 1989; 30:1305.

68. Lipsy RJ, Fennerty B, Fagan TC. Clinical review of histamine-2 receptor antagonists. Arch Intern Med 1990; 150:745.

69. Williams R et al. Multicenter trial of sucralfate suspension for the treatment of reflux esophagitis. Am J Med 1987; 83(suppl 3B):61.

70. Hetzel DJ et al. Healing and relapse of severe peptic esophagitis after treatment with omeprazole. Gastroenterology 1988; 95:903.

71. Winnan J, Auella J, Callachan C, McCallum RW. Double-blind trial of metoclopramide versus placebo-antacid in symptomatic gastroesophageal reflux. Gastroenterology 1980; 78:1292 (abstract).

72. Verlinden M. Review article: a role for gastrointestinal prokinetic agents in the treatment of reflux oesophagitis? Aliment Pharmacol Ther 1989; 3:113.

73. Krupp S, Rosetti M. Surgical treatment of hiatal hernias by fundoplication and gastropexy (Nissen repair). Ann Surg 1966; 194:927–934.

74. Larrain A, Csendes A, Pope CE II. Surgical correction of reflux: an effective therapy for esophageal strictures. Gastroenterology 1975; 69:578–583.
75. Morton LS, Fromkes JJ. Gastroesophageal reflux disease: diagnosis and medical therapy. Geriatrics 1993; 48:60–66.
76. Bott S, Prakash C, McCallum RW. Medication-induced esophageal injury: survey of the literature. Am J Gastroenterol 1987; 82:758.
77. McCord GS, Clouse RE. Pill-induced esophageal strictures: clinical features and risk factors for development. Am J Med 1990; 88:512–518.
78. Kikendall JW et al. Pill-induced esophageal injury: case reports and review of the medical literature. Dig Dis Sci 1983; 28:174–182.
79. Hey H et al. Oesophageal transit of six commonly used tablets and capsules. Br Med J 1982; 285:717.
80. Kikendall JW. Pill-induced esophageal injury. Gastroenterol Clin North Am 1991; 20:835–846.
81. Evans KT, Roberts GM. Where do all the tablets go? Lancet 1976; 2:1237–1239.
82. Delpre G, Kadish U, Stahl B. Induction of esophageal injuries by doxycycline and other pills: a frequent but preventable occurrence. Dig Dis Sci 1989; 34:797.
83. Semble EL, Wu WC, Castell DO. Nonsteroidal antiinflammatory drugs and esophageal injury. Semin Arthritis Rheum 1989; 19:99–109.
84. Bonavina L et al. Drug-induced esophageal strictures. Ann Surg 1987; 206:173.
85. Eras P, Goldstein MJ, Sherlock P. *Candida* infection of the gastrointestinal tract. Medicine 1972; 51:367–379.
86. Scott BB, Jenkins D. Gastro-oesophageal candidiasis. Gut 1982; 23:137–139.
87. Kodsi BE et al. *Candida* esophagitis: a prospective study of 27 cases. Gastroenterology 1976; 71:715–719.
88. Ginsburg CH, Braden GL, Tauber AI, Trier JS. Oral clotrimazole in the treatment of esophageal candidiasis. Am J Med 1981; 71:891–895.
89. Howiler W, Goldberg HI. Oesophageal involvement in herpes simplex. Gastroenterology 1976; 70:775–778.
90. Galbraith JC, Shafran SD. Herpes simplex esophagitis in the immunocompetent patient: report of four cases and review. Clin Infect Dis 1992; 14:894–901.
91. Seamen WB, Ackerman LV. The effect of radiation on the esophagus: clinical and histologic studies of the effects produced by the betatron. Radiology 1957; 68:534–541.
92. Berthrong M, Fajardo LF. Radiation injury in surgical pathology. II. Alimentary tract. Am J Surg Pathol 1981; 5:156–178.
93. Palmer ED. Dysphagia lusoria: clinical aspects in the adult. Ann Intern Med 1955; 42:1173–1180.
94. Birnholz JC, Ferrucci JT Jr, Wyman SM. Roentgen features of dysphagia aortica. Radiology 1974; 111:93–96.
95. Pearson RH, Bessell EM, Bowely NB. Compression of oesophagus by tortuous dilated aorta. Br Med J 1981; 282:1032–1033.
96. McMillan IKR, Hyde I. Compression of the oesophagus by the aorta. Thorax 1969; 24:32–38.

97. Moertel CG. Alimentary tract cancer: the esophagus. In Holland J, Frei E, eds. Cancer Medicine. Philadelphia: Lea & Febiger, 1982.

98. Muehrcke DD, Kaplan DK, Donnelly RJ. Oesophagogastrectomy in patients over 70. Thorax 1989; 44:141.

99. Pearson JG. Value of radiation therapy. JAMA 1974; 227:181–183.

100. Dancygier H, Classen M. Endoscopic ultrasonography in esophageal diseases. Gastrointest Endosc 1989; 35:220.

101. Muehrcke DD, Kaplan DK, Donnelly RJ. Oesophagogastrectomy in patients over 70. Thorax 1989; 44:141.

102. Nakayama K. Surgical treatment of esophageal malignancy. In: Bockus H, ed. Gastroenterology. Philadelphia: Saunders, 1974:310–312.

103. Peura D, Heit H, Johnson L, Boyce HW. Esophageal prosthesis in cancer. Am J Dig Dis 1978; 23:796.

104. Barr H et al. Prospective randomised trial of laser therapy only and laser therapy followed by endoscopic intubation for the palliation of malignant dysphagia. Gut 1990; 31:252.

105. Ponsky JL, Gauderer MWL. Percutaneous endoscopic gastrostomy: a nonoperative technique for feeding gastrostomy. Gastrointest Endosc 1981; 27:9–11.

106. Pearson JG. The value of radiotherapy in the management of esophageal cancer. AJR 1969; 105:500–513.

4

Gastrointestinal Disorders of the Stomach and Duodenum in the Elderly

Bradley A. Connor
The New York Hospital–Cornell Medical Center, New York, New York

I. INTRODUCTION

The last two decades have witnessed many changes and advances in the field of gastroenterology. Perhaps the most significant and far-reaching of these changes and advances, in terms of diagnosis, therapeutics, and general management of patients with gastrointestinal disorders, have occurred in the areas of gastritis and peptic ulcer disease.

Since the mid-1970s we have seen the development and refinement of endoscopy as a diagnostic and therapeutic tool. From somewhat cumbersome fiberoptic prototypes to the sleek videoendoscopic models in use today, the endoscope has opened up our understanding of and ability to treat upper gastrointestinal disorders.

In addition, the development of histamine H_2 receptor antagonists and more recently proton pump inhibitors has revolutionized the treatment of peptic ulcer disease, rendering ulcer surgery nearly obsolete.

More recently the discovery of *Helicobacter pylori* as the most important determinant of gastritis and peptic ulcer disease has opened up further areas of possibility with respect to treatment and prevention of peptic ulcer and cancer of the stomach.

How this quantum leap in diagnosis, treatment, and preventive intervention has affected the elderly is of particular relevance as the elderly account for a disproportionate share of gastritis, peptic ulcer, and gastric cancer morbidity and mortality.

37

II. PHYSIOLOGIC CHANGES WITH AGING

A. Acid Secretion

Contrary to the popular notion that gastric acid secretion decreases with aging, recent work has suggested that rates of basal gastric acid secretion, meal stimulated as well as gastrin-17 stimulated, are actually higher in the elderly than in younger subjects. An increasing body of evidence has allowed us to examine the original data in a more critical light. Interpretation of the data to suggest that acid secretion decreases with aging is erroneous. The data are somewhat conflicting, and not every study has shown a decrease in acid secretion with aging. Most of the studies have been retrospective analyses performed many decades ago and have failed to take into account factors such as the incidence of atrophic gastritis in the population studied.

Most studies included patients with various medical and surgical problems rather than healthy elderly volunteers and studies did not consider potential effects of serum gastrin alterations or the effects of *H. pylori* infection on data obtained. In a Finnish study decreased acid secretion was associated with a very high incidence of atrophic gastritis in the elderly of the country of Finland. When Finns where studied without atrophic gastritis, acid secretion did not decrease in men and actually went up in women.

In a study by Goldschmiedt et al. (1), in which 41 healthy persons were studied prospectively for the effects of age on basal food-stimulated and gastrin-17-stimulated gastric acid secretion and pepsinogen concentrations, older subjects were found to have higher mean basal, meal-stimulated, and gastrin-17-stimulated acid secretory rates than younger subjects as well as increased basal pepsinogen concentrations. Age-related differences in acid secretion were especially prominent in men, and age-related differences in pepsinogen concentrations were more prominent in women. The higher acid secretion could not be explained by body size or a higher incidence of *H. pylori*. In fact, *H. pylori* infection had an independent negative effect on acid secretion. Goldschmiedt et al. (1) concluded that age was associated with increased gastric acid secretion, especially in men, and that *H. pylori* infection is associated with lower acid secretory rates. As *H. pylori* infection increases with age, so does the incidence of atrophic gastritis. These two factors may account for the apparent decrease in acid secretion with age. Once they are factored out, acid secretory rates usually increase with age, at least up to the ninth decade, and may relate to an increase in ulcer incidence in the elderly in Western countries.

Many of the older gastric secretory studies suggest that gastric hydrogen production is not reduced as a function of age per se. In 20% of the population over age 70, hypochlorhydria is present most likely as a result of atrophic gastritis. In the remainder (80%), acid production is no different from young adults. In studies from Finland, elderly subjects with normal gastric mucosa by biopsy had as much acid production as younger subjects with normal gastric mucosa. Thus, acid output decreases only with a concomitant increase in the incidence and severity of atrophic gastritis.

B. Gastric Motility

Although reports are conflicting, gastric motility and gastric emptying appear to decrease with age; however, studies using radiolabeled solid and liquid phase meals showed that it is primarily the vagally mediated liquid emptying that is slowed. Antral solid phase emptying appears to be the same in the young and the old.

In a study of the effect of age on gastric emptying of a dual radioisotope marked liquid solid phase meal in a healthy population with no gastrointestinal complaints, there was no significant difference in solid food emptying, but a delay in the liquid emptying was noted in the elderly. Major reported delays in gastric emptying in the elderly are most probably not due to normal changes with aging but probably due to associated diseases or medications rather than aging itself. The validity of many of the older studies is subject to question because of the use of sick, elderly patients such as inpatients, or those on medications. Some of the observations of gastric emptying are also confounded by inaccurate measurements of gastric emptying and the possibility of the influence of acid on gastric emptying and the high incidence of atrophic gastritis seen in some of the studied populations. Solid phase emptying is noted to be slowed by acid, and achlorhydria is more common in populations with atrophic gastritis.

C. Effects of Aging on Gastroduodenal Mucosal Prostaglandins

Endogenous gastroduodenal mucosal prostaglandins are felt to prevent peptic ulcer disease, and the incidence of peptic ulcer disease is known to increase with age. Recent work studying the effects of aging on gastroduodenal mucosal prostaglandin levels has shown a decline in these concentrations with aging. Cryer et al. (2) studied 46 healthy adults (35 younger, 11 older), obtained mucosal biopsies endoscopically from the fundus, antrum, duodenal bulb, and postbulbar duodenum, and by radioimmunoassay they measured prostaglandin F2 alpha and E2 concentrations. Older patients were found to have significantly lower prostaglandin concentrations in both stomach and duodenum. Additional studies measuring several different prostaglandin concentrations such as 6 keto PGF 1 alpha, PGF 2 alpha, PGE 2, and PGD showed that these prostaglandin concentrations significantly declined in patients greater that 70 years of age compared to younger patients. Additional work by Cryer et al. (3) showed no effect on gastroduodenal prostaglandins by alcohol, gender, endoscopic appearance or *H. pylori* status but found that cigarette smoking was an additional factor influencing gastroduodenal mucosal prostaglandin concentrations. Elderly smokers had a 70% to 80% reduction in prostaglandin concentrations. Elderly individuals who ingest drugs that reduce mucosal prostaglandin synthesis (such as aspirin or nonsteroidal antiinflammatory drugs; NSAIDs) have a greater risk of developing life-threatening peptic ulcer disease than do to younger persons.

D. Gastrointestinal Proliferation and Aging

Data in animal and human models show increased cell proliferation as well as diminished response to injury with aging. The gastric mucosa, like the gastrointestinal tract in general, is characterized by rapid proliferation and by cells that demonstrate differentiation from immature stem cells to terminal differentiated mature cells.

Much of our knowledge of gastric cellular proliferation comes from roden work done within the last decade. Taken together, the results indicate that aging is associated with increased gastric mucosal proliferative activity. Many of the markers of cell proliferation are increased in aged rodents compared with younger animals.

A reduced response to injury also appears to be a feature of the aging stomach. The administration of hypertonic saline to aged animals appears to result in more severe mucosal and submucosal damage as compared to younger animals. It can be concluded that the extent of gastric mucosal damage produced by hypertonic saline is higher in aged rats and the magnitude of stimulation of mucosal proliferative activity is lower. This suggests that aging increases the susceptibility of gastric mucosa to injury while diminishing its regenerative capacity. The incidence of gastric and duodenal ulcer noted to increase with age could be partly attributed to an increased susceptibility of the gastric mucosa to various damaging agents together with an impediment of the repair process.

Do proliferative changes result in atrophic gastritis, pernicious anemia, or even gastric metaplasia and cancer? Aging is associated with an increased incidence of precancerous lesions in the gastrointestinal tract. Is the hyperproliferation seen with aging in some way responsible? This remains to be evaluated.

III. GASTRITIS

A. Classifications

Gastritis is perhaps the most common gastrointestinal disorder of the elderly. Gastritis as a term, however, needs to be defined. The term gastritis means different things to different people. Unfortunately this has led to confusion. As a result, true understanding of gastritis is only now beginning to emerge. Gastritis to clinicians may be synonymous with acid peptic disease or nonulcer dyspepsia. Endoscopists may refer to the visual appearance of gastric erythema or loss of normal folds as gastritis. Some pathologists define gastritis as an increase in inflammatory cells in the mucosa. Other pathologists require a loss of glandular tissue to make the definition. Furthermore, at least a half a dozen nomenclatures for the description of gastritis exist, and there is much confusion surrounding etiology, morphology, and natural history of this disorder.

Because one pathologist's "autoimmune gastritis" is another's "type A gastritis" and one pathologist's "chronic gastritis" is another's "hypersecretory gastritis," a veritable Tower of Babel has emerged in communications about this most prevalent of gastrointestinal illnesses. This confusion and the subsequent discovery of *Helicobacter pylori* and its role as a etiologic agent of gastritis have prompted clinicians, pathologists, and investigators alike to arrive at a consensus for the description of gastritis.

Any classification of gastritis must take into account the following factors: anatomic, endoscopic, histologis, and etiologic. The anatomic location of gastritis has been found to have important prognostic implications representing a different natural history of the disorder. Gastritis of the antrum has been distinct from gastritis of the body, and the topographic location of gastritis has been one factor in all classification schemes at least since the advent of endoscopic biopsies. Endoscopic appearance may give us further information, such as the presence of erosions, erythema, and submucosal hemorrhage. It should be noted that endoscopic appearance may not correlate with histology, and in fact most histologic gastritis has no characteristic endoscopic appearance. Histologically a predominance of acute or chronic inflammatory cells may be noted. The inflammation may be superficial or may extend down into the deep glandular levels and may be associated with atrophy. In addition, intestinal metaplasia may be a histologic feature. Etiologically, autoimmune gastritis, the type leading to pernicious anemia, is associated with gastritis of the corpus. Other etiologies include chemical gastritis such as from nonsteroidal antiinflammatory drugs, aspirin, alcohol, or bile reflux. The most important etiologic agent of gastritis has within the past decade been found to be a gastric bacterium, *Helicobacter pylori.*

The standard classification of gastritis begins with the work of Whitehead et al. (4), who described a morphologic designation (antrum or corpus) and a grade of gastritis. Inflammation limited to the level of the gastric pits and surrounding lamina propria has been designated chronic superficial gastritis. When there is a loss of specialized glands, this is termed chronic atrophic gastritis and is designated either mild, moderate, or severe. When severe atrophic gastritis was associated with intestinal metaplasia and a decrease in inflammatory cells, the term gastric atrophy has been applied. Strickland and Mackay in 1973 defined the topographic groups, type A and type B (5). Type A refers to chronic atrophic gastritis of the corpus associated with parietal cell antibodies. Type B is strictly antral gastritis. Glass and Pitchumoni (6) designated the types A/B to refer to a mixed antral and corporal gastritis.

Kekki et al. (7) combined topography and morphology, and their grading is based on the loss of normal glands in each gastric compartment. Chronic gastritis without a loss glands regardless of the depth of inflammation is referred to as superficial gastritis. A loss of glands is referred to as atrophic gastritis and again is graded mild, moderate, or severe. Phenotype A refers to gastritis of the corpus, phenotype B gastritis of the antrum; phenotype A/B is both. Kekki's group suggest that chronic gastritis is a progressive disease which starts as a diffuse superficial gastritis in the young and progresses to a specific atrophic phenotype with age. This is based on longitudinal studies in the Finnish population.

Correa et al. (8,9) modify the existing topographical nomenclatures by replacing alphabetic terms with etiologic. Gastritis of the corpus or type A they call autoimmune chronic gastritis. Gastritis of the antrum of type B they call hypersecretory gastritis and suggest that this is the type associated with duodenal ulcer. An environmental chronic gastritis or multifocal pattern compares with previously described types A/B. This is a type of chronic gastritis most common at the junction of the antrum and the corpus and is seen in populations with an increased risk of gastric ulcer and gastric cancer.

B. *H. pylori* Gastritis

Correa et al. modify their nomenclature to account for atrophy and the discovery of *Helicobacter pylori*. They designate a nonatrophic chronic gastritis as chronic superficial gastritis, which they feel is the initial pattern for all forms of chronic gastritis and a diffuse antral gastritis (DAG) which compares with the hypersecretory associated with *Helicobacter pylori*. In addition, they describe a diffuse corporal or autoimmune type A gastritis and a multifocal atrophic gastritis (MAG) which compares with his environmental gastritis and leads to intestinal metaplasia. Yardley (10) accentuates the development of metaplasia and describes metaplastic atrophic gastritis MAG-A (which is the Correa autoimmune) and metaplastic atrophic gastritis or MAG-B (which is the environmental gastritis) as well as a chronic nonspecific gastritis which is superficial and antral associated with *Helicobacter pylori.*

Once *Helicobacter pylori* had been recognized as the predominant etiology of chronic gastritis, a divergence in opinion became apparent. Some investigators believed in the "single pathway" theory of chronic atrophic gastritis in that except for autoimmune, all gastritis begins with *Helicobacter pylori.* Others such as Yardley (10) and Stolte and Heilmann (11) disagree, and believe chronic atrophic gastritis and metaplasia results from divergent pathways, the predominant one being *Helicobacter pylori,* however. In any event, by 1990 it became apparent that differences in nomenclature and differences in opinion on the importance of etiology and natural history made it clear that a uniform standard system was necessary for the description of gastritis. At the ninth World Congress of Gastroenterology in Sydney, Australia, in 1990, a working party was convened to devise a new system of nomenclature. The Sydney system became a working matrix employing three limbs of description: etiology, topography, and morphology. No longer were alphabetic or functional descriptions used, and three forms of gastritis were recognized: acute, chronic, and special. Recommendations for the diagnosis of gastritis involved a message to the endoscopist to biopsy from both compartments the antrum and corpus as the two compartments have differing roles in the nature history of gastritis.

1. Morphology

Five morphologic parameters were identified: inflammation (chronic inflammatory cells), activity (neutrophils), atrophy, metaplasia, and numbers of *H. pylori.* Each morphologic feature is graded mild, moderate, or severe. The morphologic parameters allow a quantitation of progression and response to therapy and correlate with the outcome of the illness.

2. Topography

Refers to corpus, antrum, or pan-gastritis.

3. Etiology

H. pylori is recognized as an etiologic agent. This diagnosis may be made histologically when antibody status is known. Autoimmune gastritis may be diagnosed, and if a medication history is available, such as the use of NSAIDs, this information is incorporated into the diagnosis. It should be noted that etiologic factors break down as follows: 80% of gastritis is *Helicobacter pylori* associated, 3–5% is autoimmune, and 15% is "idiopathic," which involves other gastritides or chemicals such as NSAIDs, aspirin, bile reflux, and alcohol.

So the completed classification involves a prefix of etiology, a morphologic description, and topography (e.g., *H. pylori*-associated chronic gastritis of the antrum). The advantages of the Sydney system are its flexibility and the use of simple morphologic terms. It provides a reference matrix and eliminates semantic confusions. It also correlates with the natural history of gastritis in that although *H. pylori* is the initial insult in 80% of gastritis, some gastritis becomes atrophy and metaplasia; in others it is associated with peptic ulcer and yet in others gastric cancer.

Criticism of the Sydney system has its most vocal advocates in Correa and Yardley (9). Their concern is that the "single pathway" theory of gastritis is incorrect, and an example of this is what they call multifocal atrophic gastritis which is patchy gastritis primarily of the antrum that involves extensive metaplasia. This type of gastritis is associated primarily with gastric ulcers and cancer rather than duodenal ulcer, and they invoke the work of Stemmerman (12), who found that aspects of the environment other than *H. pylori,* such as diet or cigarettes, may affect the presence of intestinal metaplasia. This type of atrophic gastritis is more common in the developing world and with lower socioeconomic status and is also been more commonly in this country with aging. To support the contention that there are multiple pathways, they cite African studies showing a very high prevalence of *H. pylori* in the population with a very low prevalence of intestinal metaplasia. Could this relate to virulence factors or specific strains of *H. pylori*?

Rubin (13) attempts to reconcile the differences between the Sydney system and the criticisms of Correa and Yardley (9). He believes the gastritis associated with *H. pylori* results in duodenal ulcer in the white middle-class Americans; this he calls a diffuse antral gastritis (DAG). A focal gastritis which is atrophic involving loss of glands and intestinal metaplasia he terms multifocal atrophic gastritis (MAG). This is more common in developing countries and with a lower socioeconomic status and has an even higher incidence of *H. pylori* than DAG. This type is associated with gastric ulcer and gastric cancer, and, in addition to antral biopsies, he recommends biopsying at the angulus because the changes are most common at this junction between pyloric gland and fundal gland tissue.

The following are noted to increase with age with respect to chronic gastritis: 1. incidence of chronic gastritis; 2. incidence of chronic atrophic gastritis; 3. incidence of intestinal metaplasia; 4. incidence of gastric ulcer; 5. incidence of gastric cancer; 6. incidence of autoimmune gastritis; 7. incidence of pernicious anemia; 8. incidence of elevated parietal cell antibodies; 9. incidence of *Helicobacter pylori* (this incidence is noted to decline once intestinal metaplasia becomes established, probably because *H. pylori* does not survive in this histologic milieu).

Chronic gastritis is seen more commonly in the older population but should by no means be considered a natural consequence of aging. To the contrary, chronic gastritis has been shown to be a dynamic disease process, beginning with superficial gastritis, chiefly *H. pylori* associated with progressing usually slowly over years or decades to chronic atrophic gastritis. Most histologically documented chronic gastritis is asymptomatic. It appears that chronic, superficial antral gastritis in some cases is hypersecretory and is associated wtih duodenal ulcer. In other cases it remains chronic superficial gastritis for many years appearing not to progress at all. In still other cases a progression to chronic atrophic gastritis is seen with further progression to multifocal atrophic gastritis and intestinal metaplasia and associations with gastric ulcer and gastric cancer. The factors involved in progression and transformation from chronic superficial gastritis are unknown.

The changes of chronic gastritis leading to gastric atrophy progress with age, and a concomitant proximal migration of the fundic/pyloric junction is seen with age in affected patients. The exact incidence of chronic gastritis in the elderly is difficult to assess. In the 1960s, many workers showed a relationship between the prevalence of chronic gastritis and age but not all studies agreed. Palmer in 1954 (14) showed normal gastric biopsies in 27 of 30 persons over 60 years of age. Andrews et al. (15) studied 24 asymptomatic Australians between the ages of 64 and 87 and showed that 23 of 24 had varying degrees of chronic atrophic gastritis. So age is certainly not the primary factor affecting the gastric mucosa. This has been further recognized by Bird et al. (16) in showing nearly normal histology in one-third of patients over the age of 80 and in four of seven patients over 90 years of age. Thus, there is no direct link between histology and age. The autoimmune type of chronic gastritis (corporal gastritis) appears to start at a later age and progresses more rapidly to atrophy. The association of this type of gastric atrophy with cancer is apparent but less so than with multifocal atrophic gastritis (or *Helicobacter*-associated gastritis).

Type A gastritis or autoimmune gastritis is associated with parietal cell antibodies, and intrinsic factor antibodies may be found in up to 30%. Many in this group ultimately develop overt or latent pernicious anemia. In addition, serum gastrin levels are elevated in almost every case of type A gastritis but are normal in type B gastritis. The elevation of gastrin is attributed to the uninhibited release secondary to achlorhydria and an increase in functional G cell mass. Patients with autoimmune gastritis seropositive for parietal cell antibodies in general show antral sparing from the gastritic process, basal hypergastrinemia, and an increased gastrin secreting cell mass. The degree of gastrin elevation is quite variable, but there is a correlation between basal serum gastrin levels and age in these patients.

Autoimmune gastritis is characterized by autoantibodies to parietal cells and intrinsic factor. The levels of these autoantibodies are highest in full-blown pernicious anemia. In addition, reduced acid secretion is noted and impaired vitamin B_{12} absorption, hypergastrinemia, and normal antral biopsies. The incidence of autoimmune gastritis appears to be less than 25% that of nonautoimmune gastritis. The incidence of autoimmune gastritis rises with advancing age, as seen by longitudinal studies. In its most advanced form, pernicious anemia is noted related to a failure of intrisic factor secretion and vitamin B_{12} absorption. The risk of gastric cancer appears to be two to three times that of the general population. The risk is not as high as that seen in chronic antral gastritis.

Korman et al. (17) show increasing parietal cell antibodies with increasing age. Other population studies have determined the prevalence of fundic atrophic gastritis by histologic examination of gastric biopsy specimens. Siurala et al. (18) reported a 28% prevalence rate in 142 randomly selected subjects, ages 16–65 years, living in rural Finland. Villako et al. (19) report a 20% prevalence rate in 155 randomly selected subjects ages 16 to 69 living in the rural Soviet Union. Both of these studies report a significantly greater prevalence of fundic atrophic gastritis with increasing age.

In a study from the Netherlands by Kreuning et al. (20), 50 healthy volunteers aged 20–58 were examined by biopsy, and 28% had fundal atrophic gastritis, also noted to increase with age. In this study the incidence of 31% is higher than in the other studies, probably reflecting the greater age of the population. Furthermore, in this particular study there is a significant association between age and prevalence of atrophic gastritis despite the narrow age range of 60 to 99 years in this particular sample population.

The chronic sequelae and course of chronic gastritis during a 30-to-34-year bioptic follow-up study is reported by Ihamaki et al. (21). The general trend during the follow-up period of more than 30 years was the formation of new cases of gastritis and progression of existing ones. There were nearly two dozen patients who despite the long follow-up period up to a high age (mean 68 years) still retained morphologically completely normal conditions in both the antrum and the body. On the whole, however, the follow-up results suggested gastritis as a progressive disease until the geriatric age when there is a healing tendency of antral changes.

In duodenal ulcer disease, none showed atrophic changes in the body mucosa, and the process was usually arrested at the stage of superficial gastritis. The body mucosa remained essentially unchanged with age and implies that the acid-secreting layer of body glands will remain unchanged and capable of secreting normal amounts of acid up to a high age.

Two types of peptic ulcer are seen with chronic gastritis. In multifocal atrophic gastritis, gastric ulcers predominate; with diffuse antral gastritis, duodenal ulcers predominate. Although *H. pylori* is the predominant etiologic agent in chronic gastritis, other environmental factors may influence *H. pylori*–infected gastritis. For example, among white middle-class Americans, diffuse antral gastritis predominates. In the developing world and among the elderly in this country, multifocal atrophic gastritis is more common and a higher incidence of intestinal metaplasia is seen. This may of course reflect the fact that *H. pylori* infection is one of childhood in the developing world and the time course to multifocal atrophic gastritis may be a factor in its higher prevalence in the developing world. If *H. pylori* infections occur later in life in this country, then we would expect mainly the elderly to have the chronic changes of the time course necessary for chronic atrophic gastritis.

C. *Helicobacter pylori* Gastritis

1. Overview

This gram-negative microaerophilic curved bacillus was first discovered in stomach biopsies by Marshall and Warren in 1982 (22). The prevailing belief at the time was that the stomach was sterile; the hostile acid environment made it inhospitable for any microbial growth. Because early attempts at culture were unsuccessful, the discovery was initially ignored as insignificant. However, over the Easter holiday in 1982, culture plates were left in a closed laboratory and when Dr. Marshall returned after the long weekend, growth was noted. This made further characterization possible, and the results were initially reported in 1983. The organism was initially called *Campylobacter pyloridis* or gastric *Campylobacter*-like organism (CLO). The name was changed to *Campylobacter pylori* in 1987, but it soon became apparent that the organism was different from known *Campylobacter,* and the organism was renamed *Helicobacter pylori* in 1989. The organism is spiral, which adapts to motility in a viscous gastric mucus layer. Cell wall lectins (binding proteins) allow selective binding to mucous and epithelial cells. The organism attaches tightly to the epithelial cell, "attachment pedestals" form and the organism causes localized cell damage by enzyme production. Urease is broken down to ammonia and phospholipases, which may act as irritants to the gastric mucosa.

Helicobacter pylori survives in the acid environment and can be cultured from gastric fluid of pH less than 2.0. Survival occurs by its ability to metabolize urea and generate ammonia. These may be important virulence factors. The fact that *H. pylori* is urease positive forms the basis of one of the diagnostic tests for its presence. The urease may be inhibited by certain heavy metals, such as bismuth.

The pathogenesis of *H. pylori* occurs by a disruption of the hydrophobic gastric mucous layer. Cellular tight junctions may be disrupted by *H. pylori* attachment moieties, and there is chemotaxis of neutrophils into the mucosa causing local tissue damage and an antibody response.

Once acquired, *Helicobacter pylori* produces persistent infection. It is truly a slow bacterium in that infection may last years, decades, and probably for life. All infected persons develop chronic superficial gastritis. Although the bacteria live offshore, antigens are found in the lamina propria which elicit an antibody response. Substances produced are chemotactic for mononuclear cells and neutrophils which lead to chronic superficial gastritis. With time, permanent changes in the structure and function of epithelial glands led to atrophic gastritis in some persons.

One of four possible outcomes is likely from *H. pylori* infection. In most persons *Helicobacter pylori* infection remains a clinically silent phenomenon. The infection may lead to low-grade gastritis, which may be clinically silent and have no further progression. Second, a bacterial-induced inflammation may alter the normal gastrin hydrochloric acid pH homeostasis, leading to an ulcer diathesis. Third, progressive atrophic gastritis may result in the development of gastric ulcer. Fourth, gastric atrophy and intestinal metaplasia may result with gastric adenocarcinoma the long-term sequela of this condition.

The epidemiology of *H. pylori* infection has been well studied. The organism has a worldwide distribution. It is ubiquitous and rivals the oral cavity microbe *Streptococcous mutans* as the most common worldwide bacterium. Population studies show that the prevalence of *H. pylori* increases with age. It is found equally in men and women. There appears to be no animal or environmental reservoir, but person-to-person transmission may occur. Virulence factors are as yet incompletely described, and why and how *H. pylori* interacts with traditional risk factors for ulcer disease such as cigarettes, aspirin, NSAIDs, and alcohol is unknown.

Recent work on associations with blood group antigens has been described. It is known that the acquisition of *H. pylori* occurs mostly in childhood in developing countries. The prevalence of *H. pylori* increases with age. The age-related increase in *H. pylori* infections may be due to the fact that it is a chronic lifelong infection or to the cohort effect in which exposure to *H. pylori* was more prevalent in the past and as a consequence the increased prevalence of infection in older persons reflects more common infection rates a generation ago.

Ethnic differences are also noted in the United States. Healthy Hispanic and black populations have seropositivity rates severalfold higher than comparable white populations. *H. pylori* infection is more prevalent in lower socioeconomic groups. In developed countries the infection is uncommon in children, but 50% of adults will be seropositive by age 60. In developing countries the organism appears to be acquired in childhood, and 50% of adults will be seropositive by age 20.

The data on incidence suggest an annual incidence of 1–2%. In the study of white male physicians by Parsonnet et al. (23) the annual seroconversion rate was 0.49%. It seems that although the prevalence of the infection is high, the incidence is low among adults in developed countries. Follow-up studies after treatment also support the finding of low incidence in infection in developed countries. In the Netherlands, new *H. pylori* infections did not occur during a mean of 11 months of follow-up of 22 patients who cleared the infection.

The prevalence of *H. pylori* infection is higher in developing countries. The prevalence rates rise with increasing age; however, there appears to be a plateau or decline above age 60. This may relate to inhospitable histologic milieu for continued survival of *H. pylori* (i.e., intestinal metaplasia) or other factors such as increase frequency of antibiotic use in the elderly.

Age and acquisition of infection may impact disease outcome. With advanced age *H. pylori* may disappear from the stomach.

2. Diagnosis

There are now several methods of making a specific and accurate diagnosis of *Helicobacter pylori.* Sensitivity and specificity of these tests are approximately equal. The question of when to use which tests relies primarily on the specific clinical or research problem that needs to be addressed. In a patient undergoing endoscopy, antral biopsies may be obtained for a rapid urease test, histologic examination, or culture. It would be unnecessary to obtain a blood sample for serology in a patient already undergoing endoscopy. Serologic tests are most appropriate in studying large populations for prevalence of the organism and may be of limited usefulness in determining response to treatment. Methods of detecting *H. pylori* can be direct or indirect. Histologic examination is a direct method of identification. Indirect methods rely on detecting a characteristic of the bacterium such as the ability to break down urea or the response of the host's immune system to the presence of the bacteria such as a serologic test.

a. Histology. Microscopic detection relies on the identification of curved rods adjacent to surface epithelium. Routine H&E stain of gastric biopsies can be used by experienced pathologists to detect the organism;

however, the ability to see *Helicobacter* is improved by using stains such as Warthin-Starry stain or a routine Giemsa stain. Each specimen has a sensitivity of around 90%, so two biopsy specimens are taken from the antrum. It has been advised to avoid the immediate prepyloric and distal lesser curvature areas because of the high incidence of intestinal metaplasia in these areas.

Despite the fact that there is an uneven distribution of the organism throughout the mucosa, in a somewhat patchy fashion, a number of studies have addressed the problem and shown that only a minority of cases (approximately 10%) from a positive patient will be completely free of the organism. As a result, sampling errors are thought to be only a minor problem in histologic diagnosis so that if two antral biopsies are obtained, this should be sufficient to make a diagnosis.

The advantages of using histology as a diagnosis are the additional ability to assess the gastric mucosa for evidence of inflammation, thus tying together *Helicobacter* with its primary pathogenic response. In addition, the biopsy provides a permanent record of the presence of the organism. The disadvantages of histology are the need for endoscopy and the cost involved in this procedure and subsequent histologic evaluation.

False-negative results may occur when patients have taken medication that inhibits *H. pylori*. Such medications include bismuth, antibiotics, omeprazole, and sucralfate. It is advisable to postpone elective endoscopy for 2–4 weeks when patients have taken either bismuth or antibiotics, and for up to 1 week in patients who have been on sucralfate or omeprazole.

b. Culture. Diagnosis by culturing *Helicobacter pylori* has been found to be quite difficult. This results from difficulty in handling the specimens carefully. If the specimen is let dry, it is often impossible to culture. A suggested method of preparation would be to crush or mince the specimen immediately and place it in a nonbacteriostatic saline for transport up to 1 hour. The organism grows in blood agar or chocolate agar in a moist microaerophilic environment at 37°C.

The identification of *H. pylori* is based on colony morphology which appears as a typical "water spray" appearance, 1- to 2-mm translucent colonies. Plates are examined at 48, 72, 96, and 120 hours. Further identification is confirmed by gram stain showing gram-negative rods and by urease, catalase, and oxidase positivity.

The disadvantages of culture include the need for endoscopy, the cost, and the high false-negative rate due to handling or recent antibiotic or bismuth use. Culture appears to add little to the sensitivity of the histologic examination. One important application of culture, however, would be in determining antibiotic susceptibility profiles in patients who have been resistant to antibiotic eradication therapy. It may be useful in patients who have failed therapy or who have resistant organisms.

c. Rapid Urease Test. The rapid urease or CLO test takes advantage of a characteristic of the *Helicobacter pylori* bacterium—that is, the production of urease. When urease catalyzes the breakdown of urea to ammonia and bicarbonate, the reaction causes an increase in the pH of the surrounding medium which can be detected with a colorimetric indicator. The CLO test is a mounted gel disk which contains urea, phenolphthalein, and a bacteriostatic agent. If *Helicobacter pylori* is present, urea is split, releasing ammonia, which raises the pH of the gel indicator and turns it from yellow to red. The sensitivity and specificity is well over 90%, and positive results are usually seen on the same day. Seventy-five percent of tests that will ultimately turn positive will do so within 20 minutes, making this a very useful endoscopic "bedside" diagnosis before the patient leaves the endoscopy suite. Excepting the cost of endoscopy, the test is inexpensive, but sampling error may result in a rare false-negative. The disadvantage is that it requires the use of endoscopy.

d. Breath Test. Breath tests measure the actual presence of *H. pylori* in the stomach by detecting its urease enzyme. Breath tests are highly specific, very sensitive, and noninvasive. The test urea has been labeled with a carbon isotope either carbon 13 or carbon 14, which is administered orally. In infected individuals the urea is metabolized to ammonia and labeled bicarbonate; the latter is excreted in the breath as labeled carbon dioxide. This excretion can then be quantified. In the original description by Graham et al. (24), carbon 13 label was used, breath collected for 1 hour, and most radiolabeled ^{13}C detected within 20 minutes. This is a nonradioactive isotope but does require mass spectrometer for detection. Carbon 14 is available for the same purpose; it is radioactive but requires only a scintillation counter. Although the carbon 14 is a radioisotope, it has been estimated that a single upper GI series produces more bone marrow exposure than 100 carbon 14 breath tests.

Breath tests can indicate cure of *H. pylori* 4 weeks after antibiotic therapy, and false negatives may occur in patients who have taken bismuth or antibiotics in the few days before the test. The disadvantage is the need for specialized equipment and, in the case of carbon 14, the radioactivity. In addition, the breath tests occasionally fail to detect treatment failures in cases where the bacterial load is diminished but not eradicated.

e. Serology. Serologic tests rely on the fact that spontaneous cure of *H. pylori* is uncommon. As a chronic infection *H. pylori* elicits both a local and a systemic immune response. These antibodies persist in a stable fashion over time. Serologic tests detect IgG and or IgA directed at various outer membrane antigens unique to *H. pylori*. Antibody titers will fall after *H. pylori* eradication, and most tests will give a negative results 1 year after effective eradication.

Several serologic tests are commercially available to diagnose infection with *H. pylori*. They are accurate and inexpensive and include latex agglutination, complement fixation, enzyme-linked immunosorbent assay, and Western blot tests. They have excellent sensitivity and specificity and low cost, and have now been widely used for diagnosis. Some have advocated using *Helicobacter pylori* serology as a CBC for epigastric distress.

3. *Therapy of* H. pylori

Much work has been done to refine the therapeutic approach to *H. pylori* infections. Initial enthusiasm for the effectiveness of bismuth compounds waned after it was discovered that these compounds merely suppress the gastric bacteria rather than eradicate them. However, bismuth had a very prominent role in the initial "triple therapy" used to eradicate *Helicobacter pylori*. Bismuth salts work as topical antimicrobial agents against *H. pylori* in the gastric mucosa. Within 1 hour after ingestion bismuth granules can be demonstrated surrounding nonviable detached organisms. Mechanism of action is unclear, but it is assumed that bacterial enzyme activity is interrupted. Unfortunately, infection recurs quickly following discontinuation of bismuth. Their chief usefulness has been as part of triple therapy including metronidazole in all cases and a second antibiotic, usually tetracycline or amoxicillin. Several studies that have confirmed an 80–90% eradication rate with a low incidence of side effects using this regimen.

Most work has demonstrated the paramount importance of nitroimidazoles such as metronidazole or tinidazole in the successful eradication of *Helicobacter pylori*. However, exposure to these agents selects out resistant strains which then may predominate, and, since resistance can develop after a single dose, persons previously exposed to nitroimidazoles are likely to have resistant organisms. This resistance is particularly prominent in parts of the developing world, where nitroimidazoles are used to treat parasitic infections such as amebiasis.

Nitroimidazoles such as metronidazole are never used alone in therapy because of the possibility of resistance. The second antibiotic (tetracycline or amoxicillin) has limited usefulness as monotherapy; however, when combined with metronidazole it is efficacious. It has recently been found that substituted benzimidazoles such as omeprazole or lansoprazole are able to suppress *Helicobacter pylori* as well and have been substituted for bismuth in many of the newer treatment regimens. There has been a move in the direction of shorter regimens for treatment moving from more cumbersome 2- to 3-week regimens initially described for treatment. Ten-day and even

1-week regimens have been found effective in eradication of *Helicobacter pylori.*

Helicobacter pylori infection is now operationally defined as eradicated if the organism cannot be detected 4 weeks after therapy has stopped. Eradication of *H. pylori* infection changes the natural history of gastric or duodenal ulcers; the disease is cured and the risk of recurrence is virtually eliminated. In a study by Graham (24), triple therapy antibiotics plus bismuth along with H_2 receptor antagonists was found superior to H_2 receptor antagonists alone for duodenal ulcer healing. In addition, treatment of *Helicobacter pylori* infection has been found to prevent long-term recurrence of gastric or duodenal ulcers.

Conservative recommendations on treatment have also been broadened recently to include treatment of most patients with *H. pylori* infections. In a consensus conference recently convened by the NIH, guidelines for the treatment of *H. pylori* infections were proposed.

In approaching the aging patient with *H. pylori* infection there are several questions to ask yourself. What is the disease you wish to avert? What other risk factors for this disease does the patient have? What are the likely toxicities of therapy? What is the likelihood of benefit by eliminating infection? What alternatives to *H. pylori* eradication are there? When these questions are addressed, logical decision making is forthcoming with respect to treatment options.

IV.   PEPTIC ULCER DISEASE IN THE ELDERLY

A.   Introduction

Peptic ulcer disease is more serious in the elderly and presents in an atypical manner. Despite great advances in the fields of diagnosis and therapy, elderly patients with peptic ulcers are typically managed in a relatively conservative way. Whereas other age groups seem to have benefited more from the technology and therapeutics, the elderly still have a disproportionate share of morbidity and mortality from this illness.

B.   Epidemiology

In general, morbidity and mortality from peptic ulcer disease are declining. Several studies including office-based, inpatient hospital-based, surgical series, and mortality studies show peptic ulcer disease declining in the general population. However, there is a rise in the incidence of peptic ulceration observed in the elderly. Hospital admissions for peptic ulcer disease have declined in all age groups except the elderly, where the proportion over age 65 has increased. There is a much higher incidence of perforation, bleeding, and peptic ulcer disease mortality among the elderly. Over 80% of peptic ulcer–related deaths in the United States occur in the over-65 age group. Why the increase in peptic ulcer disease in the elderly, and furthermore why the increase in complication rate? Several factors have been implicated. There is an increase in life expectancy and as a result there is a larger number of elderly in our population. The risk of peptic ulcer disease appears to rise with age and in parallel to the rise in *H. pylori* incidence. Gastric ulcer is responsible for the majority of complications and deaths from peptic ulcer in the elderly. In the developed world gastric ulcer is primarily a disease of old age.

The clinical presentation of peptic ulcer disease in the elderly is atypical. Classic ulcer symptoms are rarely reported. The absence of pain in the presence of an ulcer occurs in a third of elderly patients who present with bleeding ulcers and in more than half of the patients using NSAIDs. The elderly present more frequently with bleeding, perforation or anemia as the first sign of peptic ulcer disease. Gastric and duodenal ulcers tend to be larger. Gastric ulcers in the elderly tend to occur more proximally in the stomach.

C. NSAIDs as a Cause of Peptic Ulcer Disease

It is generally agreed that NSAIDs are associated with peptic ulcer disease, and the elderly appear to be at particular risk. The pathophysiology of NSAID ulcers relies on understanding two modes of NSAID damage: topical action, producing superficial damage; and systemic action, which produces ulcers. The topical effects of NSAIDs that produce superficial damage rely on the fact that in the acidic environment of gastric juice, weak acids are un-ionized and freely penetrate the gastric barrier. When these compounds encounter the neutral pH of gastric mucosal cells they yield a hydrogen ion, and negatively charged ions are unable to exit the cell. Weak acid NSAIDs are thus concentrated from the acidic gastric juice into mucosal cells, amplifying potentially damaging effects. Within minutes, petechiae and superficial erosions are produced. These lesions can cause occult bleeding and, rarely, chronic iron deficiency anemia, but usually not clinically significant GI bleeds.

The more clinically important effect of NSAIDs, the production of ulcers, can occur with systemic NSAID administration in the absence of acute superficial damage seen with topical administration. With enteric-coated NSAIDs and enteric-coated aspirin the topical superficial damage is reduced because of decreased gastric exposure, but there is no evidence to suggest that the ulcer risk is reduced. It is very important to realize that the absence of superficial mucosal injury with a given NSAID preparation does not necessarily predict the absence of an ulcer risk. It is believed that the systemic action of NSAIDs that produces ulcers is the reduction of mucosal prostaglandin production. All NSAIDs share the ability to inhibit cyclooxygenase, the rate-limiting step in the production of prostaglandins from precursors. Mucosal prostaglandin is widely believed to maintain mucosal integrity. In addition, NSAIDs inhibit mucosal bicarbonate secretion and mucous secretion and reduce mucosal blood flow. NSAIDs also prevent the increase in cell replication observed at the ulcer margin, an action that may delay mucosal repair and ulcer healing.

An understanding of the relationship between ordinary peptic ulcers and NSAID ulcers is beginning to emerge. Whereas most peptic ulcers associated with *Helicobacter pylori* are accompanied by antral gastritis, only about 50% of NSAID-associated gastric ulcers are associated with gastritis or *H. pylori*. These observations support the conclusions that NSAIDs are an independent cause of ulcers and that NSAIDs do not cause gastritis. When gastritis is seen, *Helicobacter pylori* is probably present. NSAIDs can exacerbate an underlying ulcer diathesis, and it has been suggested that *Helicobacter pylori* or the associated gastritis may predispose NSAID-induced ulceration, but data do not show that acute NSAID-induced injury is exacerbated simply by the presence of *Helicobacter pylori*.

Most of the studies that show an increased risk of ulcer complications from NSAIDs have demonstrated this risk in elderly individuals. Is this related to the fact that the elderly probably have more exposure to NSAIDs, or is it related to the fact that elderly individuals tolerate their ulcer complications less well than younger individuals? In a controlled study age was a distinct risk factor for aspirin-induced ulcer hospitalization even when pill consumption was comparable across age groups. Age was also the most important single predicator for ulcer complications in the rheumatoid arthritis ARAMIS database. This study also suggested that patients with rheumatoid arthritis are more susceptible to NSAID mucosal damage than patients with osteoarthritis. The rate of hospitalization and for upper GI problems in patients with rheumatoid arthritis is 1.4%, compared with 0.4% in patients wtih osteoarthritis.

The pathophysiology underlying an increased risk of ulceration with NSAIDs in the elderly has not been established. The question of duration of exposure and dose dependency with NSAIDs has been addressed. Griffin and co-workers (25) note that the risk of NSAID complications is greatest within the first month of therapy. Experimental and clinical studies show that the ulcerogenic effects appear to be dose dependent; however, the risk may still be increased with very low doses of NSAIDs because they reduce gastric mucosal prostaglandins. Nonacetylated salicylates such as salsalate appear to be less ulcerogenic than other NSAIDs.

Corticosteroids may potentiate the ulcer risk when added to NSAIDs; Piper et al. (26) show that the relative risk for upper gastrointestinal hemorrhage in patients who are on both steroids and NSAIDs was 10.6-fold above that found with NSAIDs alone. In addition, monitoring patients from the ARAMIS database also indicates that the concurrent use of prednisone enhances the risk of hospitalization from ulcer disease. These data argue for avoiding this combination, especially in elderly patients.

Quite often the first sign of an NSAID ulcer is a dramatic event such as a major GI bleed or perforation. NSAIDs may contribute to the different clinical spectrum of peptic disease by increasing the bleeding tendency and by decreasing the sensation of visceral pain. The finding of less pain associated with duodenal ulcer may delay the onset of recognition until a later stage in the ulcer diathesis, such as when ulcers bleed. This might also correlate with the high prevalence of giant duodenal ulcers among older people. Most patients with giant duodenal ulcer had either no history of pain or pain of short duration only. Most of the patients with giant duodenal ulcer presented with bleeding. Permutt and Cello (27) said that rebleeding occurred within 48 hours of admission in approximately 40% of elderly patients, a significantly greater percentage than in the young. Mortality rates were correspondingly higher as well. The percentage of patients with perforations taking NSAIDs increased in those aged 65 or above, especially women. This is independent of numbers of patients taking NSAIDs. No association is seen between NSAID ingestion and perforated peptic ulcer in those under 65. In fact, the largest number of prescriptions for NSAIDs is written for women under age 65 in the United Kingdom. Thus the elderly, particularly women, appear to be especially susceptible to the effects of NSAIDs.

Discontinuation of NSAIDs is most effective as therapy for NSAID-induced peptic ulcer. Lancaster-Smith et al. (28) show gastric ulcer healing rates with 8 weeks of ranitidine 95% in those who have stopped NSAIDs as compared to 63% who continued the NSAIDs. Duodenal ulcers in those who continued NSAIDs healed 84% of the time, versus one 100% healing in those who stopped the NSAIDs. Similar results were seen with 8-week famotidine trials. More profound acid suppression, such as seen with omeprazole, may be more effective in healing ulcers during continued NSAID use. Walan et al. (29) suggest that gastric ulcer patients who continued using NSAIDs were observed to have rapid ulcer healing with omeprazole, equivalent in efficacy to ranitidine therapy in patients who stopped using NSAIDs.

Other work has shown that treatment with omeprazole is very effective as an antiulcer drug if NSAIDs are continued. If NSAIDs are stopped, any antiulcer therapy is effective. In addition to considerations of therapy in patients who have developed NSAID-induced ulcers, an additional question is how to prevent these complications in the elderly individual who has a need for NSAIDs. The question must be addressed whether an antiinflammatory effect is necessary or simply an analgesic effect is required. Recent studies show acetaminophen to be as effective as ibuprofen for short-term symptomatic relief of osteoarthritis pain. Obviously with rheumatoid arthritis antiinflammatories would be more appropriate therapy.

In addition to the nonacetylated salicylates, newer NSAIDs such as nabumetone (Relafen) may be employed. Nabumetone is a nonacidic prodrug which has no cyclooxygenase inhibitor effects. Its nonacidic structure avoids mucosal ion trapping and subsequent topical injury. Metabolites do not appear to significantly inhibit gastric prostaglandin synthesis. This type of prodrug may be more useful to some patients at risk of NSAID injury, but further study is called for.

The question of whether to give NSAIDs along with antiulcer agents is raised. In normal volunteers ranitidine protected only the duodenum from NSAID injury in endoscopic studies in rheumatoid arthritis patients. Another study showed omeprazole protecting 85% of subjects from extensive gastric erosions or ulceration. Of the agents marketed as cytoprotective, sucralfate has found to play no role in the prophylaxis of NSAID injury. Misoprostol, a synthetic prostaglandin, augments the depleted mucosal defense factors and has proven efficacy for prevention of gastric and duodenal ulcers in NSAID users. Whether misoprostol decreases clinical endpoints of hospitalization, GI bleeding, perforation, and death is unclear.

D. Clinical Features of Peptic Ulcer Disease

A difference in clinical presentation among elderly peptic ulcer patients is noted. Symptoms are more poorly defined. Familiar pain characteristics such as epigastric gnawing and burning may not be present in the elderly. Symptoms when present are often vague and poorly localized. Occasionally, a peptic ulcer that is bleeding intermittently or acutely may present as an acute cardiovascular or cerebral event such as angina or myocardial infarction due to anemia from GI blood loss.

Because the symptoms may be atypical and poorly localized, consideration for early endoscopy should be made when clinically appropriate. The risk of endoscopy in the elderly has been shown in several studies to be no greater than that in the younger patient population. Some concern was raised about intravenous sedation; especially with some of the newer benzodiazepines, appropriate dosing needs to be adhered to along with available resuscitative equipment and pulse oximetry monitoring.

1. Gastric Ulcer

A feature of gastric ulcers in the elderly is that more proximally situated gastric ulcers are noted in the elderly than in younger individuals. This is probably due to the increasing incidence of chronic gastritis with age and the proximal migration of the pyloric fundic junction which occurs with advancing age. High gastric ulcers tend to be large and sometimes penetrating. They tend to heal slowly and are prone to recur. There is a high frequency of complications and mortality. Giant ulcers, those with diameters of greater than 3 cm, in the stomach represent a severe form of ulcer diathesis. It may be difficult to distinguish benign gastric ulcer from ulcerating gastric carcinoma. Gastric ulcers must be biopsied to rule out underlying malignancy and must be followed for healing on medical therapy. The geriatric ulcer is the disease of later life with peak incidence in the sixth decade. The peak incidence of giant gastric ulcers is 5–10 years later than for gastric ulcers in general. The highest incidence in females is in the seventh decade, and the highest incidence of males is in the eighth decade. Characteristics include atypical pain. Although the majority are benign, there is a greater likelihood of malignancy as the size increases. Medical therapy of benign giant gastric ulcer is usually effective and not associated with an excessive incidence of complications. The presence of a giant gastric ulcer is not an absolute indication for surgery, as it had been previously felt to be. Gastric ulcers represent the most common site of upper gastrointestinal bleeding in the elderly. In studies by Llewellyn and Pritchard (30) of 552 acute admissions for GI hemorrhage, 18% were found to be taking NSAIDs at the time of the bleed. Forty-nine percent were found to have gastric or prepyloric lesions, compared to 20% in the non-NSAID group.

Sipponen et al. (31,32) report that patients with chronic gastritis had a tendency to develop gastric ulcers 14 times that of patients of similar age without gastritis. This has been related to *Helicobacter pylori* infection. These studies also support the concept that the size of gastric ulcers in older patients is appreciably larger than in younger patients. Their studies also did not find a delay of healing specfically based on age.

2. Duodenal Ulcer

Giant duodenal ulcers, those greater than 2 cm, have been reported with increasing frequency in the elderly. These ulcers may penetrate and perforate more frequently. Evidence suggests that the incidence of duodenal ulcer disease is declining in developed countries and that the male/female ratio has also been declining. In developed countries duodenal ulcers are more common than gastric, the incidence of ulcer disease increases with age, ulcers are more common in urban than rural areas, and they are also more common in lower socioeconomic classes. There is familial aggregation in duodenal ulcer disease with up to 50% of patients having a positive family history. Subjects with blood group O and subjects who are nonsecretors of blood group substances have an increased risk of developing duodenal ulcer disease. The incidence of duodenal ulcer increases with increasing age, paralleling the age-related increase in the prevalence of *H. pylori* infection in developed nations.

Duodenal ulcers tend to present atypically in the elderly, and pain is not the major symptom of activity. Upper gastrointestinal bleeding is more common in this age group, and there is a greater incidence of concurrent gastric ulcer and duodenal ulcer. Because of the high incidence of painless peptic ulcer disease and the increased likelihood of bleeding, a different approach to diagnosis and a higher index of suspicion must be entertained, especially in those patients on NSAIDs or aspirin.

Much of the information on duodenal ulcer in the elderly has derived from inpatient studies. This obviously misses the greatest proportion of the elderly. In addition, almost all of the clinical trials with new therapeutic modalities in peptic ulcer disease exclude the elderly from their database. Permutt and Cello (27) studied duodenal ulcer disease in hospitalized elderly patients. Theirs was a retrospective study of 168 patients admitted to a municipal hospital over a 3-year period. Patients were separated into two groups—elderly patients of greater than or equal to the age of 60, and a young patient group less than 60. Nearly one-third of the duodenal ulcer patient population was age 69 or older. This higher incidence of the elderly admitted with duodenal ulcer may reflect increase in life expectancy of elderly patients with lifelong peptic ulcer disease, a decrease in duodenal ulcer in the younger population, or an actual increasing prevalence of duodenal ulcer in the elderly. Permutt and Cello (27) found no difference between the two groups in the use of aspirin or NSAIDs. Alcohol use was found to be significantly lower by a significantly lower percentage of the elderly patients compared to the younger group. A difference in the critical presentation of the two age groups was noted in that a smaller percentage of the elderly had symptoms of epigastric pain—42.6%, versus 64% of the young. Melena was the most common initial presenting symptom in the elderly, occurring in 61.1% of the patients.

E. Complications

In a study by Levrat et al. (33), complications were experienced by almost half of all patients, over age 70 with peptic ulcer. Complications are not uncommonly the initial manifestation of peptic ulcer disease in the elderly. Comorbidity may increase mortality rate, which may reach 30%. In this age group greater than 75% of all ulcer operations are performed on an emergency basis. Since the advent of H_2 blockers, perforated duodenal ulcer accounts for approximately 5–10% of hospital admissions related to ulcer disease. The age distribution of this surgical emergency has shifted upwards toward elderly persons. Perforated duodenal ulcer has been reported to be associated with a higher operative mortality in the elderly. A trend of increasing admission rates with ulcer perforation and rising ulcer mortality, particularly from duodenal ulcer, has been noted among elderly women. Admissions for ulcer perforation have continued to fall in younger people during this same period of time. The very old appear to be at particular risk of ulcer perforation or death either because of inherent susceptibility or the impact of other environmental influences. It has been suggested that the cohort of people born before the end of the 19th century have a particular susceptibility to peptic ulceration which has remained throughout their lives. This of course may be related to high rates of childhood exposure to *Helicobacter pylori.*

In a classic study by Elashoff and Grossman (34) on trends in hospital admissions and death rates from peptic ulcer in the United States from 1970 to 1978, a 26% decline in hospital admission rates of peptic ulcer occurred during this time period, but the percentage of persons over age 60 hospitalized with duodenal ulcer increased from 27% to 37% and with gastric ulcer from 40% to 48%. An office-based survey of physicians from 1958 to 1984 noted a decline in office visits for peptic ulcer disease in all age groups except for elderly women, who showed an increase in gastric ulcer.

1. Gastrointestinal Hemorrhage

Elderly patients who bleed from peptic ulcers are more likely to continue to rebleed, require an operation, and die as a result of the GI bleed. Bleeding is the most common complication of peptic ulcer disease in the elderly. The elderly who bleed are 4 to 10 times more likely to die from such a bleed than younger patients.

In recent studies of upper GI hemorrhage in octogenarians the overall mortality rate was 25%. Some studies suggest that gastric ulcer has a greater tendency to bleed, but whether mortality rates from bleeding gastric ulcers are higher is unclear. In rebleeding the key prognostic indicators are hypotension and stigmata of recent hemorrhage such as visible vessel or sentinel clot. When these stigmata are present the risk of rebleeding increases to almost 80% and mortality rates are between 29% and 60%.

Hypovolemia due to a large first bleed is the best indicator for predicting further bleeding. Studies examined 70 patients over age 75 with bleeding peptic ulcers. The overall mortality rate was 17.6%, and operative mortality rate was 61%. Surgical intervention is sometimes delayed by the use of nonoperative endoscopic therapies such as bipolar electrocoagulation, hemostasis or heater probe coagulation, or laser photocoagulation. The mortality rate for bleeding gastric ulcers is twice that of bleeding duodenal ulcers; 30% mortality rates are noted, and half of the bleeding episodes occur in absence of prior symptoms.

Half of gastric ulcer fatalities after bleeding in a series by Jensen et al. (35) had symptoms for less than 4 weeks. Recurrent hemorrhage in-hospital is noted up to one third of gastric ulcers; 30% of these patients were 75 years of age or older. Mortality rates were stable regardless of therapy. There are no consistent reports of efficacy of H_2 receptor antagonists on the incidence of rebleeding in gastric ulcer.

Giant gastric ulcers over 3 cm in diameter typically seen in individuals over age 60 are associated with more common complications of hemorrhage. Other causes of upper gastrointestinal hemorrhage in the elderly include the ulcer of Dieulafoy or exulceratio simplex, which may cause massive upper gastrointestinal hemorrhage in the elderly. This is a dilated gastric artery with an overlying mucosal defect typically located within 2 cm of the gastroesophageal junction. Hemorrhage usually requires surgery but has also been treated with electrocautery or laser.

One important difference between old and young patients with GI bleeding is that the elderly are more likely to die during their hospital stay. Seventeen percent of admissions followed by Cooper et al. (36,37) ended in death, 11% as a result of hemorrhage. In a large national cooperative study mortality rates of patients over 60 were significantly higher than those in patients under 60. Risk factors for mortality from GI bleeding in the elderly when peptic ulcer is the cause of the bleed include serious comorbidity, the use of NSAIDs, and the requirement of more than 5 units of transfused blood.

2. Perforation

Perforation is the second most common emergency complication of peptic ulcer. The presentation may be subdued. There may be delays in seeking medical attention due to a lack of overt physical findings and an underestimation of the significance of the presenting complaints. Prior history of ulcer is often lacking. An absence of previous peptic ulcer disease is noted in 25–33%, so the index of suspicion must be high. Pain may be subdued or muted, and symptoms of other organ systems such as cardiovascular may predominate and take attention away from the abdomen. Free air may be absent on X-ray. The majority of perforations require prompt surgical intervention, and mortality rates are as high as 30–50%. The surgical approach is often conservative simple closure rather than definitive ulcer operation. Perforation of gastric ulcers occurs only 20% as commonly as perforation of duodenal ulcers in the elderly. The mortality is fivefold greater with gastric ulcers. A higher proportion are women among older patients with perforation compared to younger age groups, up to 40% in some series. Mortality rates reach 50% in patients over 75 years of age. Highest mortality rates are in ulcers of the body and fundus, but perforation is more common in the distal stomach.

3. Obstruction

Gastric outlet obstruction has decreased dramatically in the United States but is still seen in developing countries. The majority are due to deformity with fixed fibrosis secondary to duodenal ulcer usually with a lower mortality than other complications.

F. Treatment

The elderly have been excluded from most clinical trials of new antiulcer drugs, a standard exclusion criteria being age 70 or over. So the great benefit of clinical experience with medications before their release usually has no bearing on the elderly age group. Questions unanswered until well after new drug release include: Does age influence response of peptic ulcer to medical therapy? Do ulcers heal less rapidly in the elderly?

Several studies have confirmed the efficacy of H_2 receptor antagonists such as ranitidine in the treatment of duodenal ulcer in the elderly. In the United States the over 65-year-old group constitutes 12% of the population, but it accounts for half of all hospitalizations for peptic ulcer disease and 80% of peptic ulcer mortality. An attempt to study the efficacy of an H_2 receptor antagonist (ranitidine) in the elderly was undertaken by Koop et al. (38) specifically in response to the fact that patients over 70 years of age are excluded from clinical trials. Over 2,000 outpatients with active duodenal ulcer were studied with respect to efficacy of healing and relapse rates in patients on treatment doses and maintenance doses of the ranitidine. In this study the efficacy of therapy was evaluated in patients older than 65 years of age compared to younger patients. It was concluded that the healing of acute duodenal ulcer was delayed in the elderly irrespective of ulcer size or the use of NSAIDs.

Simon et al. (39) did not find any significant effect of age in duodenal ulcer patients treated with either 300 mg nizatidine or 300 mg ranitidine, but differences in relapse rates were reported. Duodenal ulcers recurred slightly less in old age, and smoking did not affect the relapse rate in old age, which contrasts with results in patients below 65 years of age in whom smoking is a major risk for DU recurrence. Limited data on gastric ulcer seemed to show an opposite tendency since gastric ulcers seem to recur faster in the elderly than in younger patients. It should be emphasized that these results were obtained during continuous ranitidine administration. It remains possible that a different course of duodenal ulcer recurrence in the elderly occurs in the natural or spontaneous course of this disease. There is no increased incidence of side effects with ranitidine compared with the placebo group.

Antisecretory drugs are logical in the elderly as gastric acid secretion should be normal. Battaglia et al. (40) also showed slow healing of peptic ulcer on full H_2 ranitidine therapy in the elderly. They found that alcohol and NSAID consumption probably accounted for a slower healing. A second study by Pilotto et al. (41) showed two dosing regimens of omeprazole, 20 mg vs. 40 mg, to be both safe and effective in elderly patients for short-term ulcer therapy. No difference in healing rates are noted between the two doses, and 20 mg/day is the recommended choice for acute phase omeprazole therapy in the elderly.

G. Specific Considerations in Therapy

Antacids have been found to achieve good ulcer healing rates, but they require frequent dosing and the sodium content may be a problem in the elderly. H_2 receptor antagonists are available in liquid preparations, and once-daily dosing makes them convenient. Cimetidine is known to interfere with the elimination of lidocaine, nifedipine, propranolol, theophylline, clonidine, and coumadin, and intravenous cimetidine with impaired renal function may cause CNS effects. However, the overall incidence of side effects in the elderly is low. In one study IV cimetidine was given to 1,196 hospitalized patients (387 aged 70 and older), and the incidence of side effects possibly due to the drug was only 3.4%. The incidence of CNS reactions in those aged 70 or older was low. The CNS reactions commonly associated with cimetidine were also found with ranitidine.

Clinically significant drug interactions occur in the elderly on ranitidine. CNS symptoms such as confusion and lethargy are uncommon but may occur with any of the H_2 blockers. Because the elderly are often on multiple medications, drug interactions are an important consideration. Famotidine has been studied in the elderly and found to be safe and efficacious. Sucralfate has been used because of a lack of systemic absorption. This makes it particularly attractive for the elderly. However, some difficulty with swallowing of the large tablets and inconvenient four-times-daily dosing have made this somewhat problematic. A new liquid preparation of sucralfate has eliminated the former problem. The synthetic prostaglandins such as misoprostol inhibit gastric acid secretion as well as increase mucosal defense. They do not appear to be as effective as H_2 blockers in healing ulcers; however, the administration of these agents appears to have great benefit in preventing NSAID-induced gastric ulcers. They are most useful as prophylaxis in elderly woman taking NSAIDs, especially those with previous gastric ulcers or concomitant illness that may increase the morbidity of bleeding ulcers.

Proton pump inhibitors, which are substituted benzimidazoles, such as omeprazole, act by inhibiting the hydrogen/potassium ATPase pump of the parietal cell and have been found to be safe and efficacious in the elderly.

Other therapeutic modalities include therapeutic endoscopy, which has now been more widely used to control bleeding. A number of endoscopic therapies are now standard practice. Thermal modes such as electrocautery, heater probe, or laser as well as injection of alcohol, epinephrine, or other agents are capable of controlling bleeding from ulcers and reducing the frequency of rebleeding.

In patients who are *Helicobacter pylori*–positive, the consideration of using antibiotics either as a substitute or in addition to H_2 receptor antagonists or other acid inhibitory medications is raised. What is the rationale for treatment regimens aimed at eradicating *H. pylori*? If the goal is to prevent ulcer recurrences, this is a logical course of action.

Maintenance therapy with H_2 blockers in those who are *H. pylori*–negative or in those who you choose not to treat with antibiotics is an appropriate course of action. Long-term maintenance is often given to the elderly who have had relapses or complications, or who would be at particular risk for another ulcer or serious outcome. Maintenance therapy should be considered for those who have had two or more recurrences yearly, ulcer complications, concomitant medical conditions, or increased operative risk if surgery is required. This would be true for many elderly patients. However, it should be kept in mind that the elderly are often asymptomatic and symptomatic recurrences may not be a good guide for maintenance therapy.

V. GASTRIC CARCINOMA

A. Gastric Adenocarcinoma Following Ulcer Surgery

Peptic ulcer surgery, specifically partial gastrectomy, has been associated with an increased risk of gastric carcinoma with time. Sequential analysis of the gastric mucosal morphology after partial gastrectomy shows that early postoperative changes include those of reflux gastritis. Long-term intestinal metaplasia intervenes and varying degrees of dysplasia become prevalent. These appear to be precursor lesions of the intestinal type of gastric cancer. At this stage cell kinetic studies show increased proliferative activity. Thus the long-term effects of bile reflux gastritis appear to predispose to metaplastic changes in the gastric stump.

It is well documented that after gastric surgery the stomach mucosa is abnormal. There is a high proportion of diffuse gastritis with and without atrophy. In a prospective endoscopic study of 63 patients 15–27 years after partial gastrectomy Savage and Jones (42) note varying degrees of gastritis, intestinal metaplasia, and dysplasia in all cases. In a large endoscopic study, gastritis, intestinal metaplasia, and cystic dilatation of the glands were most severe at the gastrojejunostomy. Other investigators have made similar observations. Morson (43) states that all of these histologic lesions should be regarded as premalignant.

Cohort studies identify an increased risk of stomach cancer beginning 20 years or more following gastric surgery. A recent cohort study by Fisher et al. (44) confirms in a group of male veterans the increased risk for developing gastric cancer in those undergoing gastrectomy for benign disease. They find that the increased risk is not delayed for 20 years. Partial gastrectomy for peptic ulcer disease, as with any surgical approach to peptic ulcer, is a rarity nowadays since the advent of effective medical therapy for peptic ulcer. However, because of the large cohort of individuals who underwent this surgical procedure two or more decades ago (and this of course includes the elderly), it has been suggested that surveillance may be appropriate for this subgroup of patients. Fisher et al. (44) studied a cohort of 15,983 men demonstrating a 90% increase in gastric cancer risk among males 1–20 years after gastric surgery for benign disease.

It has been felt that there is an increased risk specifically with the Billroth II procedure because of the continuous reflux of secondary bile acids into the gastric stump of anastomosis. In addition to persistent reflux of bile, luminal bacterial flora may overgrow, converting nitrates consumed in the diet to nitrites, which are known precursors of a carcinogenic N-nitroso compound. Correa et al. (8,9) propose that surgically induced atrophy or gland loss establishes a precancerous microenvironment that predisposes to carcinoma. Other workers have attempted to follow a cohort of patients who have undergone gastric resection. Terjesen and Erichsen (45) found a 1.2% incidence of gastric carcinoma occurring 9–28 years after Billroth II resection. Domeloff et al. (46,47), in studying 676 gastric resections, found a 2% incidence of remnant cancer. Papachristou et al. (48), using a matched control study, examined 1496 patients with gastric cancer and 1496 patients with other GI tumors. The overall incidence of medically treated peptic ulcer was similar in the two groups, but the incidence in surgical treatment for peptic ulcer is three times greater in the gastric cancer group. Stalsberg and Taksdal (49) report a sixfold greater incidence of previous surgery for benign gastric disease in patients operated on 25 years or more before death than in matched controls, but Kivilaakso et al. (50), using a matched control autopsy approach, found no increase in risk.

How does one guide the management of patients with previous gastric surgery for peptic ulcer disease? In a study of 504 gastrectomy patients by Offerhaus et al. (51), it is concluded that large-scale surveillance of postgastrectomy patients is not justified. Perhaps a subset within the post-gastrectomy population which may be at a higher risk should be under surveillance, and this might include those who are *Helicobacter pylori–*

positive. Suggestions have been made that any patient in whom new upper GI symptoms develop more than 10 years after partial gastrectomy should undergo endoscopy with biopsy of the gastric mucosa adjacent to the anastomosis.

B. Gastric Adenocarcinoma and *Helicobacter pylori* Infection

Significant associations have been found between *H. pylori* infection and noncardia gastric cancer. Results of serologic studies support the hypothesis of a relationship between H. pylori infection and the development of noncardia gastric adenocarcinoma. It has been speculated that superficial chronic gastritis progresses to chronic atrophic gastritis, which is a precursor lesion for gastric cancer.

Epidemiologic studies show that countries with a high rate of gastric cancer tend to have high rates of chronic gastritis. *H. pylori* infection appears to result in a precancerous condition from a chronic inflammatory stimulus. Environmental factors long postulated to play a role in the pathogenesis of gastric cancer have found a potential answer in the form of *Helicobacter pylori*. The first observations in humans of gastric organisms resembling *H. pylori* were in gastric specimens obtained after surgery for gastric carcinoma. The prevalence of *H. pylori* infection increases with age. This age pattern is also apparent in gastric cancer. Patients with noncardia gastric adenocarcinomas have a significantly increased risk of having *H. pylori* infection.

Gastric carcinoma, especially the intestinal type, is considered to occur as the end result of the sequence of gastric mucosal lesions. These changes have been summarized by Correa et al. (8,9) as superficial gastritis, atrophic gastritis, intestinal metaplasia, dysplasia, and carcinoma. The pattern in the stomach is referred to as multifocal atrophic gastritis beginning at the incisura and fanning out proximally and distally, especially along the lesser curvature. *H. pylori* infection appears to have been prevalent since an early age and is more prevalent in the high-risk populations. Severe atrophic gastritis with intestinal metaplasia represents a risk lesion for gastric adenocarcinoma at the population level but may be too nonspecific to be of any value in surveillance in the individual patient.

The incidence of carcinoma of the cardia appears to be increasing worldwide as the incidence of carcinoma elsewhere in the stomach is decreasing. The incidence of *H. pylori* appears to be declining in the United States, and noncardia cancer also appears to be declining. Cancers of the cardia and esophageal adenocarcinomas are increasing in incidence. Unlike distal stomach carcinomas, these adenocarcinomas are generally accompanied by normal fundic gland mucosa, and their *H. pylori* prevalence is in the same range as that of controls. The mean age of these patients is the 60s. As the more distal gastric carcinoma incidence is decreasing, there has been a steady increase in cardia cancer to the point now where it represents approximately 50% of all gastric cancer in white males. This seems to be related to adenocarcinomas of Barrett's epithelium.

A recent report of regression of gastric lymphoma after eradication of *Helicobacter pylori* is intriguing. A primary low-grade B-cell gastric lymphoma with mucosa-associated lymphoid tissue has been found to regress and disappear following eradication of *Helicobacter pyrlori.* The paradox of lymphoma arising in the stomach, which normally contains no organized lymphoid tissue, has been explained by observations that mucosa-associated lymphoid tissue appears in the stomach in response to infection by *Helicobacter pylori* and that the organism is present in over 90% of gastric mucosa associated with lymphoid tissue lymphomas. It has been proposed that *H. pylori* evokes immune response and in doing so stimulates tumor growth. An initial report demonstrated six patients with primary gastric low-grade B-cell MALT lymphoma who were treated with eradication of their lymphoma by successful eradication of their *H. pylori* infection.

Results of surgery on elderly patients with gastric carcinoma show no problem with surgical treatment, and more complications, morbidity, and mortality relate to preexisting medical illnesses than the specific cancer or factors related to the cancer. There is also no age dependency with respect to prognosis. Japanese studies lend credence to the idea that patients in the seventh and eighth decades of life should not be denied surgical intervention simply because of age. Age alone should not be a factor in determining whether operation is indicated. Morel et al. (52) report that surgery is a safe and valid option for patients over the age of 80 with gastrointestinal malignancies.

Increased frequency of postoperative complications in the elderly is related to comorbidity. Provided that curative total gastrectomy is performed, the long-term survival rate of the elderly is not significantly lower than that for young patients. Bittner et al. (53) report that the 5-year survival rate after curative total gastrectomy was 19.4% for the elderly and 14.5% for the young. Coluccia et al. (54) report 5-year survival rates of 8.3% for the elderly, 4.3% for young patients. They found no significant difference in survival rates between the two age groups. In a series by Bandon et al. (55), the 5-year survival rate after curative total gastrectomy is 48.6% for elderly and 49.4% for young patients. When considering the indications for total gastrectomy, elderly patients should not be regarded as unsuitable solely because they are aged.

In summary, then, gastric cancer is a disease of the aged, and in the elderly symptoms of gastric cancer are often minimal or nonspecific. Large-scale endoscopic screening in the elderly is probably not warranted, but patients who are at increased risk, especially those with lifelong *Helicobacter pylori* infection, might be candidates for screening. In any event, a high index of suspicion for gastric carcinoma needs to be entertained, and one should have a low threshold for early diagnostic endoscopy. As Ogilvie stated in 1938, "In carcinoma of the stomach, antacids are the undertaker's best friend." The same may be said today about H_2 blockers and proton pump inhibitors. Empiric therapy with these agents is probably not warranted in the elderly, but prompt and early diagnostic endoscopy should be performed.

C. Gastric Polyps

Four types are identified: adenoma, hyperplastic polyp, foveolar hyperplasia, and inflammatory polyps. Transitional forms between different groups are sometimes seen. The mean age of the patients is increased in this order: inflammatory polyp, foveolar hyperplasia, hyperplastic polyp, and adenoma, suggesting that the different groups are not separate entities but may represent related stages in the morphogenesis of gastric polyps. Hyperplastic inflammatory polyps may spontaneously disappear.

Carcinoma is associated with adenomas. Adenomas are considered neoplastic; the other types are not. The sequence of events may begin with inflammation of the mucosa and progress through hyperplastic overgrowth and disorganization of the gastric foveolae and in some cases end in neoplasia. Gastric polyps and chronic gastritis commonly coexist. Inflammatory gastric polyps and polyps of hyperplastic origin are dynamically labile, and spontaneous regression of these polyps is possible. Most carcinomas associated with polyps are of the intestinal type, suggesting that malignant growth starts from intestinalized glands and indicating adenoma carcinoma sequence in the stomach. Gastric adenomas are found to be more frequent in the aged with a rate of 0.1% in the third decade but 3.7% in the ninth decade on gastroscopic examination. Gastric cancers may coexist with gastric adenomas and are more frequent in male than in female patients.

The frequency of gastric adenomas in different age groups reveals a tendency to increase markedly with aging, especially above the fifth decade. This may have some relation to atrophic changes and especially to intestinal metaplasia of the gastric mucosa among the aged.

In patients with inflammatory polyps the location of the polyp coincides with the location of the gastritis changes. In some patients with hyperplastic polyps or foveolar hyperplasia in which severe atrophy of body mucosa was found, polyps had also been seen in normal or slightly changed antral mucosa in up to 50% of cases. Also detected was a consistent increase in the rate of progression of body gastritis in the order of inflammatory polyps, foveolar hyperplasia, and hyperplastic polyps. This finding, together with the increase in the mean age in the same order, suggests that perhaps there is a single process that starts as inflammation and foveolar hyperplasia and develops into a hyperplastic polyp.

It appears that the pernicious anemia type of gastritis (type A) is closely related to gastric polyps of hyperplastic origin. Also noted is an increase in the prevalence of intestinal metaplasia and epithelial dysplasia in stomachs with polyps as compared with controls. An association is reported between gastric carcinoma as well. Type A gastritis is associated with achlorhydria, low serum pepsinogen I levels, hypergastrinemia, circulating parietal cell and intrinsic factor antibodies, and low intrinsic factor secretion. Gastric polyps are found more frequently than expected in connection with type A gastritis of pernicious anemia. The polyps are hyperplastic and foveolar hyperplasia. In roughly half of these cases carcinomas are found in the gastric mucosa separate from the polyps, which might indicate an increased occurrence of premalignant alteration such as atrophic gastritis. The incidence of gastric polyps and gastric cancer is related to age, and a 2% incidence of gastric carcinoma during follow-up studies has been noted at seven times the expected incidence. Some controversy remains, however, about the gastric cancer risk in pernicious anemia. There is a dispute over the magnitude of the risk and indeed whether it exists at all. Gastric atrophy of pernicious anemia does predispose to malignancy, but the level of risk appears to be substantially lower than suggested by earlier studies.

REFERENCES

1. Goldschmiedt M, Barnett CC, Schwarz BE, Karnes WE, Redfern JS, Feldman M. Effect of age on gastric acid concentrations in healthy men and women. Gastroenterology 1991; 101:977–990.
2. Cryer B, Redfern JS, Goldschmiedt M, Lee E, Feldman M. Effect of aging on gastric and duodenal mucosal prostaglandin concentrations in humans. Gastroenterology 1992; 102:1118–1123.
3. Cryer B, Lee E, Feldman M. Factors influencing gastroduodenal mucosal prostaglandin concentrations: roles of smoking and aging. Ann Intern Med 1992; 116:636–640.
4. Whitehead R, Truelove SC, Gear MW. The histological diagnosis of chronic gastritis in fiberoptic gastroscope biopsy specimens. J Clin Pathol 1972; 25:1–11.
5. Strickland RG, Mackay IR. A reappraisal of the nature and significance of chronic atrophic gastritis. Dig Dis 1973; 18:426–440.
6. Glass GBJ, Pitchumoni CS. Atrophic gastritis. Hum Pathol 1975; 6:219–245.

7. Kekki M, Samloff IM, Ihamäki T, Varis K, Siurala M. Age- and sex-related behavior of gastric acid secretion at the population level. Scand J Gastroenterol 1982; 17:737–743.

8. Correa P, Haenszel W, Cuello C, et al. Gastric precancerous process in a high risk population: cohort to follow-up. Cancer Res 1990; 50:4737–4740.

9. Correa P, Yardley JH. Grading and classification of chronic gastritis: one American response to the Sydney system. Gastroenterology 1992; 102:355–359.

10. Yardley JH. Pathology of chronic gastritis and duodenits. In: Goldman H, Appelman H, eds. Gastrointestinal Pathology. Baltimore: Williams & Wilkins, 1990: 69–143.

11. Stolte M, Heilmann KL. New classification of gastritis. Lebermagen Darm 1989; 19:220–226.

12. Stemmermann GN, Nomura AMY, Guchyou PH, et al. Impact of diet and smoking on risk of developing intestinal metaplasia of the stomach. Dig Dis Sci 1990; 35:433–438.

13. Rubin CE. Histological classification of chronic gastritis: an iconoclastic view. Gastroenterology 1992; 102:360–361.

14. Palmer ED. The state of the gastric mucosa of elderly persons without upper gastrointestinal symptoms. Jam Ger Soc 1954; 2:171–173.

15. Andrews GR, Haneman B, Arnold BJ, Booth JC, Taylor K. Atrophic gastritis in the aged. Aust Ann Med 1967; 16:230–235.

16. Bird T, Hall MRP, Schade ROK. Gastric histology and its relation to anemia in the elderly. Geront 1977; 23:309–321.

17. Korman MG, Hansky J, Strickland RG. Progressive increase in the functional G cell mass with age in atrophic gastritis. Gut 1974; 14:549–551.

18. Siurala M, Lehtola J, Ihamäki T. Atrophic gastritis and its sequelae. Scand J Gastroenterol 1974; 9:441–449.

19. Villako K, Kekki M, Maaroos H-I, et al. Chronic gastritis: progression of inflammation and atrophy in a six-year endoscopic follow-up of a random sample of 142 Estonian urban subjects. Scand J Gastroenterol 1991; 26: 135–141.

20. Kreuning J, Bosman FT, Kuiper G, et al. Gastric and duodenal mucosa in "healthy" individuals. J Clin Pathol 1978; 31:69.

21. Ihamäki T, Kekki M, Sipponen M, Siurala M. The sequelae and course of chronic gastritis during a 30- to 34-year bioptic follow-up study. Scand J Gastroenterol 1985; 20:485–491.

22. Marshall BJ, Warren JR. Unidentified curved bacilli in the stomach of patients with gastritis and peptic ulceration. Lancet 1984; i:1311–1314.

23. Parsonnet J, Blaser MJ, Perez-Perez GI, Hargrett-Bean N, Tauxe RV. Symptoms and risk factors of *Helicobacter pylori* in a cohort of epidemiologists. Gastroenterology 1992; 102:41–46.

24. Graham DY, Ginger ML, Evans DG, Evans DJ, Klein PD. Effect of triple therapy (antibiotics plus bismuth) on duodenal ulcer healing: a randomized controlled trial. Ann Intern Med 1991; 115:266–269.

25. Griffin MR, Piper JM, Daugherty JR, Snowden M, Ray WA. Nonsteroidal anti-inflammatory drug use and increased risk for peptic ulcer disease in elderly persons. Ann Intern Med 1991; 114:257–262.

26. Piper JM, Ray WA, Daugherty JR, Griffin MR. Corticosteroid use in peptic ulcer disease: role of nonsteroidal anti-inflammatory drugs. Ann Intern Med 1991; 114:735–740.
27. Permutt RP, Cello JP. Duodenal ulcer disease in the hospitalized elderly patient. Dig Dis Sci 1982; 27:1–6.
28. Lancaster-Smith MJ, Jadeberg ME, Jackson DA. Ranitidine in the treatment of nonsteroidal anti-inflammatory drug associated gastric and duodenal ulcers. Gut 1991; 32:252–255.
29. Walan A, Bader JP, Classen M, et al. Effect of omeprazole and ranitidine on ulcer healing and relapse rates in patients with benign gastric ulcer. N Engl J Med 1989; 320:69–75.
30. Llewellyn JG, Pritchard MH. Influence of age and disease state in nonsteroidal anti-inflammatory drug associated gastric bleeding. J Rheumatol 1988; 15: 691–694.
31. Sipponen P, Seppälä, Äärynen M, Helske T, Kettunen P. Chronic gastritis and gastro duodenal ulcer: a case control study on risk of coexisting duodenal or gastric ulcer in patients with gastritis. Gut 1989; 30:922–929.
32. Sipponen P, Varis K, Fräki, Korri U-M, Seppälä K, Siurala M. Cumulative 10-year risk of symptomatic duodenal and gastric ulcer in patients with or without chronic gastritis. Scand J Gastroenterol 1990; 25:966–973.
33. Levrat M, Pasquier J, Lambert R, et al. Peptic ulcer in patients over sixty: experience in 287 cases. Am J Dig Dis 1966; 11:279.
34. Elashoff JD, Grossman MI. Trends in hospital admissions and death rates for peptic ulcer in the United States from 1970 to 1978. Gastroenterology 1980; 78:280.
35. Janssen CW Jr, Lie RT, Maartmann-Moe H, Matre R. The influence of age on the growth and spread of gastric carcinoma. APMIS 1991; 99:78.
36. Cooper BT, Weston CFM, Newmann CS. Acute gastrointestinal hemorrhage in patients eighty years or more. Q J Med 1988; 258:765.
37. Cooper BT, Neumann CS. Upper gastrointestinal endoscopy in patients aged eighty years or more. Age Ageing 1986; 15:343.
38. Koop H, Arnold R, Classen M, et al. Healing and relapse of duodenal ulcer during ranitidine therapy in the elderly. J Clin Gastroenterol 1992; 15:291–295.
39. Simon B, Cremer M, Dammann HG, et al. 300 mg. nizatidine at night vs. 300 mg. of ranitidine at night in patients with duodenal ulcers. A multicentre trial in Europe. Scand J Gastroenterol 1987; 22(suppl 136):61–70.
40. Battaglia G, Di Mario F, Dotto P, et al. Markers of slow-healing peptic ulcer in the elderly. Dig Dis Sci 1993; 38:1414–1421.
41. Pilotto A, Battaglia G, Vigneri S, et al. Omeprazole 20 mg/day versus 40 mg/day in elderly peptic ulcer patients: a four-week study. Abstr Eur Cong Gastroenterol 1993:A55.
42. Savage A, Jones S. Histological appearances of the gastric mucosa 15–27 years after partial gastrectomy. J Clin Pathol 1979; 32:179–186.
43. Morson BC. Carcinoma arising from areas of intestinal metaplasia in the gastric mucosa. Br J Cancer 1955; 9:377–385.

44. Fisher SG, Davis F, Nelson R, Weber L, Goldberg J, Haenszel W. A cohort study of stomach cancer risk in men after gastric surgery for benign disease. J Natl Can Inst 1993; 83:1303–1310.
45. Terjesen T, Erichsen HG. Carcinoma of the gastric stump after operation for benign gastroduodenal ulcer. Acta Chir Scand 1976; 142:256–260.
46. Domellof L, Eriksson S, Janunger KG. Late precancerous changes and carcinoma of the gastric stump after Billroth I resection. Am J Surg 1976; 132:26.
47. Domelloff L, Eriksson S, Janunger KG. Carcinoma and the possible precancerous changes of the gastric stump after Billroth II resection. Gastroenterology 1977; 73:462–468.
48. Papachristou DN, Agnanti N, Fortner JG. Gastric carcinoma after treatment of ulcer. Am J Surg 1981; 139:193–196.
49. Stalsberg H, Taksdal S. Stomach cancer following gastric surgery for benign conditions. Lancet 1971; 2:1175–1177.
50. Kivilaakso, Hakkiluoto A, Kalima TV, Sipponen P. Relative risk of stump cancer following partial gastrectomy. Br J Surg 1977; 64:336–338.
51. Offerhaus GJA, Tersmette AC, Giardiello FM, Huibregtsek K, Vandenbroucke JP, Tytgat GNJ. Evaluation of endoscopy for early detection of gastric-stump cancer. Lancet 1992; 340:33–35.
52. Morel P, Egeli RA, Wachtl S, Rohner A. Results of operative treatment of gastrointestinal tract tumors in patients over 80 years of age. Arch Surg 1989; 124:662–664.
53. Bittner R, Schirrow H, Butters M, et al. Total gastrectomy: a fifteen-year experience with particular reference to the patients over seventy years of age. Arch Surg 1985; 120:1120–1125.
54. Coluccia C, Ricci EB, Marzola GG, Molashi M, Nano MG. Gastric cancer in the elderly: results of surgical treatment. Int Surg 1987; 72:4–10.

5

Small Bowel

Michael Ruoff
New York University School of Medicine, New York, New York

Small-bowel abnormalities in the elderly could be discussed from the viewpoint of specific disorders unique to the elderly population. However, aside from vascular disorders and motility disorders, which are discussed elsewhere in the text, there are no small-bowel conditions unique to the elderly. One is more likely to encounter differences in presentation or differences in response to therapy.

Therefore small-intestinal dysfunction in the elderly is best considered from the viewpoint of the complaints offered by the patient. Some symptoms, of course, will immediately focus on the gastrointestinal tract as a potential etiology. These include bloating, nausea, emesis, alterations in the pattern of defecation and in the volume and consistency of stool, fecal incontinence, and abdominal pain.

Other signs and symptoms of small-bowel origin are more subtle. The patient might complain of weight loss, dyspnea on exertion, edema, ecchymoses, cheilosis, glossitis, bone pain, arthritis, arthralgias, fatigue, and muscular weakness. Although these findings may be caused by disorders that affect the small bowel, the physician's attention will not at first be drawn to the gastrointestinal tract as a source of pathology. Finally, abnormalities found on blood testing, such as microcytic and megaloblastic anemias, and hypocalcemia may also be caused by disorders affecting the small intestine.

I. ABSORPTION IN THE ELDERLY

It might well be anticipated that absorptive functions of the small bowel would decrease with aging, but the minor changes that have been measured in experimental studies seem to be of little functional significance. Descriptions of changes in cellular morphology and uptake of nutrients seen in some experimental animals may not be applicable to the aging human. For example, jejunal biopsies obtained from patients with a mean age of 71.5 years with no evidence of malabsorption or malnutrition had no significant difference in surface-to-volume ratio of jejunal mucosa and enterocyte height when compared to younger controls (1).

D-xylose absorption, measured by a decline in the urinary excretion of D-xylose after an oral load, can be seen with advancing age. This is more likely to be due to a decline in renal function than to the presence of malabsorption. Actual declines in absorptive function, measured by this method, probably occur only after the age of 80 (2).

Why does small-bowel absorptive function apparently not deteriorate with age? The answer seems to be in the extraordinary reserve that the small-bowel possesses. The small intestine is some 21 feet in length and has a surface area of 2 million cm^2. Some nutrients are preferentially absorbed proximally but can be absorbed distally in the face of dysfunction or resection of the proximal small bowel. Even bile salts, which are normally absorbed only in the ileum by an active transport mechanism, may traverse other areas of the intestine by passive diffusion. Thus bile salt functions are preserved, in part, even with disease or resection of the distal ileum. The transport of vitamin B_{12} occurs solely in the ileum. Resection or disease of this area of the intestine will lead to deficiency of the vitamin after an interval of several years due to significant hepatic storage of the vitamin. We can conclude that subtle abnormalities of small-intestinal function may be documented in the elderly. However, the small intestine has such an enormous reserve capacity that if a patient develops clinically significant malabsorption, a pathological disorder must be present. We must remember that elderly subjects may have reduced food intake for a variety of reasons not at all related to abnormalities of the gastrointestinal tract. It is not clear what effect even minor reductions in absorptive ability might have in patients whose intake of essential nutrients is decreased.

II. MALABSORPTION SYNDROME

Malabsorption syndrome is a disease of the small intestine. It refers to defective absorption of the main foodstuffs, carbohydrate, protein, and fat, as well as vitamins and minerals. Malabsorption can be quite selective, so that only one substance is poorly absorbed—for example, iron or calcium, or lactose in people with lactase deficiency. But usually malabsorption is more general, so that when we speak of the malabsorption syndrome we mean the clinical consequences of multiple absorption failures. Usually the presence of such multiple malabsorptions leads to diarrhea and to steatorrhea, the presence of fat in the stool.

Malabsorption can best be documented by measuring the output of fecal fat on a diet that contains at least 100 g fat per day. A 72-hour collection is obtained and the fatty acids are titrated with NaOH. the fecal fat content is usually 4 g/day and is abnormal when it exceeds 6 g/day. The mechanics of this type of collection, of course, may be more difficult in the elderly.

A simple way of screening for steatorrhea in the office is to treat a random stool specimen with acetic acid on a glass microscopic slide to form protonated fatty acids from the Mg^{++}, Ca^{++}, Na^{++}, and K^+ soaps. Finally the stool is heated with ethanolic Sudan III to stain the fat globules. If examination, in a $40\times$ field, shows over 100 stained globules that are a bit larger than a red blood cell in size, then 10 g of fat or more is being excreted in 24 hours.

III. BACTERIAL OVERGROWTH

Bacterial overgrowth is one condition that may lead to malabsorption and may occur more frequently in the elderly population. When measured by special sterile intubation techniques, the normal proximal small bowel contains less than 10^5 bacteria per ml, and these are predominantly aerobic. The presence of over 10^5 aerobic or, especially, strictly anaerobic or facultative anaerobic bacteria per ml jejunal fluid is abnormal.

In the small bowel, bacteria proliferate due to stasis, due to the introduction of excessive bacteria into the intestine, or perhaps due to abnormalities in secretory IgA or local cellular immunity. Stasis is brought about by structural changes such as strictures, adhesions, diverticula, areas of bypass, and pouches. Prolongation of the transit time through the bowel also leads to bacterial overgrowth. This can be seen with decrease or absence of the interdigestive migratory motor complexes. Intestinal pseudo-obstruction as seen in diabetes mellitus and in scleroderma will lead to stasis as well.

Decreased gastric acidity from gastritis, gastric resections, or the use of drugs that inhibit acid secretion allows viable organisms to enter the small intestine. Fistulas from the colon to the stomach or small bowel will provide a large load of organisms to the small intestine.

IV. EFFECTS OF BACTERIAL OVERGROWTH

Bacteria compete for the intraluminal nutrients and deconjugate and 7-alpha-dehydroxylate, the primary bile salts cholic acid and chenodeoxycholic acid to form the secondary bile salts deoxycholoic and lithocolic acid. This leads to less effective micelle formation because these altered bile salts are passively absorbed in the proximal intestine or are precipitated in the lumen. The absorption of fats is thus impaired. The patient may experience bloating and diarrhea with associated abdominal cramps or may present with a more subtle failure to thrive. The diarrhea is mainly due to steatorrhea, but in part is due to osmotic fluxes secondary to the malabsorption of carbohydrates.

Anaerobic bacteria can produce proteases that affect the functioning of the brush border disaccharidases (3). The bacteria are able to produce folic acid and vitamin K, so deficiencies of these two substances are not seen in the malabsorption caused by bacterial overgrowth. If there are actual mucosal changes, these are subtle and best seen with electron microscopy. There are reports of mucosal abnormalities that have returned to normal after antibiotic therapy (4). There is no actual invasion of the bowel wall. The bacteria colonize the surface mucous layer. Hypoalbuminemia, hypocalcemia, and anemia can develop. The anaerobic bacteria take up the B_{12}-intrinsic factor complex, so macrocytic anemia, peripheral neuropathy, ataxia, and mental changes can develop. Iron-deficiency anemia can occur from blood loss.

Components of the bacteria may act as antigens and form immune complexes which after absorption cause skin reactions, arthritis, and autoimmune manifestations in other organs.

V. TESTS FOR BACTERIAL OVERGROWTH

The presence of bacterial overgrowth can be reflected in abnormalities of the D-xylose absorption test because the bacteria digest the sugar and cause a reduction in blood and urine levels after an oral dose. Other test sugars such as glucose, lactose, and lactulose (a synthetic disaccharide of galactose and fructose) can be given orally and the level of hydrogen excreted is measured in the expired air. It should be noted that overgrowth of organisms that happen to be incapable of producing hydrogen would give false-negative testing with this method. A ^{14}C-xylose breath test will show early elevations in exhaled $^{14}CO_2$ due to metabolism of the sugar by the bacteria in the small bowel.

The effect of the intraluminal bacteria on the bile salts can also be used to look for bacterial overgrowth in the small bowel. If the patient is given ^{14}C-glychocolic acid by mouth, it is cleaved by the bacteria to cholic acid and ^{14}C-glycine. The ^{14}C-glycine is further metabolized to $^{14}CO_2$, which diffuses across the intestinal wall and is exhaled by the lungs. An increased amount of rapidly exhaled $^{14}CO_2$ is found when bacterial overgrowth is present. When compared with direct bacterial culture, these breath tests are highly specific but of relatively low sensitivity.

A more direct way of documenting bacterial overgrowth is to collect uncontaminated aspirates from the bowel. This can be accomplished during upper gastrointestinal endoscopy by placing a sterile suction catheter inside a sterile overtube and passing both through the suction channel of an endoscope (5). It is not totally clear if small-bowel bacterial overgrowth can occur in the absence of any overt pathology, or indeed if overgrowth itself is sufficient to present as malabsorption. In a prospective study of small-bowel bacterial overgrowth in subjects over the age of 70, five of 13 control subjects had duodenal bacterial counts over 10^5 organisms per ml (6). Studies have shown that bacterial contamination of the small bowel may be present in normal, fit elderly people who have only minor nutritional differences when compared with patients without bacterial contamination of the small bowel (7). Others have shown that elderly patients with an anatomically normal small bowel may have significant malabsorption, but the only demonstrable abnormality is a slower mean transit time through the small intestine (8). To conclude that bacterial overgrowth is causing the clinical problems, a good clinical response must follow antibiotic therapy.

VI. TREATMENT OF BACTERIAL OVERGROWTH

Therapy of malabsorption due to bacterial overgrowth can be directed against a mechanical disorder causing stasis, but surgery is an option that one would like to avoid in an elderly patient. Drugs can be used to accelerate small-bowel emptying. Cisapride, a pro-motility agent newly released in the United States, increases small-bowel motility by enhancing the release of acetylcholine at the myenteric plexus and perhaps by its action as a serotonin receptor agonist. It might be of help when intestinal motility is abnormal, but to date this orally administered agent has been released only for the therapy of nocturnal heartburn.

Domperidone is an investigational, orally administered dopamine antagonist that also stimulates intestinal motility. It does not cross the blood-brain barrier, so central nervous system side effects are rare. Octreotide, a somatostatin analog, can also be used to stimulate intestinal motility (9). The drug stimulates propagative intestinal phase 3–like activity through motilin-independent pathways. The drug is given subcutaneously. Multiple large daily doses must be avoided to prevent steatorrhea due to Octreotide's impairment of pancreatic secretion and mucosal absorption. Changes in the composition of the diet can be therapeutic. The intake of fat can be increased and will allow an improvement in nutrition at the expense of larger and more frequent stools. Vitamin B_{12}, fat-soluble vitamins, and iron supplements can be provided. Antibiotics can be used in intermittent or rotating regimens to reduce the levels of bacteria. Metronidazole, tetracycline, amoxycillin-clavulanic acid, or trimethoprim-sulfamethoxazole can be given in courses of 2–4 weeks.

VII. CELIAC SPRUE

Celiac sprue is a chronic disorder of the small-intestinal mucosa that leads to the malabsorption of nutrients. The abnormalities found in the small bowel are caused by the ingestion of wheat, rye, oats, and barley. The bowel returns to normal when these cereal grains are excluded from the diet.

Celiac disease is not an unusual diagnosis in middle or old age. When celiac sprue presents in the adult, there is a bimodal distribution with an early peak in the fourth decade in women and a later peak in the sixth and seventh decades in men. As many as 27% of patients may be diagnosed for the first time when they are over 60 years of age (10). Celiac disease is suspected in childhood when symptoms of weight loss, delayed growth, and bulky, malodorous stools develop. Older patients are more likely to manifest the underlying malabsorptive process with complaints of dyspnea and fatigue due to a hypochromic, macrocytic anemia with a low serum folate level. Bone pain and compression fractures may be secondary to degrees of osteomalacia and osteopenia beyond what might be expected for the patient's age. Ecchymoses or more significant bleeding disorders may result from hypoprothrombinemia.

Patients with celiac disease seem to have an increased incidence of other malignant tumors. Carcinomas of the nasopharynx and esophagus are increased in incidence. Malignant lymphomas, usually reticulum cell sarcomas, are found in patients with celiac disease and are more likely to occur after 15 or more years of the disease. Some authors believe that celiac patients whose diagnosis has been made when they are more than 50 years of age have a 1 in 10 chance of having a lymphoma (11). These patients must be followed closely to see if the presentation of celiac disease in this age group was precipitated by the development of a lymphoma in a previously asymptomatic or subclinical case. The most common symptom of malignancy in a sprue patient on a stable diet is weight loss. Muscle weakness, fever, and lymphadenopathy, if present, can make one suspicious of the presence of a lymphoma because these findings are unusual in uncomplicated celiac disease.

A. Pathogenesis of Celiac Disease

Celiac sprue seems to represent an abnormal immune response to the ingestion of certain cereal peptides that develops in genetically susceptible individuals. T-cell-mediated immune responses appear to be involved in the production of the intestinal damage. There are increased numbers of gamma/delta T-cell receptor (TCR) + intraepithelial lymphocytes in the jejunal epithelium of patients with celiac sprue. This T-cell population is heterogeneous and not the result of monoclonal expansion. The disorder is linked to certain alleles of the HLA-DQ loci. Up to 10–20% of first-degree relatives of patients with celiac disease are affected. The toxic peptide fractions of alpha-gliadin are absorbed by the small intestine and bind to HLA class II molecules. They are then presented by macrophages in the lamina propria to antigen-specific CD4+ T-cells. Activation of these T-cells leads to cytokine production and activation of other local immunocytes. Eosinophil degranulation and activation of complement may also contribute to the subsequent enterocyte damage. Even small amounts of dietary gluten will produce definite abnormalities of the small intestinal mucosa with increases in the crypt epithelial volume and expanded crypt intraepithelial lymphocyte population.

B. Diagnosis of Celiac Disease

Patients with celiac sprue have characteristic, although not entirely specific, changes in the appearance of the small-bowel mucosa. An endoscopist may be led to suspect the presence of celiac sprue by finding the folds in the descending duodenum to be scalloped (12), markedly reduced, or absent (13). The circular folds of Kerkring, or valvulae conniventes, are reduplications of the mucous membrane that are normally found in the second portion of the duodenum and beyond. The two layers of the fold are bound together by the submucosa and are not obliterated when the small bowel is distended. The diagnosis of celiac sprue requires the presence of diffuse villous atrophy, an increase in chronic inflammatory cells in the lamina propria, and a clinical response to dietary restriction of gluten with or without corticosteroid therapy. The tissue samples used to make a diagnosis of celiac disease had required biopsies from the small intestine with peroral suction biopsies obtained using capsules or suction tubes. This procedure is time-consuming and requires fluoroscopic guidance and radiation exposure. It has been noted recently that diagnostically useful small-bowel biopsies can be obtained from the third and fourth parts of the duodenum with a conventional gastroscope (14) and from the proximal jejunum using a narrow diameter (stricture) colonoscope passed orally.

The presence of the disease can be screened by the use of markers of permeability. In active celiac disease the absorption of large molecules such as lactulose and cellobiose is increased while the absorption of small molecules like mannitol is reduced. Two sugar differential absorption tests using cellobiose and mannitol or lactulose and mannitol have been developed as screening tests (15). Antigliadin antibodies can be measured in the blood. Combining the tests gives a sensitivity of 96% and specificity of 70.6% (16). The levels of serum IgA antigliadin antibodies may fall after treatment with a strict gluten-free diet and may be a way of following compliance (17). Other immune markers like the measurement of IgA antiendomysial antibodies with a sensitivity of 87% and specificity of 100% (18). Fecal alpha-1-antitrypsin clearance after a gluten challenge may provide a way of measuring the intestinal response to gluten challenge (19).

C. Treatment of Celiac Disease

Removal of gluten-containing foods from the diet will lead to symptomatic improvement within 4–6 weeks. Patients may respond within a week. A rare patient may require corticosteroid therapy. It is important to give the patient specific instructions concerning the details of selecting a diet. Gluten is often added to foods when they are processed and be present when not anticipated by an uninformed shopper. Since the glutin intolerance is lifelong, the dietary restrictions must be lifelong as well.

VIII. SIGNIFICANCE OF CALCIUM MALABSORPTION

Calcium absorption seems to decline with age (20). It is possible that the small intestine of an elderly patient may be less able to adjust to the diet that is deficient in calcium. Calcium salts must be ionized at an acid pH to be absorbed. This allows the calcium to dissociate from food complexes and enter into solution. Calcium ions are absorbed throughout the small intestine. Calcium absorption is reduced in the elderly because it is dependent on adequate levels of 1,25-hydroxycholecalciferol ($1,25(OH)_2D_3$). This hormone enhances the facilitated diffusion of calcium ions into the enterocyte, induces the synthesis of calbindin D (the binding protein that moves calcium through the cell), and stimulates ATP-dependent calcium ion transport out of the cell. Normally endogenous vitamin D_3 is hydroxylated in the liver to $25(OH)D_3$, which is then hydroxylated in the kidney to $1,25(OH)_2D_3$. With decreased sun exposure there is less conversion of 7-dehydrocholesterol in the skin by ultraviolet light to endogenous vitamin D_3. Renal production of 1,25-hydroxycholecalciferol is decreased in the elderly, and the response of the small bowel to the hormone may be reduced (21). With overgrowth of bacteria in the small bowel, the absorption of vitamin D_3 may be reduced.

IX. NSAIDS AND THE SMALL BOWEL

It must be remembered that the small intestine may also be affected by medications that are prescribed to the geriatric population. Users of nonsteroidal antiinflammatory drugs (NSAIDs), particularly those over the age of 60, have a three times greater risk of developing serious adverse gastrointestinal problems than nonusers (22). While the effects of these drugs on the stomach and duodenal bulb are well known, they can also cause inflammation of the small intestine in up to 70% of patients on long-term therapy (23). These patients can have diarrhea, develop hypoalbuminemia from a protein-losing enteropathy, and lose blood from intestinal inflammation. Small-intestinal strictures may develop. The strictures that are seen are thin, concentric, diaphragmatic strictures that can variably block the lumen of the bowel (24). The cause of the inflammation is not clear, but the increase in small-intestinal permeability caused by a local effect of NSAIDs on the bowel may permit damage by luminal toxins and bacteria. Thromboxane-induced vasoconstriction or platelet aggregation may also contribute to the permeability changes induced by NSAIDs.

A. Effects of Enteric-Coated Medications

When enteric-coated potassium preparations were used to reduce gastrointestinal discomfort induced by oral potassium supplementation, they were found to cause small-intestinal ulcers. The tablets released high concentrations of potassium adjacent to the bowel wall and caused spasm of the bowel vessels with subsequent ischemic necrosis. Significant fibrosis accompanied healing and led to bowel stenosis. These tablets are no longer used, but other slow-release preparations that are held up during their passage through the intestine by a stricture, or lodge in a diverticulum, could cause similar injury.

B. Small-Bowel Diverticula

Most duodenal diverticula are found in the midduodenum, on the medial wall near the papilla of Vater. The incidence of these diverticula varies from up to 20% in postmortem studies to a few percent on upper gastrointestinal series. Studies have shown a positive correlation between age and duodenal diverticula (25). These diverticula are only rarely responsible for nutritional deficiencies in the elderly (26). The presence of a diverticulum in this position may make cannulation of the ampulla during endoscopic retrograde cholangiopancreatography a bit more difficult. More importantly, the presence of these juxtapapillary diverticula also seems to increase the frequency of biliary calculi (27). Thirty-five percent of patients with choledocholithiasis have a juxtapapillary diverticulum. The stones that are found are commonly pigmented. This suggests that bacterial overgrowth in the diverticulum, perhaps associated with papillary sphincer insufficiency or functional stasis in the bile duct, leads to infection of the biliary tract and secondary calculus formation. The bacterial B-glucuronidase deconjugates bile pigments and permits formation of pigmented stones.

Jejunal diverticula are formed when the mucosa herniates through the submucosa and muscularis. This occurs on the mesenteric side of the intestine at the points of entrance of blood vessels in a fashion that is similar to the formation of the false diverticula found more commonly in the colon. The sacs are atonic, without a muscular coat, so they fill during peristalsis but empty with difficulty through their narrow stomas. These diverticula are found at postmortem in up to 4.6% of cases but are seen on only some 1.5% or less of small-bowel barium studies (28). These diverticula can cause adhesions and strictures with intestinal obstruction. They can cause a volvulus, lead to enterolith formation (29), perforate with formation of a pneumoperitoneum, intussuscept, or trap a foreign body. Their role in bacterial overgrowth has been discussed.

REFERENCES

1. Corazza GR, Frazzoni M, Gatto MRA, Gasbarrini G. Ageing and small-bowel mucosa: a morphometric study. Gerontology 1986; 32:60–65.
2. Arora S, Kassarjian Z, Krasinski SD, Croffey B, Kaplan MM, Russell RM. Effect of age on tests of intestinal and hepatic function in healthy humans. Gastroenterology 1989; 96:1560–1565.
3. Riepe SP, Goldstein J, Alpers DH. Effect of secreted Bacteriodes proteases on hyman intestinal brush border hydrolases. J Clin Invest 1980; 66:314–322.
4. Haboubi NY, Lee GS, Montgomery RD. Duodenal mucosal morphometry of elderly patients with small intestinal bacterial overgrowth: response to antibiotic treatment. Age Ageing 1991; 20:29–32.
5. Bardhan PK, Gyr K, Beglinger C, Vögtlin J, Frey R, Vischer W. Diagnosis of bacterial overgrowth after culturing proximal small bowel aspirate obtained during routine upper gastrointestinal endoscopy. Scand J Gastroenterol 1992; 27:253–256.
6. Donald IP, Kitchingmam G, Donald F, Kupfer RM. The diagnosis of small bowel bacterial overgrowth in elderly patients. J Am Geriatr Soc 1992; 40:692–696.
7. Lipski PS, Kelly PJ, James OFW. Bacterial contamination of the small bowel in elderly people: is it necessarily pathological? Age Ageing 1992; 21:5–12.
8. Haboubi NY, Montgomery RD. Small bowel bacterial overgrowth in elderly people: clinical significance and response to treatment. Age Ageing 1992; 21:13–19.
9. Soudah HC, Hasler WL, Owyang C. Effect of octreotide on intestinal motility and bacterial overgrowth in scleroderma. N Engl J Med 1991; 325:1461–1467.
10. Swinson CM, Levi AJ. Is coeliac disease underdiagnosed? Br Med J 1980; 281:1258–1260

11. Cooper BT, Holmes GKT, Cooke WT. Lymphoma risk in celiac disease of later life. Digestion 1982; 23:89–92.
12. Jabbari M, Wild G, Goresky CA. Scalloped valvulae conniventes; an endoscopic marker of celiac disease. Gastroenterology 1988; 95:1518–1522.
13. McIntyre AS, Ng DPK, Smith JA, Amoah J, Long RG. The endoscopic appearance of duodenal folds is predictive of untreated adult celiac disease. Gastrointest Endosc 1992; 38:148–151.
14. Dandalides SM, Carey WD, Petras R, Achkar E. Endoscopic small bowel mucosal biopsy: a controlled trial evaluating forceps size and biopsy location in the diagnosis of normal and abnormal mucosal architecture. Gastrointest Endosc 1989; 35:197–200.
15. Juby LD, Rothwell J, Axon ATR. Lactulose/mannitol test: an ideal screen for celiac disease. Gastroenterology 1989; 96:79–85.
16. Bardella MT, Molteni N, Cesana B, Baldassarri AR, Bianchi PA, IgA antigliadin antibodies, cellobiose/mannitol sugar test and carotenemia in the diagnosis and screening for celiac disease. Am J Gastroenterol 1991; 86:309–311.
17. Hill PG, Thompson SP, Holmes GKT. IgA anti-gliadin antibodies in adult celiac disease. Clin Chem 1991; 37:647–650.
18. Volta U, Molinaro N, Fusconi M, Cassani F, Bianchi FB. IgA antiendomysial antibody test: a step forward in celiac disease screening. Dig Dis Sci 1991; 36:752–756.
19. Bai JC, Sambuelli A, Sugai E, et al. Gluten challenge in patients with celiac disease: evaluation of alpha 1-antitrypsin clearance. Am J Gastroenterol 1991; 32:312–316.
20. Bullamore JR, Wilkinson R, Gallagher JC, Nordin BEC, Marshall DH. Effects of age on calcium absorption. Lancet 1990; ii:535–537.
21. Gallagher JC, Riggs BL, Eisman J, Hamstra A, Arnaud SB, DeLuca HF. Intestinal calcium absorption and serum vitamin D metabolites in normal subjects and osteoporotic patients. J Clin Invest 1979; 64:729–736.
22. Gabriel SE, Jaakkimainen L, Bombardier C. Risk for serious gastrointestinal complications related to the use of nonsteroidal anti-inflammatory drugs: a meta-analysis. Ann Intern Med 1991; 115:787–796.
23. Bjarnason I, Zanelli G, Smith T, et al. Non-steroidal anti-inflammatory drug-induced intestinal inflammation in man. Gastroenterology 1987; 93:480–489.
24. Bjarnason I, Price AB, Zanelli G, et al. Clinicopathological features of nonsteroidal antiinflammatory drug-induced small intestinal strictures. Gastroenterology 1988; 94:1070–1074.
25. Osnes M, Løtveit T, Larsen S, Aune S. Duodenal diverticula and their relationship to age, sex and biliary calculi. Scand J Gastroenterol 1981; 16:103–107.
26. Pearce VR. The importance of duodenal diverticula in the elderly. Postgrad Med J 1980; 56:777–780.
27. Kennedy RH, Thompson MH. Are duodenal diverticula associated with choledocholithiasis? Gut 1988; 29:1003–1006.
28. Cooke WT, Cox EV, Fone DJ, Meynell MJ, Gaddie R. The clinical and metabolic significance of jejunal diverticula. Gut 1963; 4:115–131.
29. Herbetko J, Brunton FJ. Enteroliths of small bowel diverticula. Clin Radiol 1991; 43:311–313.

6

The Colon

Ellen J. Scherl
Beth Israel Medical Center and Mount Sinai Hospital, New York,
New York

Daniel Helburn
Hamden Internal Medicine, Hamden, Connecticut

I. INTRODUCTION

The clinician caring for older patients with colonic disease needs to remind them gently but firmly that they are not being "cast off" as their colon begins to fail them. The challenge to the physician is, indeed, to balance, like a gyroscope, the external psychosocial demands of aging with the knowledge of pathophysiology of colonic disease. Treating colonic disease *in the elderly* in many ways presents the greatest challenge of treating colonic diseases.

II. DIVERTICULAR DISEASE OF THE COLON

A. Definition

Diverticulosis describes a colon with herniations or blind out-pouching of mucosa and submucosa protruding through the bowel wall muscle layers, which may be symptomatic or asymptomatic. Diverticulitis describes a colon with diverticula that are inflamed. Diverticular disease describes the symptom complex that results from colonic diverticula.

B. Epidemiology

Diverticular disease is most common in middle-aged and elderly patients in the Western world. Diverticulosis may be asymptomatic in 30% of the population in Western countries by the age of 60, and in 50% of the population by the age of 70. Clinically significant diverticular disease occurs primarily in the sixth and seventh decades of life. Diverticular disease probably develops slowly over a 20-year period of time resulting from wear and tear associated with a low-fiber diet. Painter and Burkitt has stated that diverticular disease is an unusual condition in Africa. He has suggested that it takes approximately 20 years of exposure to a low-fiber diet, in areas of Africa where dietary habits are westernizing, for the disease to occur in Africans (1).

C. Pathology

Colonic diverticula arise in weakened areas of circular smooth muscle resulting from the penetration of blood vessels passing to the submucosal layer. The development of diverticula is thought to be associated with chronically high intraluminal colonic pressure, partly due to low dietary fiber which produces small stool volume.

D. Clinical Features

In uncomplicated diverticular disease, patients complain of left lower quadrant pain. The abdominal pain is preceded by a history of intermittent lower abdominal discomfort and distension associated with constipation. In some patients, there is associated right lower quadrant pain due to cecal distension. There may be a sensation of pressure or dysuria associated with bladder irritability. There may be minor rectal bleeding and mucus in the stool. Generally, patients appear in good health. However, cancer must always be excluded. Physical examination may reveal mild left lower quadrant tenderness, or a full colon which may simulate a mass raising the possibility of an abscess or carcinoma. More often the examination is unremarkable in uncomplicated diverticular disease. Laboratory evaluation may detect anemia, leukocytosis, or elevated sedimentation rate. Abdominal sonography should exclude intrinsic compression due to ovarian tumor or abscess in patients with pelvic and rectal symptoms.

Barium enema remains the best study in diagnosing the extent of diverticulitis. Barium enema should be delayed for approximately 1 week after the onset of suspected diverticulosis to allow for some resolution of inflammation, thereby reducing the possibility of perforation. *Abdominal CT scan* with oral contrast will show thickening of the bowel wall, inflammation of the mesentery, and pericolic abscess, when present. Abdominal CT scan should be reserved for patients who cannot retain the barium enema, or who have suspected intraabdominal abscesses and might be candidates for CT guided drainage. *Colonoscopy* is indicated, if rectal bleeding occurs, to detect the site of bleeding in patients with diverticulosis and to exclude colonic carcinoma. In patients with suspected diverticulitis, colonoscopy may identify inflammatory bowel disease or ischemic colitis. As with barium enema, perforation is a risk in patients with diverticulitis and should be delayed for at least 1 week after acute symptoms. *Angiography* is also helpful in determining the site of diverticular bleeding.

E. Differential Diagnosis

Ischemic colitis in the elderly may present as abdominal pain with guarding and tenderness, but more often it is associated with bloody diarrhea, contrasting with the more typical constipation of diverticular disease. Acute ischemia with necrosis presents with hypotension and shock, and may simulate perforated diverticulitis. Ischemic colitis occurs more frequently in elderly patients with major cardiovascular or thrombotic diseases.

Colon carcinoma is usually associated with weight loss and loss of appetite, and may be associated with a palpable mass on physical examination.

Inflammatory bowel disease, more commonly Crohn's disease than ulcerative colitis, does occur in segments of the colon containing diverticular disease. If concomitant inflammatory bowel disease and diverticular disease go unrecognized, the patient often suffers a more severe "malignant" course with fistula and abscess formation, with a poor prognosis. Acute diverticulitis associated with acute ulcerative colitis predisposes to toxic megacolon.

Appendicitis occurs in the elderly population, and a long appendix on a mobile cecum falling into the pelvis or the left abdomen does occur. If surgical exploration is indicated and no obvious diverticulitis is discovered, the appendix should not be overlooked (2).

Irritable bowel syndrome remains a diagnosis of exclusion. In the older patient with a long history of constipation, with or without alternating diarrhea and abdominal pain, the diagnosis of diverticular disease and carcinoma must be excluded before entertaining the diagnosis of irritable bowel syndrome.

Angiodysplasia of the right colon must be excluded in the elderly patient who presents primarily with colonic hemorrhage. The majority of such patients thought to be bleeding from diverticulosis are, in fact, bleeding from angiodysplasia of the right colon (3). The complications of diverticular disease include acute diverticulitis, abscess, diverticular mass (phlegmon), peritonitis, colovesicular or enterovaginal fistulae, obstruction, and bleeding. Symptoms often change when complications occur.

F. Management: Uncomplicated Diverticular Disease

Managing asymptomatic diverticulosis usually involves ingesting 20–30 g fiber, which will decrease the intraluminal pressure and increase transit time. High-fiber cereals, fruits, vegetables, and grains are good sources. Fiber supplements such as bran or psyllium may be used. Methylcellulose may achieve decrease in intraluminal pressure without causing secondary flatulence. Lactulose will increase transit time, but may cause flatulence and distension due to release of intestinal gas resulting from bacterial metabolism of sugar. Fiber should be increased to 20–30 g/day gradually, and the patient should understand that optimal therapeutic response may take at least 3 months. Fluid intake should be increased as well. If symptoms do not improve on a high-fiber diet with adequate fluid supplementation, cholelithiasis, peptic ulcer disease, gastroesophageal reflux, and other inflammatory conditions should be excluded. Some patients, however, do well only on a low-roughage diet, avoiding raw foods. Almost all patients do better if they avoid spices and alcohol.

G. Management: Complicated Diverticular Disease

Acute diverticulitis is often associated with fever and leukocytosis. If the diverticulitis is mild, clear fluid diet and oral antibiotics should be initiated. Diet is gradually liberalized to a low-residue solid diet. If the diverticulitis is moderate to severe, it is best treated with IV hydration and IV broad-spectrum antibiotics. If the patient fails to respond within 72 hours, surgical intervention needs to be considered for possible abscess or perforation (4). Surgical intervention should also be considered for recurrent attacks of diverticulitis or persistent left lower quadrant tenderness and leukocytosis. Either a staged Hartmann procedure or resection of the affected segment with anastomosis may be performed. Peritoneal lavage, with or without antibiotic solution, may be added to the operative approach.

Diverticular abscess presents with persistent fever, increasing leukocytosis (15,000–50,000 WBC count), worsening abdominal pain, possibly with suggestion of localized mass and signs of localized peritonitis. Surgical resection with or without a diverting colostomy (a staged Hartmann procedure) is recommended.

Purulent peritonitis usually follows rupture of a diverticular abscess, or spread of severe acute diverticulitis. Clinically, there is marked abdominal tenderness and guarding, fevers, leukocytosis, and bacteremia progressing to hypotension, tachycardia, and finally septic shock. In elderly patients this clinical presentation may either suggest myocardial infarction or thromboembolism, in which case these entities must be excluded. Alternatively, myocardial infarction, thromboembolism, or urosepsis may complicate severe diverticulitis/peritonitis in the elderly. While a staged resection (Hartmann's procedure) with drainage is the treatment of choice, drainage of the abdominal cavity with saline and antibiotic solution may be all the elderly patient's condition allows. Postoperative complications and mortality rise significantly in the elderly patient with peritonitis secondary to diverticular disease.

Colovesicula fistulae may present with pneumaturia, fecaluria, or mild dysuria and pyuria. Most fistulae are treated by a one-stage resection of the pelvic colon (5).

Obstruction in diverticular disease always raises the concern of carcinoma. Patients with diverticular obstruction usually have a long history of increasing abdominal discomfort and generally appear healthy, contrasted with cancer patients, who have a shorter history of abdominal symptoms associated with anorexia and weight loss. Many patients with diverticular obstruction respond the nasogastric or long tube suction, with intravenous antibiotics. Interval segmental resection can then be performed.

Bleeding (please see the section on colonic hemorrhage).

H. Surgical Decisions

Uncontrolled infection such as abscess, fistula, peritonitis, or perforation is an imperative indication for surgical intervention. Since the surgical mortality is high in the older patient, careful selection of patient is critical. Conservative management is appropriate for mild leukocytosis which is not rising steadily. There is need to exclude ischemic colitis and inflammatory bowel disease, both of which present with abdominal pain, tenderness, and fever, similar to diverticulitis, but which also present with bloody diarrhea and mucus. While patients with ischemic colitis frequently have concomitant cardiovascular diseases, cardiovascular disease also occurs with diverticular disease.

III. COLON CANCER

A. Definition

Colorectal carcinoma is second only to lung cancer as the leading cause of cancer deaths. In the United States an individual has about a 1 in 20 lifetime risk of developing colorectal carcinoma, but the risk increases with age.

B. Epidemiology and Etiology

The majority of colorectal cancers occur in persons over the age of 40. While colorectal carcinoma is not exclusive to the geriatric population, recent reviews of operated patients show that two-thirds are over the age of 60 and one-quarter are over the age of 70. The sigmoid colon is the most common primary site of colon carcinoma. As the age of onset increases, however, right-sided tumors become more common. The importance of this disease will become more of an issue as the aging population continues to grow (6). Factors believed to increase the incidence of colon cancer include *personal or family history of colorectal carcinoma, familial polyposis, inflammatory bowel disease*, and the presence of *adenomatous polyps*. There seems to be an association with increasing age, obesity, high-fat low-fiber diet, and low calcium intake (7).

C. Clinical Presentation

Abdominal discomfort, weight loss with or without associated anorexia, and recent change in bowel habits should always be evaluated and should not be considered part of the aging process until other diagnoses have been excluded. Because elderly patients tend to have medical problems, their symptoms tend to be minimized or ignored. Social isolation and financial constraints may limit their participation in screening programs. Age itself is not a determining factor for survival. The 5- and 10-year cure rates following resection are approximately the same for patients in their seventh, eighth, and ninth decades of life (8).

D. Differential Diagnosis

Approximately 1% of colorectal carcinoma patients have chronic ulcerative colitis (9). Patients with colonic Crohn's disease also have an above average risk of developing colorectal carcinoma (10).

E. Screening Guidelines

The most recent guidelines of the American Cancer Society (ACS) recommend fecal occult blood testing annually and sigmoidoscopy every 3–5 years in asymtomatic people over the age of 50 (11). Modified screening for individuals at higher risk for developing colorectal carcinoma is also suggested (12). Patients with a personal history of *previous colorectal cancer, adenomatous polyps*, or *inflammatory bowel disease* are at greater risk for colorectal cancer. Once colonoscopy has cleared the colon of adenomatous polyps, repeat colonoscopy should be performed in 3–5 years. If clear of polyps at that time, it should be performed again in 5 more years (13).

IV. MANAGEMENT
A. Surgical Treatment

Many if not most patients with diagnosed colorectal carcinoma will have an operable cancer intended for cure. Even patients with incurable cancer should be considered for palliative resection, when medically stable, to prevent or delay anemia and/or obstruction, and to reduce the risk of invasion to adjacent organs. Preoperative CT scan is important. The need for IVP can be determined from the CT scan. Either complete colonoscopy or barium enema should be performed to exclude synchronous colorectal cancer. Endoscopic ultrasonography is available which is useful in assessing the depth of invasion of small rectal tumors. Sigmoidoscopy, with or without ultrasonography, is important in determining whether low anterior resection or abdominal peritoneal resection is necessary. A rectal tumor with the lower edge above 8 cm from the anal verge in a woman, or above 9–10 cm from the anal verge in a man, is treatable by primary resection (lower anterior resection) rather than abdominal peritoneal resection with colostomy.

Elderly patients with colorectal carcinoma may have preexisting cardiopulmonary disease and typically require preoperative cardiologic assessment, hydration, and antibiotics. Not only should these patients be hospitalized prior to surgery, but the surgeon and anesthesiologist should work closely together and should educate the patient and their family about realistic postoperative expectations. The morbidity and mortality associated with resection of colorectal carcinoma in the elderly is acceptable even with the presence of advanced disease as long as there is adequate preoperative assessment of the patient's risks based on cardiopulmonary and general physiologic status (14). If the patient is a poor operative risk, then laser photocoagulation with tumor ablation provides a palliative approach for both obstruction and hemorrhagic manifestations of colorectal carcinoma.

B. Adjuvant Therapy

Adjuvant therapy involves chemotherapy following primary tumor resection in an attempt to prevent recurrence. Very few adjuvant therapies have successfully decreased the overall mortality from the disease. In elderly patients this becomes important because these patients, with multiple medical problems, tolerate the toxicity of adjuvant therapy poorly. The National Institutes of Health Consensus Conference recently concluded that Stage III patients unable to enter a clinical trial should be offered adjuvant 5 FU/Levanithole unless medical or psychosocial contraindications exist (15). Oral supplemental calcium as adjuvant therapy may be beneficial (16).

C. Treatment of Metastatic Cancer

A recently reported regimen with significant benefit in pancreatic carcinoma has been tried in the treatment of metastatic liver disease from colon carcinoma. This regimen of 5 FU, Leukovorin, Mitomycin C-, and Dipyrimadole is associated with minimal toxicity (17).

D. Postoperative Follow-up

After colorectal surgery, initial follow-up screening colonoscopy should be performed at 3–6 months and annually thereafter. If the 1-year postoperative examination of the colon is negative, some endoscopists recommend follow-up at 2- to 3-year intervals thereafter. After a curative resection, an elevated postoperative CEA usually normalizes within 6 weeks. Postoperative CEA should be followed at each visit. All patients should have an annual chest X-ray.

E. Management of Recurrence

If postoperative CEA elevation is confirmed by repeat analysis, CT scan of the abdomen, pelvis, and chest should be performed. MRI may be more informative if pelvic recurrence of rectal carcinoma is suspected. Improvements in surveillance and operative technique have enabled some patients with isolated intrahepatic, intraabdominal, or pulmonary metastases to benefit from curative resection (18).

Chemotherapy and radiation therapy are beneficial to patients with recurrent colorectal carcinoma. Radiation therapy is the treatment of choice for accessible solitary metastases in bone, brain, or presacral area. Contact with family members and social workers encourages communication which will favorably affect the patient's postoperative course and needs at some. Elderly patients require special assistance in handling and caring for their colostomy, and this instruction should begin while the patient is hospitalized. Intractable pain associated with colorectal carcinoma secondary to invasion of the lumbosacral plexus may not respond well to opiates and requires a multidisciplinary effort. Again, psychosocial intervention is helpful to both the patient and the family.

The collaborative effort of physicians, nurses, social workers, psychologists, and family members in supporting and understanding patients with colorectal carcinoma enables them to continue to lead purposeful lives while enhancing their sense of self-esteem.

V. COLONIC HEMORRHAGE

A. Definition, Differential Diagnosis, Clinical Features, and Management

The most frequent presentation of colonic bleeding in the elderly is occult blood in the stool, followed by bright red blood coating the surface of the stool, seen in the toilet bowel or on cleaning the perianal area. The latter usually indicates local anal pathology. These anal lesions usually heal quickly, and there may not be signs of recent hemorrhage 2–3 days after the bleeding episode. Blood mixed with the stool, with or without mucus, usually suggests a colonic or rectal lesion such as colonic tumor or colitis. Large amounts of blood with little or no stool suggest bleeding from diverticular disease or angiodysplasia, two common disease entities in the elderly population.

Other common sources of colonic bleeding in the aged include diverticulosis, carcinomas, polyps, angiodysplasia, ischemic colitis, and radiation colitis. Inflammatory bowel disease is a less common in the elderly. Aortoduodenal and aortoileal fistula in elderly patients who have undergone aortic graft placement for aortic aneurysm repair is a rare cause of lower GI bleeding but does occur.

Bleeding may be exacerbated or unmasked by anticoagulation therapy or idiopathic or atrogenic thrombocytopenia. Some patients who have undergone antibiotic therapy may have prolonged coagulation due to malabsorption of vitamin K. After resuscitation and stabilization of a patient with major lower GI bleeding, diagnosis should be made with colonoscopy when possible. Colonoscopy will yield a diagnosis in 80–90% of patients with lower GI hemorrhage.

Sometimes colonoscopy provides the additional advantage of being therapeutic (19). GI bleeding from colon carcinomas in the elderly may be treated nonoperatively either if the patient is a poor surgical risk or if the tumor is inoperable. Endoscopic laser therapy both controls bleeding and may ablate the tumor mass (20). Sigmoidoscopy is indicated in any patient with lower GI hemorrhage. Barium enema may be helpful in cases where the colon is narrowed by diverticular stricture. However, it should generally be discouraged in lower hemorrhage due to its failure to detect angiodysplasias, and its interference due to retained barium should angiographic studies or future colonoscopy become necessary.

If barium enema is performed, sigmoidoscopy should be performed to adequately investigate the rectum. Anoscopy remains the procedure of choice for investigating hemorrhoids, fissures, and other anal pathology. Angiography is helpful in massive GI bleeding, often immediately preceding emergency surgery. Slow or intermittent hemorrhage may be detected by radionuclide scans. Technetium-99m-labeled red blood cell scan is more accurate than technetium-99m sulfur colloid scans. Small-bowel enteroscopy may be helpful in defining bleeding of obscure origin (21). If initial workup fails to establish a cause for bleeding and the bleeding stops, it is necessary to follow the patient carefully for recurrence. Too often the elderly patient is discharged and returns several months later with a major, life-threatening hemorrhagic episode. This is especially true in the elderly patient with herald bleeding due to an aortoenteric fistula.

B. Angiodysplasia

In elderly patients angiodysplasia is a common cause of lower GI bleeding. Typically, the lesions occur in the right colon and ileum and appear as 0.5–1.0 cm fat or slightly tufted red areas. They are submucosal arteriovenous malformations. Angiodysplasia is associated with cardiovascular disease, especially of the aortic valve. Acute presentation of angiodysplasia is either hematochezia, or maroon or melenic stool. Chronic bleeding may present with either anemia and/or guaiac-positive stool. Diagnosis is made either by colonoscopy or by angiography. Endoscopic therapy consists of laser photocoagulation or electrocoagulation. Rebleeding occurs in 10–30% of cases, and therefore colonoscopic follow-up is appropriate. Right hemicolectomy may be curative (?), and should be reserved for patients who have continued bleeding uncontrolled by endoscopic methods and have no evidence of ileal angiodysplasia ileoscopy and/or angiography.

C. Diverticular Disease

Diverticular bleeding usually causes mild to moderate hemorrhage in association with diverticulitis. Occasionally, acute massive hemorrhage from colonic diverticula occurs in the absence of preceding symptoms of diverticulitis. Typically, there is a history of acute hematochezia in association with clots. Massive diverticular bleeding typically stops spontaneously in 80% of patients. Rebleeding is rare if the patient has had no further bleeding after 24 hours from the initial bleeding episode.

Colonoscopy is the diagnostic procedure of choice in most cases of colonic bleeding. However, in diverticula bleeding, positive findings are infrequent. Barium enema is useful in defining anatomical extent of diverticulosis but has limited value in determining a bleeding site. Intraoperative endoscopy is also not diagnostic in diverticular bleeding. Angiography is the only accurate method to document the actual bleeding site.

Success of angiography depends on the rate of bleeding at the time of the study. Because bleeding is intermittent in massive diverticular bleeding, timing in angiography is key. Also, bleeding from a diverticulum may not be shown on angiogram. When active bleeding is documented angiographically, vasopressin infusion is associated with cessation in the majority of patients. If bleeding continues despite vasopressin infusion, arterial embolization may be attempted. Although embolization is successful, many clinicians are reluctant to use embolization because of the increased risk of infarction. Surgical resection is reserved for patients with continued hemorrhage. Segmental resection, when the source of bleeding has been identified angiographically, is associated with a lower risk and less postoperative long-term diarrhea than subtotal colectomy. When the bleeding site is unidentified, subtotal colectomy is the procedure of choice.

D. Ischemic Colitis

Ischemic colitis may cause either acute or chronic lower GI bleeding and, occasionally, bloody diarrhea in the elderly. Although atherosclerotic occlusion of the inferior mesenteric artery occurs frequently in the elderly, it is a rare cause of ischemic colitis. Ligation of the inferior mesenteric artery during abdominal aortic surgery is the usual etiology. Nonocclusive ischemic colitis occurs more frequently and is caused by hypoperfusion due to cardiogenic shock. Digitalis and dehydration may contribute. Sudden onset of explosive bloody diarrhea is typical presentation. Alternatively, the presentation may be subtle, with delayed onset of mild bloody diarrhea. Clinically, localized tenderness in the presence of bloody diarrhea is the distinguishing feature of ischemic colitis. Stricture formation is likely to occur if bloody diarrhea persists beyond 4–6 weeks, and often requires resection and anastomosis. Persistent leukocytosis and fever suggest possible perforation. The development of a palpable mass, persistent fever, and leukocytosis suggests an abscess which, if not drained, may eventually rupture. If rupture does occur, then segmental resection with interval reanastomosis is recommended.

Diagnosis may be suggested by abdominal X-rays which show characteristic "thumbprinting" due to submucosal edema and hemorrhage. Early endoscopic findings reveal dusky-violet and hemorrhagic patches of mucosa; later, ulcerations with or without exudate are seen. The rectum is usually spared in nonocclusive ischemic colitis. Occlusive ischemic colitis due to ligation of the inferior mesenteric artery usually extends into the rectum. While the risk of perforation is not high, the endoscopist is cautioned against aggressively defining the limits of the lesion.

Therapeutic management includes putting the bowel at rest with either a clear liquid diet or intravenous fluids. Antibiotics may also be used, although their efficacy is not well documented. If perforation occurs, segmental resection with an interval anastomosis is recommended.

E. Anorectal Bleeding

Hemorrhoids and anal fissures may cause lower GI bleeding, characterized by bright red blood with, or following, bowel movements. Hemorrhoidal bleeding is often painless while bleeding from anal fissures is associated with discomfort on defecation. Anal fissures are usually posterior, but occasionally anterior, in women. Other locations raise the concern of Crohn's disease, ulcerative colitis, or carcinoma in elderly patients. Anal lesions rarely cause anemia. Colonoscopy or barium enema should be performed in elderly patients to evaluate other possible sources of hematochezia or anemia.

Bulk agents to soften the stool are advised. Frequent warm baths and anesthetic ointments are helpful in managing painful aspects of anal lesions. Bleeding hemorrhoids may be treated by rubber band ligation or hemorrhoidectomy. Injection sclerotherapy, cryosurgery, infrared coagulation, and laser excision have not been shown to be superior to rubber band ligation or hemorrhoidectomy.

VI. INCONTINENCE AND CONSTIPATION
A. Definition

Incontinence is a disorder of defecation which consists of loss of bowel control. Constipation is difficult or infrequent defecation.

B. Epidemiology

Fecal incontinence increases in prevalence with increasing age. In age, a multitude of disease processes may interfere with the mechanism of continence. It may be due to physiological overload, where anorectal sphincter function is overwhelmed, as in diarrhea, uncontrolled inflammatory bowel disease, or irritable bowel syndrome. Fecal incontinence may also be due to disease, in which case *minor incontinence* consists of incontinence to flatus, liquid or partially formed stool. *Major incontinence* is defined as incontinence to formed stool. Constipation is defined as a disorder of delayed colonic emptying as well as delay or difficulty in evacuation. The paradoxical situation of overflow incontinence due to accumulation of soft stool above massive fecal impaction should be considered.

C. Clinical Features
1. Incontinence

In robust or frail elderly patients fecal incontinence is a distressing personal and social burden resulting in dependence, loss of dignity, and loss of self-esteem. In patients who are demented or dying, incontinence limits the patient's acceptability by family, although the patient may be unbothered by the social implications. The most disruptive type of incontinence to the aware elderly patient is unfelt loss of stool. Sphincteric impairment may be due to neurologic events such as CVA or multiple sclerosis, or to metabolic conditions such as diabetic neuropathy or thyrotoxic myopathy collagen vascular diseases such as scleroderma or polymyositis, or anorectal surgery such as hemorrhoidectomy or fistulectomy. Radiation injury may also be associated. Incontinence associated with fecal impaction is treated with disimpaction followed by attempt at bowel habit retraining. The patient is instructed to defecate after a specific meal, in order to take advantage of the gastrocolic response. If the patient fails to defecate for 3 successive days, an enema should be used (24). Bowel retraining may reduce the likelihood of further impaction with incontinence. Physical examination will often reveal weakness of internal and external sphincters if the patient is asked to "bear down" as in defecating. In some patients with incontinence, biofeedback training or even surgery may be of value.

2. Constipation

Most clinicians accept a definition of constipation as less than three bowel movements a week. Commonly, the patient complains of straining at bowel movement. The stool is often hard, scylabous, or ribbonlike in irritable colon and in obstructing lesions. Large, bulky stool that is difficult to pass occurs in colonic atony. The patient with chronic, severe, intractable constipation may be evaluated with anorectal motility and defacography.

There is no one treatment for constipation. Dietary fiber is a mainstay. Wheat bran increases stool size and weight. Fruits and vegetables achieve a similar effect. If anorectal motility is normal, *bowel habit retraining* may be helpful. The patient is encouraged to attempt to have a bowel movement daily, within 10 minutes after a given meal, usually breakfast, in order to take advantage of the gastrocolic reflex. If unsuccessful after 10 minutes, enema or suppositories are given.

Wetting agents such as dioctyl sodium or sulfosuccinate soften the stool by acting as "detergents." The effect is helpful in patients with hard stool, but this can actually make rectal evacuation more difficult in the elderly patient.

Lubricants, such as mineral oil, retard water absorption and can make the stool softer and larger. Aspiration pneumonia and depletion of fat soluble vitamins are possible complications. Following disimpaction, the patient is instructed to take 1–3 tbsp mineral oil between meals, two times a day. The dose is gradually reduced to a maintenance level.

Stimulant laxatives, such assenna, cascara, aloe, bisacodyl (Dulcolax), and phenolphthalein (Ex-Lax) reduce water absorption and increase secretion. These agents may damage the myenteric neurons, producing diminished effect of the laxative, and may lead to colonic atony.

A combination of a bulking agent such as psyllium plus senna (Perdiem) may be more effective than either agent alone. Milk of Magnesia produces small-bowel secretion without causing damage to the myenteric neurons. Lactulose, a nondigestible sugar, also increases secretion but may cause bloating and flatulence due to intraabdominal bacterial fermentation of sugar.

Prokinetic agents such as Cisapride may have significant effect on increasing colonic transit time. Naloxone (an opioid antagonist) has also been used in treating constipation. *Biofeedback* in some patients with functional anorectal sphincters may be helpful. *Surgery* such as abdominal colectomy and ileoproctostomy for patients with colonic inertia should be considered only after motility studies of the esophagus, stomach, and small bowel have established that dysmotility is limited to the colon.

D. Megacolon

Colonic inertia (atonic constipation) is not uncommon in the elderly. Ogilvie's syndrome refers to pseudo-obstruction which is associated with a specific event such as a serious cardiovascular compromise, orthopedic surgery, or spinal cord injuries. The entire colon appears dilated, and stool in the rectal ampulla is hard. Often fecal impaction with overflow incontinence occurs in conjunction. Therapy in laxative-induced megacolon consists of a program of replacing laxatives with gradual increasing dietary fiber. Cisapride (Naloxone) and cholinergic medications such as urecholine may be helpful.

Ogilvie's syndrome or megacolon complicated by volvulus is best treated by colonoscopic decompression. During colonoscopy, continuous suction is applied in an attempt to decompress the megacolon and reduce the volvulus. The need for surgical management of megacolon is rare. On occasion, however, diverting ileostomy or colostomy is necessary for patients who fail to decompress colonoscopically.

REFERENCES

1. Painter NS, Burkitt DP. Diverticula disease of the colon: a 20th century problem. In: Smith AN, ed. Diverticula Disease of the Colon, Vol 4 (1) Clinics in Gastroenterology. London: WB Saunders, 1975; 3–21.
2. Smith A. Diverticula disease of the colon. In: Phillips S, Pemberton J, Shorter R, eds. The Large Intestine: Physiology, Pathophysiology and Disease. New York: Mayo Foundation, 1991; 549–577.
3. Casarella WJ, Kanter JE, Seaman WB. Right-sided colonic diverticula as a cause for acute rectal hemorrhage. N Engl J Med 1972; 286:450–453.
4. Wald A. Colonic diverticulosis. In: Winawer S, ed. Management of Gastrointestinal Disease. New York: Gower Publishing, 1993; 34.2–34.18.
5. Rodkey GV, Welch CE. Changing patterns in surgical treatment of diverticula disease. Ann Surg 1984; 200:466–477.

6. Block G. Colon cancer: diagnosis and prognosis in the elderly. Geriatrics 1989; 44(5):45–53.
7. Catalano M, Levine B. Cancer of the colon and rectum. Clin Geriatr Med 1991; 7(2):331–346.
8. Rosemurgy A, Block G, Shihab F. Surgical treatment of carcinoma of the abdominal colon. Surg Gynecol Obstet 1988; 167:399–406.
9. Lennard-Jones J, Melville DM, Morson BC. Precancer and cancer in extensive ulcerative colitis: findings among 401 patients over 22 years. Gut 1990; 31:800–806.
10. Hamilton SR. Colorectal carcinoma in patients with Crohn's disease. Gastroenterology 1985; 89:398–407.
11. American Cancer Society. Cancer Facts and Figures, 1994. Atlanta: American Cancer Society, 1994:9.
12. Burt RW, Bishop DT, Lynch HT. Risk and surveillance of individuals with heritable factors of colorectal carcinoma. WHO Collaborating Center for the Prevention of Colorectal Cancer. Bull WHO 1990; 68:655.
13. Winawer AJ, Zauber AG, O'Brien MJ, et al. Randomized comparison of surveillance intervals after colonoscopic removal of newly diagnosed adenomatous polyps. N Engl J Med 1993; 28:908.
14. Fitzgerald S, Longo W, Vernavaa DG. Advanced colorectal neoplasia in the high risk elderly patient: is surgical resection justified? Dis Colon Rectum 1993; 36:161–166.
15. Moertel C, Fleming TR, McDonald JS. Levanithole and fluorouracil for adjuvant therapy of resected colon carcinoma. N Engl J Med 1990; 322:352–358.
16. Lipkin M, Newnark H. Effect of added dietary calcium on colonic epithelial cell proliferation in subjects at high risk for familial colonic cancer. N Engl J Med 1985; 313:1384.
17. Isacoff WH, Botnick L, Rose C. Treatment of patients with locally advanced pancreatic carcinoma with continuous infusion of 5 FU, calcium, leukovorin, mitamycin C- and dipyrimadole. Proc Am Soc Clin Oncol 1993; 12:255.
18. Hughes KS, Simon R, et al. Resection of the liver for colorectal carcinoma metastasis: a multi-institutional study of indications for resection. Surgery 1988; 103:278–288.
19. Brand EJ, Sullivan BH, Sivak MD, et al. Colonoscopy in the diagnosis of unexplained rectal bleeding. Ann Surg 1980; 192:111–113.
20. Grant D, Scherl E, Waitman A, Chateau F. Laser therapy and vascular abnormalities. Silvus S, ed. Therapeutic Gastrointestinal Endoscopy. New York: Igaku Shoin, 1990:151–174.
21. Waye LB Jr. Small bowel enteroscopy: a comparison of findings with push and sonde enteroscopy in 81 patients with G.I. bleeding of obscure origin. Gastro Intest Endosc 1988; 34:207.
22. Woolrich A. Inflammatory bowel disease in older age. In: Korelitz B, Sohn N, eds. Management of Inflammatory Bowel Disease, St. Louis: Mosby Yearbook, 1992.
23. Brandt LJ, Dickstein G. Inflammatory bowel disease: specific concerns in the elderly. Geriatrics 1989; 44:107–111.

100

24. Goodel W. Nervous rectum. JAMA 1988; 11:5–7.
25. Cerulli M, Nikoonanesh T, Schuster M. Progress in biofeedback conditioning for fecal incontinence. Gastroenterology 1979; 76:742–746.
26. Gillick MR. Choosing Medical Care in Old Age: What Kind, How Much, When to Stop. Cambridge, Mass: Harvard University Press, 1994:208.

7

Anorectal Diseases of the Elderly

Henry Ferstenberg
Albert Einstein College of Medicine, Bronx, and Beth Israel Medical Center, New York, New York

The anorectal area increases in importance as a person gets older. The fixation on "normal" bowel habits leads the elderly to perform many ritual acts such as oral intake of laxatives as well as usage of various types of enemas and suppositories. Many conditions result from use and abuse of these preparations. On the other hand, certain diseases tend to become more prevalent in the elderly.

This chapter deals with this important aspect of a human's later life.

I. ANORECTAL ANATOMY

The rectum is the end organ of the gastrointestinal tract commencing at the level of the third sacral vertebra and terminating just proximal to the dentate line. The anus is the terminal portion of the intestinal tract that begins where the rectum ends and continues for 4–5 cm (Fig. 1).

Various muscle groups line and surround the anorectal complex, forming tubes, slings, and wraps of contractile fibers. The involuntary internal sphincter is a continuation of the rectal smooth muscle and is found just proximal to the dentate line. Meanwhile, the voluntary external sphincter is a group of skeletal muscles that surround the anal canal.

The blood supply to this area involves three sets of vessels. The most cephalad is the superior rectal artery which comes off as the end artery of the inferior mesenteric artery and splits into two segments. The middle rectal arteries come off the internal iliac, and the inferior rectal arteries come off the internal pudendal arteries arising from the internal iliacs.

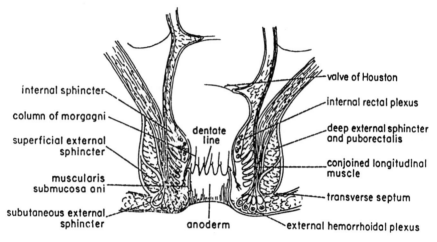

internal sphincter

column of morgagni

superficial external
sphincter

muscularis
submucosa ani

subutaneous external
sphincter

dentate
line

anoderm

valve of Houston

internal rectal plexus

deep external sphincter
and puborectalis

conjoined longitudinal
muscle

transverse septum

external hemorrhoidal plexus

Figure 1   The anorectal anatomy.

The venous drainage of the anorectal complex is extensive and rich. The returning blood exits via both the systemic and portal systems. The inferior and middle rectal veins empty into the internal iliac vein and thus into the systemic system. The superior rectal vein empties into the portal system via the inferior mesenteric vein. Further venous anastomosis occur between the three hemorrhoidal venous systems in the rectal submucosa forming various venous plexi.

Lymphatic drainage is rich and empties via the superior rectal artery to the inferior mesenteric artery, and laterally to both the superficial and deep inguinal nodes.

The anus and rectum are innervated by the sympathetic, parasympathetic, and somatic systems. The external anal sphincter and anal canal lining are supplied by somatic nerves.

The sympathetic fibers are derived from the first three lumbar segments of the spinal cord. The parasympathetic fibers emanate from the second, third, and fourth sacral nerves (nervi erigentes), and together form the pelvic plexus.

II. ANORECTAL PHYSIOLOGY

The anorectal complex is the end organ of an elongated gastrointestinal route. The pressure gradient composed of motor activity and contractile waves in the rectum results in a barrier to caudal progression of feces until

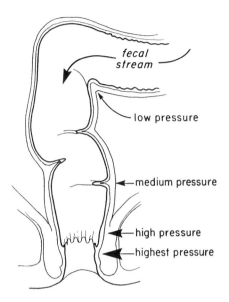

Figure 2 Physiological reservoir function.

the retentive mechanisms of the rectosigmoid are overcome (Fig. 2). The distal rectum is normally in a collapsed state with its Houston valves and rectosigmoid angle holding back the fecal load. The lateral angulation of the sigmoid colon tends to be accentuated with fecal filling.

The external sphincter, a striated muscle, adapts to various stimuli. At rest, the sphincter muscle mechanism shows tetanic activity. Coughing, deep breathing, and sneezing result in increased tone while micturition decreases tone. On the other hand, rectal distension by feces, gas, or both will increase sphincter tone with small volumes, but will cause urgency and the need to defecate with large volumes. The external sphincter reflex contraction, synchronous with the internal sphincter relaxation, maintains continence when the stimulating material reaches the distal rectum. This mechanism allows the individual time to decide on the appropriate action in regard to the nature of the stimulating material. Therefore, this allows voluntary contraction of the internal sphincter with concomitant compliance mechanisms by the colon to adjust for intrarectal volume.

III. ANAL INCONTINENCE

Incontinence can be classified into true, partial, or overflow. It may be associated with diarrhea, constipation, lack of flatus control, fecal soiling, or fluid feces.

Overlow incontinence occurs when there is relaxation of the anal sphincter as the rectum fills to its capacity, as in fecal impaction, with liquid feces and mucus leaking. True incontinence implies external and internal sphincter impairment, whether caused by sensory or mechanical deficit or both. Partial incontinence is the passage of flatus, fluid feces or mucus per anus without either voluntary contraction or the patient's knowledge or both.

The treatment of elderly patients with incontinence lies in treating the initiating cause. Alleviation of diarrhea and constipation will often obviate more aggressive care such as 1. Thiersch operation that narrows the anal ring by a foreign body implant of a silastic wire or teflon; 2. colostomy, whether sigmoid or transverse loop, to divert the fecal stream; 3. sphincteroplasty, to mobilize the ends of the external sphincter and make the anal canal 1 finger snug.

IV. RECTAL PROLAPSE (PROCIDENTIA)

Rectal prolapse is the protrusion of the entire thickness of rectal wall across the anal sphincter. Altemier (1) classified the condition into three types: Type 1 is a protrusion of the redundant mucosal layer (false prolapse most often associated with prolapsing hemorrhoids); type II is an intussusception without an associated cul-de-sac (pouch of Douglas) sliding hernia; and type III is a sliding hernia of the cul-de-sac, which occurs in the majority of cases.

The predisposing factors in rectal prolapse are straining associated with intractable constipation or diarrhea, numerous past pregnancies, pelvic operations, and neurologic diseases.

Treatment of rectal prolapse relates to resolution of the initial causes in type I: straining at stool, constipation, diarrhea, and/or hemorrhoids. Type II and III prolapses may be treated with the Ripstein procedure (Fig. 3) where the rectosigmoid is fixed to the sacrum by a sling. This prevents the rectum, which has lost its lateral attachments, to become a straight tube, intussuscept, and prolapse. Therefore, essentially, the operation restores the posterior curve of the rectum and maintains this position during defecation. Another therapeutic means to correct type III procidentia is abdominal proctopexy and sigmoid resection where a segment of sigmoid colon is removed and the rectum fixed to the sacrum (Fig. 4).

In medically unstable patients with type II or III rectal procidentia, the Thiersch operation (Fig. 5) encircles the anal orifice with a nonirritating silver wire. The palliative procedure can be done under spinal, epidural, or local anesthesia. The wire provokes a mild to moderate fibrotic reaction that reinforces the atonic sphincter and at the same time mechanically

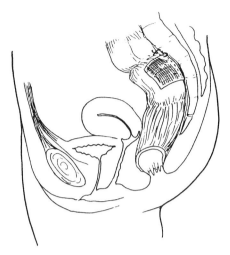

Figure 3   The Ripstein repair.

supports and contains the prolapse. The most common complications of the Thiersch procedure are fecal impaction and infections.

V. HEMORRHOIDS

All humans are born with hemorrhoids. This plexus of veins found at and about the anorectal area increases in size with age. This highly specialized

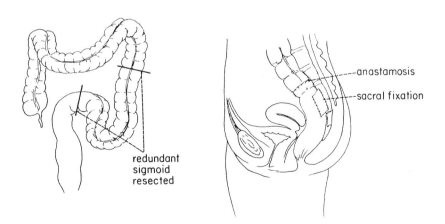

Figure 4   Abdominoproctopexy with accomanying sigmoid resection.

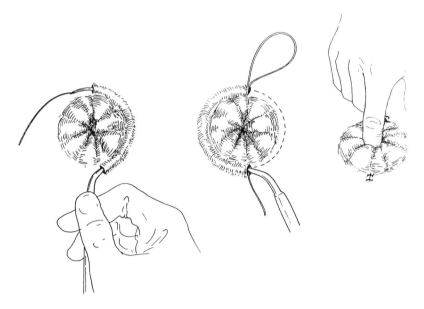

Figure 5 The Thiersch operation.

vascular padding or cushion slides down (internal hemorrhoids) in the anal canal with defecation. Hemorrhoids may be symptomatic or asymptomatic.

Internal hemorrhoids are found at the dentate line. Their relative positions are left lateral, right anterolateral, and right posterolateral. During defecation, the internal hemorrhoids tend to become engorged with blood, thereby cushioning and dilating the anorectal opening and canal.

As the population is aging, the frequency of enlarged hemorrhoids is increasing. Constipation leading to stretching of the internal hemorrhoid cushions results in further engorgement. This situation proceeds to dilation and engorgement of the smaller external hemorrhoids. Furthermore, the tendency for prolapse of the hemorrhoids increases with time, and the normally lax rectal mucosa tends to be dragged downward with the prolapsing, blood-laden, congested hemorrhoids. It is essential to remember that chronically congested, prolapsed internal hemorrhoids lying outside the tonic anal sphincter may lead to strangulation, thrombosis, gangrene, and abscess formation. Hemorrhoidal plexus abscess formation may lead to a localized pararectal, infralevator, and supralevator abscess, as well as phylephlebitis.

Elderly patients with chronic constipation and hemorrhoidal problems are frequently treated with suppositories, ointments, enemas, and quite often, oral laxatives. At first, manual massage and manual replacement are tried, when spontaneous reduction of these prolapsed hemorrhoids does not occur. Without reduction, the eventual outcome is surgery. Remember, surgical intervention does not remove the underlying causes of hemorrhoids.

In the elderly, treatment of diarrhea, constipation, and intestinal inflammation, such as inflammatory bowel disease and diverticulitis, may ameliorate and resolve hemorrhoidal problems. In the elderly, it is "essential" that prior to any assumption that hemorrhoids are the cause of rectal bleeding, a complete gastrointestinal workup is performed to ascertain that there is no other cause for bleeding. Surgical treatment of hemorrhoids, thrombosed or prolapsed, should be instituted only after a barium enema or a full colonoscopy is performed.

The treatment of external hemorrhoids is quite simple. The treatment is usually nonoperative and consists of bulk-forming agents, sitz baths, and correction of diarrhea. The most important treatment is the reassurance that, more often than not, external hemorrhoids spontaneously resolve. Operative intervention is reserved for thrombosed external hemorrhoids with removal of clot, when moderate to severe pain is present or when the

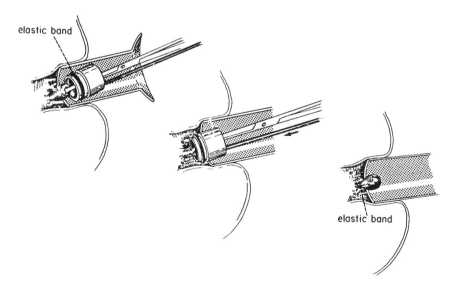

Figure 6   Internal hemorrhoids: rubber band ligation.

external hemorrhoid is part of a mixed hemorrhoid complex (elements of internal and external hemorrhoids).

On the other hand, the treatment of internal hemorrhoids is diversified. Internal hemorrhoids often present with bleeding, prolapse, and sometimes pain. Medical therapy for diarrhea, constipation, and other gastrointestinal diseases may be attempted prior to any surgical intervention. The aim is to avoid straining on defecation, whether diarrhea or constipation is present.

Rubber band ligation (Fig. 6) of internal hemorrhoids yields good results. This markedly reduces hemorrhoid size by submucosal rectal venous plexus atrophy and mucosal scarring.

Cryotherapy, infrared photocoagulation, and manual dilation of the anal canal have also been tried with some degree of success. Yet, the best results have been obtained with formal hemorrhoidectomy (Fig. 7). Properly excised, internal hemorrhoids do not return to plague the patient. There is minimal inpatient time, prompt and fairly rapid healing, and minimal soiling and incontinence. There is no anal canal manipulation nor dilatation needed when a carefully planned internal hemorrhoidectomy is performed. A 1–2% complication rate includes postoperative bleeding, localized abscess, anal stricture, and fecal or flatulence incontinence. Further surgery may be required should these occur.

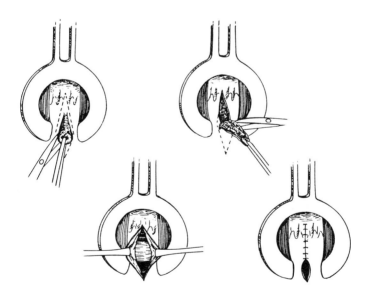

Figure 7   Hemorrhoidectomy.

VI. FISSURE IN ANO

Anal fissures are cracks or linear ulcerations in the anoderm epithelial lining that yield discomfort, spasm, and pain much disproportionate to the size of the cuts themselves. An anal fissure occurs with equal incidence in males and females; 90% are in the posterior midline. The fissure extends from just distal to the dentate line up to the anal verge. The fissure may present in the form of a localized discomfort or pain, itching, bleeding, and a mucoid discharge.

Causes of anal fissures in the elderly include constipation, diarrhea, straining at stool, inflammatory bowel disease, and local trauma such as enema abuse.

Fissures tend to heal with conservative management by first treating the primary cause and then administering local wound care. This directed care includes sitz bathes, salves, stool softeners, bulk-forming foods or agents, and increasing oral intake of fluids. Surgery is reserved for those who fail medical therapy. Surgery involves a sphincterotomy (Fig. 8), which reduces internal sphincter spasm and increases anal canal diameter. The end result is a decrease in resistance to the passage of stool, less anal trauma, and thereby fissure-in-ano healing. The other operative choice is fissurectomy with eventual sectioning of various amounts of the sphincter mechanism.

Surgical intervention for fissure in ano is marked by several complications including bleeding, abscess formation, prolonged postoperative pain, incon-

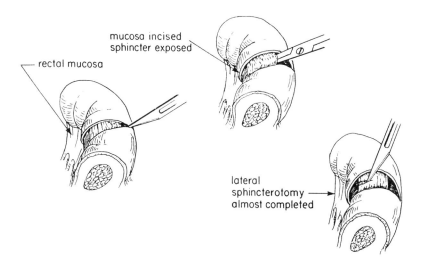

Figure 8 Lateral sphincterotomy.

tinence of flatus and/or fecal material, and hemorrhoidal prolapse. A good result is obtained in 95% of patients. Only 2% of the elderly whose primary cause (constipation, diarrhea, inflammatory bowel disease, and straining at stool) has not been corrected will continue to have anorectal disturbances.

VII. FISTULA IN ANO

Fistula in ano (Fig. 9) is a chronic tract formed between the perineal skin and the cephalad portion of the anal canal, the pectinate line. The fistula is a consequence of a pararectal inflammation and abscess that eventually penetrates and perforates the perineal floor. The inflammatory process commences at the anal crypts where the anal glands empty. The anal ducts become obstructed with liquid or solid stool. This impacted foreign material and occasional localized trauma with eventual inflammation lead to stasis with bacterial overgrowth and infection. The diagnosis is made by physical examination, anoscopy, and/or sigmoidoscopy. These endoscopic proce-dures assess the anatomy, find the internal opening, and evaluate for other diseases that produce fistulous abscesses and a fistula in ano.

Fistulas in ano have quite specific relationships to the anorectal sphinc-teric mechanism as described by Parks (2).

Treatment of a fistula in ano is most often surgical since medical therapy alone rarely leads to healing. Various techniques have been proposed. The only relative contraindication to opening a fistula in ano is established incontinence. Total transection of the anorectal ring causes complete incon-tinence. Meanwhile, the partial severance of the sphincteric muscle will lead to a weak sphincter with varying degrees of incontinence.

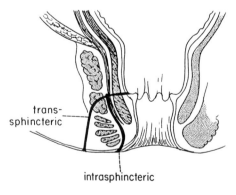

Figure 9   Fistula in ano.

Postoperative care involves first of all good surgical technique with proper alignment of tissues. Healing by granulation occurs from the depth of the wound to the surface. Sitz baths, bulk-forming agents, pain medications, and noncompressive dressings play a role in proper healing. Results of this therapy vary with the experience of the surgeon, type of fistula in ano, and postoperative care, with recurrence rates averaging 5%.

Fistula in ano may also be treated by simply "filleting open" the fistula (fistulotomy) (Fig. 10) or by placing a wire (a seton) (Fig. 11) through the fistula. The seton forms an ever tightening loop. The materials used have been metallic or nonabsorbable suture material that are left in place for several months. The progressively slow transection with scarring allows slow healing with preservation of the sphincteric mechanism.

VIII. ANORECTAL INFLAMMATION

Ulcerative proctitis may afflict the elderly with bloody, mucus-laden, debilitating diarrhea that may be continuous or episodic. The diarrheal stools may lead to dehydration, anemia, a feeling of tenesmus, and a generalized weakness. Proctosigmoidoscopy will yield a diagnosis. The management is almost exclusively medical, comprising corticosteroid enemas or supposito-

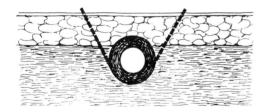

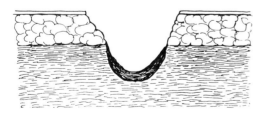

Figure 10 Fistulotomy.

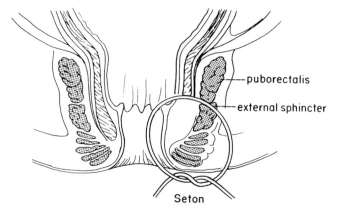

Figure 11   Seton treatment of fistula in ano.

ries, antidiarrheal compounds, oral salicylic–based medications, and low-residue diets.

Crohn's disease may involve any part of the alimentary tract. When it involves the rectum, there is an increased frequency of fistulas, fissures, and localized abscesses at and about the anorectal region. Management should be medical with oral antibiotics, antidiarrheal preparations, oral salicylates, and corticosteroids both orally and in the form of enemas and suppositories.

Irradiation proctitis may occur in both sexes as a result of localized ischemia. In females, external or internal radiation for gynecological malignancies will secondarily cause radiation proctitis. Meanwhile, irradiation of the prostrate gland will also lead to proctitis. The damage done by radiation to the end of the alimentary tract may present as rectal bleeding, diarrhea, mucous discharge, rectal pain, and tenesmus. Once again, the diagnosis is established by proctosigmoidoscopy.

The treatment is most often medical with low-residue diets, corticosteroid suppositories or enemas, and soothing sitz baths. Surgical intervention in the elderly, with ostomy diversion, is often performed to remedy debilitating symptoms such as bloody mucoid diarrheal stools. A more aggressive approach with abdominal perineal resection may be required in patients exsanguinating or with secondary tight strictures unresponsive to dilatation. Endoscopic Therapy of bleeding points by Laser or coagulation has also been used.

IX. BENIGN NEOPLASMS OF THE RECTUM

A. Hyperplastic Polyps (Metaplastic)

Small, pale, mostly sessile polyps are found in the rectosigmoid area. Histologically, they show tubular lengthening and depletion of goblet cells. They are asymptomatic and often associated with mild rectal irritation. Their malignant potential is essentially zero.

B. Adenomatous Polyps

Adenomatous polyps represent intraluminal growths, pedunculated or sessile, that protrude from the rectal mucosal surface. They may be histologically classified as tubular adenoma (75%), tubulovillous adenoma (15%), or villous adenoma (10%).

It is felt by most clinicians that these polyps have a malignant potential dependent on histologic type: 5% for tubular adenoma, 22% for villotubular adenomas, and 40% for villous adenomas. When accounting for size, a 1-cm or smaller polyp has a negligible chance of carcinoma. A 1- to 2-cm polyp has approximately a 10% chance of malignant transformation, but for polyps larger than 2 cm, there is a 50% likelihood of invasive carcinoma. When carcinomatous transformation occurs, penetration of the muscularis mucosa is the hallmark of malignant invasion. The muscularis mucosa contains the ever important lymphatics through which spread occurs. In the eldery, rectal polyps sometimes present as frank rectal bleeding.

REFERENCES

1. Altemeier WA, Cutbertson WR, Showergerdt, CJ, Hunt J. Nineteen years experience with the one stage perineal repair of rectal prolapse. Ann Surg 1971; 173:993.
2. Parks AG. Pathogenesis and treatment of fistula-in-ano. BMJ 1961; 1:463.

8

Motility Disorders in the Elderly

Jeffrey S. Gamss
Beth Israel Medical Center, New York, New York

Disorders of gastrointestinal motility are common and often unrecognized. More than half a million visits to physicians' offices for functional bowel disorders are made yearly by the elderly (1). These conditions are usually chronic and difficult to treat. Successful management often depends on a good physician-patient relationship. Motility of the digestive system is complex. An understanding of normal physiology is often the key to management.

Aging in itself has little effect on the motility of the gut. There is some evidence that there may be minor changes in gastric emptying. In the small intestine, studies suggest that there may be slower postprandial activity. It is doubtful that these changes have any significant clinical effect. Colonic motor activity is unchanged with aging alone. Motility disorders seen in the elderly are more closely related to systemic diseases and medications. Prolonged immobility alone can have profound effects on transit time (2).

Normal physiology and disorders of motility in the stomach, small intestine, and colon will be discussed here. Esophageal and anorectal dysmotility is discussed elsewhere.

I. GASTRIC MOTILITY

The function of the stomach is to store food and to deliver it as chyme to the small intestine. From a motility point of view, the stomach can be divided into two functional units: 1. The fundus and the proximal body regulate the emptying of liquids. In the resting state, the fundus is contracted. Upon swallowing, mediated by the vagus nerve, it relaxes to accom-

115

modate the ingested meal. Large volumes can be accommodated with minimal elevation in pressure (3). 2. The distal body and antrum serve as a grinding organ and pump. Antral contractions, also under vagal control, mix solid food with gastric juices. Larger particles are triturated by being pushed against a closed pylorus, thus being moved to and fro for further grinding. These contractions occur three times a minute, and are mediated by slow waves emanating from the gastric pacemaker located on the greater curvature, near the junction of the fundus and antrum. When solids are reduced to particles less than 1 mm in size, they pass through the pylorus into the duodenum (3). The pylorus has two major functions. It regulates emptying of solids by allowing only particles less than 1 mm to pass, and it prevents enterogastric reflux. Duodenal contractions clear gastric chyme downstream in order to reduce duodenal pressure, allowing further gastric emptying (3).

Normal gastric emptying is dependent upon many factors. Coordinated fundic, antral, pyloric and duodenal activity are essential. Truncal vagotomy with pyloroplasty or proximal vagotomy, with no drainage procedure, may be associated with delayed emptying of solids and accelerated emptying of liquids. Various substances, including glucose, fat, and amino acids such as phenylalanime and tryptophane, may slow gastric emptying by their action on small bowel receptors. They stimulate the release of CCK, which is responsible for the delayed gastric motility. Other hormones such as peptide YY, enteroglucagon, and possibly neurotensin may also be responsible agents. There are also duodenal receptors for pH and osmolarity. Low pH and high osmolarity of chyme slow gastric motility. An understanding of these principles will allow effective dietary manipulation.

II. DISORDERS OF GASTRIC EMPTYING

Gastroparesis is defined as a motility disorder of the stomach resulting in impaired transit of intraluminal contents from the stomach into the duodenum in the absence of mechanical obstruction (4). Symptoms include early satiety, postprandial bloating, nausea, vomiting, and abdominal pain. Patients may vomit food ingested hours previously. The pain is usually not severe, but rather a vague discomfort. Physical examination is often normal. A succussion splash may be present in severe gastric stasis.

There are many causes of gastroparesis. The most common are idiopathic, diabetes, prior gastric surgery, and drugs.

Idiopathic gastroparesis may account for more than half of all cases of gastroparesis in all age groups. The disorder is more frequent in women. It sometimes seems to follow an influenza infection. Since the vast majority of cases occur in younger patients, a thorough search for other causes must be made in the elderly before attributing symptoms to this condition.

Diabetic gastroparesis is probably due to a defect in the autonomic innervation of the stomach. These patients frequently have other kinds of neuropathy, such as orthostatic hypotension and peripheral neuropathy. Delayed gastric emptying is present in up to 75% of insulin-dependent diabetics. It should be suspected in diabetic patients who complain of nausea, bloating, or early satiety. Patients with diabetic gastroparesis may have marked fluctuation of blood glucose despite being compliant with diet and insulin doses. Hyperglycemia has been shown to cause delayed gastric emptying. Optimal control of blood glucose can improve gastric motility. Likewise, improved gastric motility can improve glycemic control.

Any surgical procedure involving a vagotomy may lead to gastroparesis. Vagotomy will often lead to more rapid emptying of liquids and delayed emptying of solids. Biliary procedures involving a Roux-en-Y diversion and vagotomy may cause gastroparesis and other upper gastrointestinal symptoms in nearly half of the patients.

It is important to recognize the effects that medications can have on GI motility. The elderly are frequently treated with a wide array of medications that can cause nausea and vomiting by central effects or by delaying gastric emptying. The most frequent culprits causing gastroparesis are antidepressants, which have an anticholinergic effect, and narcotics. Patients on these medications will frequently complain of nausea and bloating. Electrolyte depletion, often caused by drugs, is also known to delay gastric emptying.

In evaluating gastroparesis patients, a detailed history is vital. Many systemic diseases, such as diabetes mellitus scleroderma, and amyloidosis, can cause dysmotility. A history of peptic ulcer disease suggests the possibility of mechanical obstruction, due to either an active antral or a pyloric channel ulcer, or due to scarring and deformity from previous ulcers. The patient's drug history is significant, since certain drugs can lead to an easily reversible emptying disorder. Metabolic disorders, such as chronic renal failure, may cause chronic nausea and vomiting without delayed gastric emptying. Psychiatric disorders may manifest themselves as eating disorders leading to nausea and vomiting, with normal gastric emptying.

On physical examination, emphasis should be placed on assessing the patient's nutritional and hydration status. Complete neurological examination is essential. Careful attention must be given to the possibility of raised intercranial pressure. Evidence of autonomic dysfunction, such as orthostatic hypotension, peripheral neuropathy, and myopathic disorders should be sought. Significant abdominal findings include previous scars, masses, tenderness, distension, a succussion splash, and fecal occult blood. Examination of the extremities may reveal signs of connective-tissue disease.

Laboratory tests should include CBC, sedimentation rate, biochemical analysis, and thyroid function tests. An abdominal X-ray should be done to exclude the possibility of small-bowel obstruction. The next step is directed at excluding mechanical obstruction of the stomach. An upper GI series or endoscopy may reveal peptic ulcer disease or neoplasm.

At the time of upper endoscopy a biopsy for *Helicobacter pylori* is worthwhile. Active *H. pylori* infection resulting in gastritis may be a cause of chronic nausea. A small-bowel series is needed to exclude small-bowel pathology. An ultrasound or abdominal CAT scan may be neeeded to exclude an intraabdominal mass and to exclude biliary and pancreatic disorders. A radionuclide solid-phase gastric emptying study may confirm that delayed emptying is present. Radiolabeled eggs or chicken liver is used. Medications affecting gastric motility must be discontinued 48 hours prior to the test.

In research centers, antroduodenal manometry and electrogastrography using cutaneous electrodes are used to detect gastric dysrhythmias. The normal rhythm is three cycles per minute. Dysrhythmias such as tachygastria, bradygastria, tachy-bradygastria, and flatline have been described.

The treatment of chronic nausea and vomiting due to gastroparesis depends on the severity of presenting symptoms. Patients with severe nausea and vomiting may have signs of dehydration and poor glycemic control. Treatment may include hospitalization, IV hydration, careful control of blood glucose, and IV administration of prokinetic drugs. Most patients, however, can be managed on an outpatient basis.

Usually, minor dietary modifications are sufficient. Patients should be instructed to eat small, soft meals that are low in fat and fiber, and to avoid nondigestible solids. High-calorie liquid supplements may be needed in more severe cases. In a small number of patients with markedly severe gastroparesis, jejunal feedings may be needed. This is best accomplished with a surgically placed J tube, preferably via laparoscopic surgery.

Nausea and vomiting can be treated with antiemetics. Prokinetic agents are used to improve gastric emptying (5). Metaclopramide, a dopamine antagonist, increases gastric contractions, improves antroduodenal coordination, and has a central antiemetic effect. Adverse side effects include agitation, drowsiness, and tremor. Irreversible tardive dyskinesia has been reported in the elderly after long-term use. Due to the introduction of newer prokinetic agents with fewer adverse effects, the usage of metaclopramide is on the decline and will likely have limited use in the elderly.

Domperidone, a benzamidazole derivative, is awaiting approval for use in the United States. It is a dopamine antagonist with effects similar to those of metaclopramide. It rarely crosses the blood-brain barrier and therefore rarely causes CNS and extrapyramidal side effects. This agent may be uniquely useful in patients with abnormal motility due to levodopa therapy for Parkinson's disease. It can antagonize the perhipheral dopamin- ergic effects and not interfere with the central effects of levodopa.

Cisapride was recently approved for use in the United States. It is a benzamide derivative. It facilitates release of acetylcholine from cholinergic nerves in the myenteric plexus (6). It has effects throughout the GI tract. As opposed to metaclopramide and domperidone, it has activity in the jejunum and colon. It does not have antiemetic effects. Trials are under way to determine if the prokinetic effect of cisapride will persist with long- term use. Side effects are few and include loose stools and headaches.

The antibiotic erythromycin acts as an agonist of motilin receptors in the antroduodenal area. It increases amplitude and frequency of antral contractions, and it improves antroduodenal coordination (7). IV infusion of erythromycin accelerates gastric emptying in diabetic and postsurgical gastroparesis. Oral doses of erythromycin have been shown to accelerate gastric emptying. Results of long-term effects are pending. It is likely that the major role of erythromycin will be in acutely decompensated gastropare- sis. Side effects include abdominal cramping and nausea.

Opiate receptor antagonists such as naloxone HCl have shown some benefit in patients with gastroparesis. Larger trials are awaited. CCK recep- tor antagonists are being studied, since it is known that CCK inhibits gastric emptying.

Surgical intervention has a limited role in gastroparesis. A surgical jeju- nostomy may be placed (preferably via laparoscopy) in severely decompen- sated patients. Near total or total gastrectomy and Roux-en-Y gastrojeju- nostomy may lead to improvement in patients with chronic postsurgical gastric atony. Before recommending extensive surgery, it should be recog- nized that many patients may have no benefit, especially if the motility problem extends into the small bowel. Electrical pacing of the stomach via surgically implanted electrodes on the serosal surface of the stomach may be done in the future.

III. SMALL-INTESTINE MOTILITY

The motor function of the small bowel is responsible for mixing and propel- ling chyme toward the colon (8). After eating, the material is propelled in the intestine by a slow wave originating in the interstitial cells of Cajal at the junction of the outer longitudinal and inner circular layers of the muscularis mucosa. The frequency of the slow wave in the duodenum is about 12 per minute, falling stepwise along the intestine to about seven per minute in the ileum.

Net caudad movement of chyme is accompanied by extensive stirring and mixing. There are two distinct types of contractions: 1. Sleeve contractions produce shortening of the small intestine and are primarily responsible for mixing of interstitial contents. 2. Ring contractions, or perastaltic contractions, are primarily responsible for propulsion (8).

Prominent changes in the pattern of motility occur in relation to eating. During the fed state, ring contractions occur at an incidence of 30–70% of the maximum possible frequency. During the fasting state there is a cycle of three phases of motility. Phase 1 is a period of complete rest, without any contractions, lasting up to 80% of the cycle. Phase 2, lasting up to 20% of the cycle, is comprised of random contractions. Phase 3, lasting up to 5% of the cycle, occurs approximately every 1.5 hours. Between meals, ring contractions occur at maximal frequency and migrate along the gut. They are presumably responsible for clearing the intestines of bacteria and cellular debris. This pattern is frequently referred to as the migrating motor complex.

Regulation of small-bowel motility is complex. It involves the central nervous system, enteric nervous system, and various circulating hormones. Somatostatin, substance P, and others may initiate the migrating motor complex while feeding, insulin, CCK, and gastrin interrupt it. The contractile force is governed by the enteric hormones cholecystokinin and motilin.

IV. MOTILITY DISORDERS OF THE SMALL INTESTINE

Abnormalities of intestinal motility can lead to constipation, diarrhea, pseudo-obstruction, and malabsorption. Increased slow waves in hyperthyroidism result in diarrhea. Decreased slow waves in hypothyroidism result in constipation. Absence of the migrating motor complex, the intestinal housekeeper, can result in bacterial overgrowth and malabsorption, whereas increased frequency of the migrating motor complex in thyrotoxicosis may lead to diarrhea.

Small-intestinal motility disorders are now recognized more often than in the past. The disorder may be caused by dysfunctional intestinal smooth muscle, by abnormalities of the intrinsic and extrinsic nervous system, and possibly by abnormal levels of gastrointestinal hormones or neurotransmitters. There is an entire gamut of motility disorders. The disturbance may be manifested either as hypomotility or as uncoordinated hyperactive motility.

The acute absence of functional bowel activity is called ileus. It may mimic intestinal obstruction. Patients may have extreme abdominal distension, and there may be radiographic findings of air-fluid levels. It is commonly seen in the postoperative period. It may also occur in patients with severe infections and in patients who have an acute deterioration of a chronic illness. It is crucial not to confuse it with mechanical obstruction. Surgical exploration in patients with a functional problem can have disastrous results. Although the initial presentation in the two conditions can be quite similar, the absence of colic and the absence of peristalsis strongly suggest a functional disorder rather than mechanical obstruction.

The most extreme form of chronic intestinal hypomotility is called chronic intestinal pseudo-obstruction. It is defined as intestinal dilatation without obstruction (9). This syndrome represents the end of the spectrum of hypomotility disorders, and it is the most difficult form to manage. Attempts at treatment have been met with great disappointment. Newer treatment modalities may offer new hope. The acute form of functional obstruction predominantly involving the colon has been called Ogilvie's syndrome. A syndrome of polypneuropathy, ophthalmoplegia, leukoencephalopathy, and intestinal pseudo-obstruction has been named POLIP syndrome. The functional obstruction is due to visceral neuropathy.

Clinical features of intestinal dysmotility include nausea, bloating, vomiting, and generalized discomfort. The symptoms are usually precipitated by a meal, which may cause crampy pain and distension. Depending on the severity of the disorder, symptoms may be intermittent or they may occur daily. Many patients lose weight as a result of malabsorption due to bacterial overgrowth.

The physical examination may be normal in patients with mild dysmotility. In more severe cases, the abdomen may be distended, tympanitic, and tender. Bowel sounds are usually hypoactive and infrequent. Borborygmi may be present in some patients.

The etiology of chronic small-bowel dysmotility can be divided into primary and secondary disorders (10). Primary disorders include myopathic and neuropathic disorders. In the elderly the secondary causes are far more common. They include connective tissue and intestinal smooth-muscle disease, endocrine abnormalities, drug therapy, paraneoplastic syndromes, and miscellaneous causes.

Scleroderma is a disease of connective tissue that involves the skin and frequently the digestive tract leading to fibrosis. The small bowel is involved in approximately 40% of patients. As the disease progresses, degeneration of smooth muscle occurs. Bacterial overgrowth is common and may lead to malabsorption.

Patients with diabetes frequently have autonomic neuropathy. The small bowel is involved in up to 20% of patients. Intestinal transit may be slow, rapid, or normal. Diarrhea is a frequent problem. It is poorly understood and difficult to treat. Suggested mechanisms include motor abnormalities, a secretory process, bile acid malabsorption, and, rarely, bacterial overgrowth (11).

A recent onset of pseudo-obstruction, especially in a patient with a history of cigarette smoking, should raise the suspicion of oat cell carcinoma. It is often accompanied by a neurogenic bladder and other autonomic disturbances.

Several neurological conditions may be complicated by intestinal dysmotility. Parkinson's disease and antiparkinsonian medications have been associated with chronic functional obstruction.

Many drugs can affect small-bowel motility. Antidepressants may slow motility via their anticholinergic effects. Narcotics may cause dysmotility through their action on receptors in the GI tract. Calcium channel blockers frequently slow intestinal motility. The effects of drugs on motility should not be overlooked in the elderly, who are frequently on multiple medications. Recognition of small-bowel dysmotility may preclude an extensive workup and prevent much suffering.

The evaluation of small-bowel motility disorders is similar to the evaluation of gastric emptying disorders. It requires a high index of suspicion and a thorough history including a careful review of medications. A careful search for collagen vascular and metabolic disorders is required. Neurological examination should include a careful search for autonomic dysfunction (12). In addition to a CBC and complete chemistry, sedimentation rate, antinuclear antibodies, and thyroid function tests may be helpful.

It is essential that mechanical obstruction be excluded. This is especially true in patients who have had previous abdominal surgery. Abdominal plain films, as well as a small-bowel series and barium enema, are usually needed. Enterocleisis can be very helpful in detecting subtle structural abnormalities in the small intestine. Delayed transit through the small bowel without evidence of an obstructive lesion is the hallmark of intestinal hypomotility. In order to avoid complications, all barium should be evacuated, even if laxatives are required.

Small-intestinal manometry can sometimes be of value in differentiating myopathic from neuropathic causes of dysmotility (9). It is only performed in specialized centers. Manometry can characterize the migrating motor complex. In neuropathic disorders there are abnormal motor patterns, whereas in myopathic disorders, the pattern is normal but the contractions are of decreased amplitude (9).

When the diagnosis of motility disorder is in doubt and small-bowel manometry is not available, esophageal manometry may be of value. Since many intestinal motility disorders involve the entire GI tract, an abnormal esophageal manometry supports a clinical suspicion.

Other studies are sometimes helpful. Radionuclide gastric emptying studies can exclude delayed gastric emptying. Transit studies using opaque markers may show a disturbance in transit mainly due to colonic involvement. Scintigraphic studies and hydrogen breath tests may sometimes add useful information.

In mild cases of intestinal dysmotility, dietary manipulation alone may alleviate symptoms and make life manageable. Smaller, more frequent meals may preclude symptoms of nausea and pain by not exceeding the capacity of the small bowel. A low-lactose, low-fiber diet is more easily tolerated. In refractory cases, total parenteral nutrition may be necessary.

Drug therapy is not as effective in intestinal dysmotility as it is in gastric emptying disorders. It may, however, be of benefit in patients with normal small-bowel musculature. Erythromycin, a motilin agonist, induces motor contractions on a short-term basis. Trials testing long-term effects are awaited. Although cisapride has activity in the small bowel, its effects on intestinal motility have been disappointing. Octreotide, a long-acting analog of somatostatin, administered subcutaneously, has been somewhat helpful in patients with scleroderma. Opiate antagonists theroretically may be of some benefit. Further studies are needed. Symptoms of bloating, nausea, and steatorrhea due to bacterial overgrowth can sometimes be relieved by oral broad-spectrum antibiotics.

Attempts at surgical correction of intestinal motility disorders have more often than not led to major disappointment. The motility disorder is usually more generalized than initially recognized. A possible exception might be the patient with an isolated megaduodenum. In patients with severe distension and pain, a venting gastrostomy or enterostomy may relieve symptoms and may lead to a decreased number of hospitalizations for nasogastric decompression. Small-bowel transplantation is now being performed, but it is experimental at this time. It may offer an option in the future for patients with severe chronic intestinal pseudo-obstruction.

V. COLONIC MOTILITY

The motility of the colon is not as well studied as is the motility of the small intestine. Transit time through the colon is slow compared to the transit time through the small intestine. The reason may be that the mucosa of the colon is smooth and therefore has a limited surface area. Slower transit time is needed in order to complete the task of absorbing fluid and electrolytes.

Most contractions of the colon are designed to facilitate antegrade flow and to delay caudad movement. The principal points of delay are the cecum, ascending colon, sigmoid colon, and rectum. In addition, intermittent propagating contractions occur periodically, and move a mass of stool distally for longer distances. This rapid progress has been called mass movement (13).

Colonic motility varies with the state of eating. There is increased activity after meals, particularly in the sigmoid colon. The stimulus is food entering the duodenum. The likely mediator is CCK. This activity has been called the gastrocolic reflex. It accounts for the bowel movement commonly occurring after breakfast. Patients with a rather heightened gastrocolic reflex report a bowel movement after every meal. This has resulted in the false belief that the food is going right through the affected person. As opposed to the small intestine, there is no true cyclical activity in the interdigestive phase. During sleep, contractions are much less common. Stress has a definite effect on motor activity in the colon. Anger and pain have been associated with increased activity. Weeping may have the opposite effect.

VI. MOTILITY DISORDERS OF THE COLON

A. Constipation

The incidence of constipation markedly increases after age 65. Between 25% and 33% of people above 65 complain of this problem (14). Constipation, however, means different things to different people. The term may be used to describe hard stools, straining with defecation, pain with defecation, or small-volume stools. Using the definition of fewer than three bowel movements in a week will decrease the true incidence of chronic constipation to less than 5% of the elderly population (15).

Constipation may be caused by many diseases. Neurogenic causes include multiple sclerosis, Parkinson's disease, spinal cord injury, and stroke. Myopathic causes include amyloidosis and scleroderma. Metabolic causes include diabetes, hypothyroidism, and electrolyte disturbances. Many drugs have been incriminated. In the elderly, in particular, this remains the one area that is most easily corrected. It behooves every physician evaluating constipation to take a careful drug history and to be aware of the drugs that are associated with constipation.

Psychosocial factors can have great influence on bowel habits. A sedentary lifestyle, decreased fluid intake, and a low-fiber diet are often factors present in the elderly, although strict scientific evidence is lacking. Ignoring the urge to defecate or an aversion to bedpans may result in constipation or more serious complications such as fecal impaction.

Constipation not easily explained by known etiologies can be classified into slow-transit constipation, referring to a diffuse motility disorder of the colon, or rectal-outlet obstruction. The latter group of disorders is discussed elsewhere. Slow-transit constipation can be identified by radiopaque marker studies. The markers can be seen on X-ray dispersed throughout the colon demonstrating decreased propulsive activity.

Proper workup of chronic constipation begins with a careful history. It is necessary to accurately document the frequency of bowel habits, character of the stool, and duration of the symptoms. Associated symptoms such as straining, abdominal pain relieved or caused by defecation, bloating or distension, and weight loss are important to consider. Drug history is essential. The habitual use of laxatives may lead to a condition termed cathartic colon.

Physical examination should include a neurological evaluation to search for signs of cerebral infarction, deficits suggestive of spinal cord injury, features of Parkinsonism, and signs of autonomic neuropathy. During abdominal examination the presence of scars should be noted. The abdomen should be palpated for masses and areas of tenderness. Rectal examination must be done to exclude the presence of a mass or fecal impaction. The stool should be checked for occult blood. It is useful to check the perineal descent during Valsalva movement. Absent or paradoxical perineal movement is associated with outlet obstruction.

Laboratory tests should include a CBC, electrolytes, calcium, fasting blood glucose, and TSH to exclude known causes of constipation.

It is essential to exclude mechanical obstruction. Rectal or colon cancer should always be considered, particularly in patients presenting with a change of bowel habits. Postischemic, postradiation, and diverticular strictures can be associated with constipation. A flexible sigmoidoscopy and barium enema or colonoscopy are usually needed in elderly patients with recent onset of constipation or change in bowel habits. A pelvic sonogram on CAT scan may be indicated when there is evidence of extrinsic compression on the colon.

Studies using radiopaque markers may be helpful in distinguishing slow colonic transit from rectal-outlet disorders. Occasionally further tests such as defecography, electromyography, and anal-rectal manometry are useful. These tests are available in specialized centers; these are usually reserved for younger patients with chronic idiopathic constipation.

The treatment of constipation must be custom-designed for each patient. Constipating medications should be avoided if possible. Increasing activity, increasing fluid intake, and increasing dietary fiber are often beneficial in the patient with normal colonic motility. Patients should be encouraged to allow adequate time to fully evacuate their bowels. A warm meal for breakfast may stimulate the gastrocolic reflex. The patient may be instructed to use the Valsalva maneuver briefly in order to initiate defecation. For those with slow colonic transit time, and particularly in bedridden patients, a high-fiber diet may lead to serious problems, and a low-residue diet is indicated.

When dietary measures and fiber supplements are not sufficient, laxatives will usually be needed. Osmotic laxatives such as lactulose and sorbitol are very effective. They may cause large amounts of colonic gas, which may limit their use. They are absolutely contraindicated in mechanical obstruction. Magnesium salts may be used. Hypermagnesemia may occur in patients with diminished renal clearance. Chronic use of irritant laxatives such as senna and cascara are usually avoided in younger patients because of fear of cathartic colon. In the elderly this reservation is often overemphasized. Mineral oil should not be used in the elderly, since there is risk of aspiration leading to lipid pneumonia. The intermittent use of suppositories or gentle enemas can be very helpful, particularly for those with rectal-outlet obstruction. Some physicians do not advise enemas for fear of perforation of the anal canal or rectum. If one is properly instructed regarding insertion, the risk is minimal. The prokinetic agent cisapride has been shown to be somewhat effective in mild to moderate slow-transit constipation. Studies with longer follow-up are needed. Cisapride has been disappointing in patients with severe slow transit. It should not be used in patients with rectal-outlet obstruction.

B. Fecal Impaction

A potentially serious complication of constipation is fecal impaction. It can usually be detected by rectal examination. An empty rectal vault does not exclude the possibility of an impaction in the sigmoid colon. Patients often complain of pain in the rectum, although bedridden and demented patients may offer no complaints. Spurious diarrhea or liquid stool leaking around a low impaction may be the presenting symptom. It is not too uncommon to see a patient being treated with antidiarrheals for spurious diarrhea.

Large fecal impactions can sometimes cause marked colonic distension and even perforation. Stercoral ulcers can bleed profusely or, rarely, perforate, leading to fecal peritonitis.

The treatment of fecal impaction is often difficult. Digital disimpaction is unpleasant for the patient and the physician. It is often associated with pain and bleeding. On occasion, it may be necessary to disimpact the patient under sedation or even anesthesia.

An impaction higher up in the colon needs to be broken by enemas, or irrigation through a colonoscope. Polyethylene glycol–containing solutions have been used to cleanse the colon from above. Distension can occur if the impaction is not partially broken. Poorly absorbed sugars such as lactulose and sorbitol can be metabolized by colonic bacteria, generating large volumes of gas; they should not be used until the impaction is cleared. Perforation, bleeding, and sepsis have been reported from vigorous disimpaction.

Care must be taken to avoid a similar impaction in the future. Proper dietary regimen and laxative use must be understood by the patient. Dietary fiber and supplements should not be given to the bedridden patient who does not drink enough fluids, or to the patient with slow transit. Antidiarrheals should not be given for a prolonged period of time without proper monitoring.

C. Gas

Complaints relating to gas are frequently heard in the gastroenterologist's office. They include abdominal distension, excessive gas per rectum, and gas pains. The person affected rarely has excess intestinal gas (16). The complaint is usually due to hypersensitivity or a motility disorder, as seen in irritable bowel syndrome.

The normal volume of intestinal gas is around 100 ml. On a normal diet between 0.5 L and 3 L of gas is expelled daily. When fiber is eliminated from the diet, the volume of flatus can be reduced to about one-third the normal amount. Flatus is composed of several gases including carbon dioxide, hydrogen, methane, and nitrogen. The variable composition in different people is related to swallowed air, diet, and intestinal flora. Most of the gas in flatus is formed in the lower small intestine and colon, where the concentration of bacteria is the highest.

Diet plays a role in the amount of flatus produced. It is the easiest factor to modify. Hydrogen is generated by bacterial conversion of unabsorbed carbohydrates and proteins. A fiber-free diet can virtually eliminate hydrogen from flatus. Patients with malabsorption, as in bacterial overgrowth or mucosal disease such as sprue, will deliver greater amounts of unabsorbed carbohydrates and protein to the colon. This results in increased hydrogen production, leading to bloating and discomfort.

People who have low levels of a specific enzyme in the intestinal brush border needed to break down a specific carbohydrate will likewise generate greater amounts of hydrogen in their colon. The classic example is lactose intolerance, which can be documented by a hydrogen breath test. It can also be substantiated indirectly by eliminating lactose from the diet and monitoring the response.

In a similar fashion, but less well recognized, inadequate absorption of fructose and sorbitol can produce similar symptoms. Fructose is found in fruits and berries. Sorbitol is used in a large variety of candy and soft drinks. It is well recognized that beans, lentils, and peas produce excess flatus. The rich amount of oligosaccharides is a source for excess hydrogen production. Most normal people have increased breath hydrogen after ingesting wheat, corn, oats, and potatoes. Refined grains cause less production of hydrogen; rice flour does not cause increased breath hydrogen in normal individuals.

Gas in the upper GI tract is usually the result of swallowed air. Excess air swallowing in aerophagia can lead to epigastric fullness, bloating, nausea, and excessive belching. Colonic gas is mainly dependent on diet and the nature of the bacterial flora. Air trapped in the splenic flexure producing left upper quadrant pain has been termed *splenic flexure syndrome.*

The treatment of gas disorders is often disappointing. For the patient with aerophagia and upper GI tract complains, it is helpful to advise the patient to make an effort not to swallow air. Patients are advised to avoid carbonated beverages and to eat and drink slowly. Simethicone preparations may give some relief to individuals with excess gas in the upper GI tract.

Treatment of excess flatus and lower intestinal gas centers around dietary modification. Although patients usually do not have greater than normal amounts of intestinal gas, further reduction can make life more pleasant. Foods rich in dietary fiber that are useful in regulating bowel movements are often the source of increased flatus. Beans, lentils, peas, and leafy vegetables should be restricted. A 2-week trial of a lactose-free diet is helpful in determining whether further restriction is needed. Various preparations containing the enzyme lactase are available and are beneficial to the patient with mild to moderate lactose intolerance. Malabsorption of fructose or sorbitol should not be overlooked. Even the small amounts of sorbitol in sucking candies can cause significant symptoms. Eliminating these sugars for a brief period is worthwhile. If these restrictions do not lead to satisfactory results, it may be worthwhile to eliminate wheat, corn, oats, or potatoes as a trial. Rice flour and low-gluten wheat can be used as substitutes. In attempting to treat symptoms, it is wise to introduce one restriction at a time. It will allow a more positive identification of the offending agent. Activated charcoal has been used in attempts to adsorb gas. The results are usually disappointing.

A product containing the enzyme alpha-galactosidase has been introduced. It is marketed under the name Beano. It breaks linkages in oligosaccharides that human intestinal enzymes cannot break, thus providing less for the colonic bacteria to work on. Early reports are encouraging, but there are no trials establishing effectiveness and safety.

The task of providing relief of lower intestinal gas may be difficult, and requires a great deal of patient cooperation. Successful management will often lead to a grateful patient and spouse.

D. Chronic Diarrhea

Chronic diarrhea in the elderly is usually due to an underlying disorder. However, since diarrhea appears to be related to intestinal motility, it is appropriate to briefly outline the different classes of diarrhea and to discuss the evaluation and management.

The word diarrhea means different things to different people. It is frequently used to describe either an increase in stool frequency or volume, or a decrease in stool consistency. It is used to describe stool leakage or fecal incontinence. The classic definition of diarrhea is an increase in stool weight of more than 250 g in a 24-hour period. Chronic diarrhea has a duration of more than 3 months.

Diarrhea results when there is an imbalance between absorption and secretion in the intestinal tract. Approximately 9 L of fluid passes through the intestinal tract daily. Two liters comes from diet, and 7 L comes from secretions of the intestine and pancreas. Approximately 1 L of fluid is delivered to the colon where, it is further reduced to 100–200 ml. The normal colon can absorb up to 6 L of fluid daily. Diarrhea results when the ileal output is too great for the colon to handle or when the colon is diseased and cannot perform its normal function.

Diarrhea can be categorized into four separate groups for ease of discussion (17). In reality there is usually a combination of mechanisms. The basic categories are osmotic diarrhea, secretory diarrhea, mucosal abnormality leading to decreased absorption, and motility disorders.

It is not clear whether chronic diarrhea can result from abnormal intestinal motility alone. It is likely that disorders of motility are accompanied by net secretion of fluid. Hyperthyroidism, however, seems to cause diarrhea by increasing the frequency of the migrating motor complex.

The evaluation of chronic diarrhea in the elderly begins with a thorough history. First, the physician must determine if the patient truly has diarrhea. The patient's medication list must be reviewed. Magnesium-containing antacids and other laxatives are not infrequently taken by the elderly patient complaining of diarrhea. The patient's diet must be reviewed. Unabsorbed sugars, such as lactose in people with lactase deficiency and sorbitol, may be the cause of diarrhea. Elimination diets when followed carefully can often pinpoint the culprit. The patient on enteral feeding solutions often has diarrhea. The likely mechanism is an increased osmotic load. Diluting the feeding solution often relieves the problem.

The pattern of diarrhea is important to note. Nocturnal diarrhea usually signifies organic disease, whereas functional diarrhea rarely wakes the patient from sleep.

When the diagnosis of chronic diarrhea is established, it is necessary to exclude inflammatory conditions as the source. Fecal leukocytes and red blood cells are the hallmark findings.

Diabetics may have diarrhea due to several mechanisms. Neuropathy leading to sympathetic denervation can result in increased secretion and decreased absorption. Clonidine, an alpha-2 adrenergic agent, may be helpful for this condition. Motility disorders of the small bowel and colon have been described, and these may play a role.

Bacterial overgrowth can occur in diabetics, in patients with scleroderma, and in patients who have undergone gastric surgery or intestinal surgery involving bypasses or Roux-en-Y procedures. It may result in deconjugation of bile salts, which may lead to fat malabsorption or to an increased concentration of colonic bile acids inducing colonic secretion.

Effective treatment of chronic functional diarrhea depends on its cause. Management of the underlying disorder often leads to resolution of the diarrhea. Dietary management can be helpful. A low-residue diet may help some patients. Avoidance of caffeine, fat, and spices often gives symptomatic relief. Low doses of loperamide or a trial of cholestyramine is often used. Irritable bowel syndrome has been defined as a functional gastrointestinal disorder with recurrent symptoms of abdominal pain usually relieved by defecation, and an irregular pattern of defecation (18). Characteristic features include small volume stools with either diarrhea, constipation, or alternating constipation and diarrhea. Affected persons usually develop a pattern to their symptoms. Changes in a particular pattern may indicate concomitant disease. Sleep is rarely disturbed by irritable bowel syndrome. Weight loss, fever, vomiting, or bleeding argue against this diagnosis. Laboratory findings are generally normal. Anemia, luekocytosis, elevated sedimentation rate, or fecal occult blood are evidence of other disorders such as malignancy, infection, or inflammatory disease.

Irritable bowel syndrome is a generalized motor disorder that can affect the entire GI tract. Psychosocial factors, stress, food, and drugs are among the stimulae that can produce symptoms. Studies have suggested that altered pain perception may also play a role (19).

Although irritable bowel syndrome may be less common in the elderly than in younger people, it is nonetheless highly prevalent. In patients over 65 years of age, more than half a million visits to physicians are made yearly for functional bowel disorders. It is twice as likely to affect women (1). Presentation after age 60 has been said to be uncommon. It is possible, however, that the symptoms are falsely attributed to diverticular disease rather than to irritable bowel syndrome. In patients reporting symptoms later in life, it is imperative to exclude other diseases such as colon cancer, diverticulitis, and ischemic colitis. In addition to blood, urine, and stool tests, all elderly patients presenting with symptoms should undergo colonoscopy or barium enema.

An important step in treatment is educating the patient. It is important to stress that the syndrome is not progressive and that it does not affect longevity. Dietary modification can be very effective. A high-fiber diet can be particularly helpful in the elderly, who more often have constipation-predominant irritable bowel syndrome. A fiber supplement can be added if diet alone is not effective.

Antispasmodics are frequently prescribed, and they should be used with great caution in the elderly. Anticholinergic effects can cause confusion, tachycardia, constipation, urinary retention, and blurred vision. They are contraindicated in patients with glaucoma, unstable cardiac disease, or gastrointestinal or urinary obstruction.

Low doses of antidepressants may be helpful, even in the patient who does not manifest symptoms of depression. Opiates may aggravate symptoms by causing gastrointestinal spasm and should therefore be avoided. Low doses of loperamide have been effective for diarrhea-predominant irritable bowel syndrome.

REFERENCES

1. Sandler RS. Epidemiology of irritable bowel syndrome in the United States. Gastroenterology 1984; 87:314–318.
2. Brockleburst JC, Kirkland JL, Martin J, et al. Constipation in longstay elderly patients: its treatment and prevention by lactulose, poloxalkol, dihydroxyanthraquinone and phosphate enema. Gerontology 1983; 29:181–184.
3. McCallum RW. Motor function of the stomach. In: Sleisenger MH, Fordtran JS, eds. Gastrointestinal Disease: Pathophysiology, Diagnosis, Management. 4th ed. Philadelphia: W.B. Saunders, 1989:675.
4. Read NW, Houghton LA. Physiology of gastric emptying, pathophysiology of gastroparesis. Gastroenterol Clin North Am 1989; 18:359.
5. Reynolds JC. Prokinetic agents: a key in the future of gastroenterology. Gastroenterol Clin North Am 1989; 18:437–457.
6. McCallum RW. Cisapride: a new class of prokinetic agent. Am J Gastroenterol 1991; 86:135.
7. Annese V, Janssens J, Vantrappen G, et al. Erythromycin accelerates gastric emptying by inducing antral contractions and improved gastroduodenal coordination. Gastroenterology 1992; 102:823–828.
8. Christensen J. Gastrointestinal motility. In: West JB, ed. Best and Taylor's Physiologic Basis for Medical Practice. Baltimore: Williams and Wilkins, 1990:614.
9. Colemont LJ, Camilleri M. Chronic intestinal pseudo-obstruction: diagnosis and treatment. Mayo Clin Proc 1989; 64:60.
10. Chokhavatia S, Anuras S. Neuromuscular disease of the gastrointestinal tract. Am J Med Sci 1991; 301:201–214.
11. Soergel KH. Management approach to diarrheal diseases. In: Winawer SJ, ed. Management of Gastrointestinal Diseases. New York: Gower Medical Publishing, 1992:1–24.

12. Camilleri M, Philips SF. Acute and chronic intestinal pseudo-obstruction. In: Stollerman GH, LaMont JT, eds. Advances in Internal Medicine, Vol 36. Chicago: Year Book Medical Publishers, 1990:287–306.
13. Christensen J. Motility of the colon. In: Johnson LR, ed. Physiology of the Gastrointestinal Tract. 2d ed. New York: Raven Press, 1987:665.
14. Sonnenberg A, Koch TR. Physician visits in the United States for constipation: 1958–1986. Dig Dis Sci 1989; 34:606.
15. Whitehead WE et al. Constipation in the elderly living at home. Definition, prevalence and relationship to lifestyle and health status. J Am Geriatr Soc 1989; 37:423.
16. Lasser RB et al. The role of intestinal gas in functional abdominal pain. N Engl J Med 1975; 293:524.
17. Spiro HM. Mechanisms of diarrhea. In: Clinical Gastroenterology. 4th ed. New York: Macmillan, 1992:353.
18. Schuster MM. Irritable bowel syndrome. In: Sleisenger M, Fordtran J. eds. Gastrointestinal Diseases. 4th ed. Philadelphia: W.B. Saunders, 1989:1403–1408.
19. Whitehead WE, Engel BT, Schuster MM. Irritable bowel syndrome: physiological and psychological differences between diarrhea predominant and constipation predominant patients. Dig Dis Sci 1980; 25:404–413.

9

Mesenteric Ischemia

Karl T. Bednarek and Wataru Tamura
Beth Israel Medical Center, New York, New York

I. INTRODUCTION

Ischemic bowel disease occurs when blood flow to any part of the intestine is interrupted. This entity has variable clinical presentations due to tremendous heterogeneity of its pathophysiology. It is extremely important to understand the pathophysiology of the different ischemic bowel syndromes, since diagnostic and therapeutic approaches are different, and prognosis is affected. Accordingly, in this chapter we provide a review on the classification and pathophysiology of intestinal ischemia.

II. CLASSIFICATION

Listed below are some important variables to consider in classifying ischemic bowel syndromes:

onset and duration of ischemia	acute/chronic
location of bowel affected	small intestine/colon
size and type of vessel involved	artery/vein/intramural vessels
mechanism of ischemia	embolus/thrombus/vasospasm

Based on these variables, the following general concepts are noteworthy:

1. Acute ischemia is much more common than chronic forms of the disease.

2. Colonic ischemia is the most common form of intestinal ischemia (50–70%), and is seen approximately twice as often as acute mesenteric ischemia (20–30%).
3. Ischemia of arterial origin is far more frequent than that of venous disease.
4. Of acute mesenteric ischemia, emboli are more frequently the cause than thromboses.
5. Nonocclusive mesenteric ischemia due to vasospasm is being increasingly recognized.

A concise classification of ischemic bowel syndromes based on clinical manifestations is as follows:

1. Acute mesenteric ischemia
     Arterial
          Superior mesenteric artery embolism
          Superior mesenteric artery thrombosis
          Nonocclusive mesenteric ischemia
     Venous
          Acute mesenteric venous thrombosis
2. Chronic mesenteric ischemia
     (intestinal angina)
          Arterial
          Diffuse atherosclerotic stenosis of the splanchnic arteries
     Venous
          Chronic mesenteric venous thrombosis
3. Focal segmental ischemia of the small bowel
4. Colonic ischemia

III. PATHOPHYSIOLOGY (1)

A. Vascular Anatomy

The vascular anatomy of the gastrointestinal tract is complex with extreme variability. However, the more constant features and principles are important in the understanding of intestinal ischemia. The blood flow to the gastrointestinal tract is derived from three main arterial trunks; the celiac artery (supplies the stomach and duodenum), the superior mesenteric artery (SMA; supplies the duodenum to the transverse colon), and inferior mesenteric artery (IMA; supplies the transverse colon to rectum). Each arterial trunk supplies its territory within the gastrointestinal tract by forming vast cascades terminating in end arterioles that each traverse the intestinal mucosa supplying the individual villi. There are connections within these networks such as superior/inferior pancreaticoduodenal arteries between the celiac artery and SMA, the arc of Riolan and the marginal artery of Drummond between the SMA and IMA, communications between the IMA and branches of the internal iliac artery in the rectum (Fig. 1). They offer a protective mechanism against ischemia through collateral circulations. Thus, intestinal ischemia occurs when there is a significant cessation of blood flow through the main arterial trunks via occlusive or nonocclusive mechanisms in the face of poor collateral circulations. Examples of areas of possible poor collateral circulations, commonly referred to as *watershed areas*, are the splenic flexure and the rectosigmoid junction.

B. Physiology of Intestinal Blood Flow

The intestinal blood flow on average receives about 30% of the cardiac output, but the majority (approximately 70%) of this is distributed to the intestinal mucosal layer, which is the most metabolically active. The small bowel receives the most, followed by colon, and then stomach.

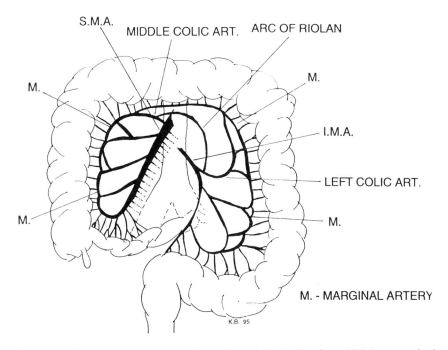

Figure 1 Vascular anatomy showing collateral circulation (arc of Riolan, marginal artery of Drummond).

Control of intestinal blood flow occurs where there is the most vascular resistance, at the arteriolar level. Very little control of blood flow occurs at the level of the arterial trunks. Additional control is achieved at the precapillary sphincter, where in the fasting state only about 20% of the capillary beds are perfused, leaving tremendous reserve for increased metabolic demands.

Although the exact control mechanism of intestinal blood flow is poorly understood, some important points are worth mentioning. Three major factors contribute—the sympathetic nervous system, humoral factors, and local factors.

1. The alpha-adrenergic system maintains vascular tone and mediates vasoconstriction; the beta-adrenergic system appears to mediate vasodilation.
2. Catecholamines, the renin-angiotensin system, and vasopressin seem to be involved in the regulation of intestinal blood flow.
3. Local decrease in pO_2, increase in pCO_2, adenosine, endothelin, and EDRF (nitric oxide) have been postulated as local factors.

C. Pathophysiology of Intestinal Ischemia

Intestinal ischemia occurs when there is a significant mismatch in metabolic demand and oxygen delivery. This can occur due to various factors. They include the hemodynamic state, the degree of atherosclerosis, the extent of collateral circulation, control mechanisms of vascular resistance, and toxic substances that can cause reperfusion injury. Since the mucosa is the most metabolically active layer and is perfused by an end arteriole without collateral circulation, ischemic injury starts from the tip of the villi. After sloughing of the villi, it is followed by edema, submucosal hemorrhage, and eventually transmural necrosis of the bowel. The clinical correlate of this process is an initial hypermotility state of the bowel resulting in significant abdominal pain that is *out of proportion to the physical findings*, at which stage the ischemia may be limited to the mucosa layer. As the ischemia progresses, bowel motility decreases and mucosal permeability increases, resulting in peritonitis, at which stage the ischemia will be transmural. The ischemic damage is further aggravated by regional vasospasm which occurs even after blood flow is restored, and by toxic substances that occur in ischemia, so-called reperfusion injury.

The key to the management of intestinal ischemia is early detection of the ischemic process with a high index of suspicion, minimizing the aggravating factors of ischemic damage. Based on etiology, the above clinical classification will be discussed individually.

IV. ISCHEMIC BOWEL SYNDROMES (2)

A. Acute Mesenteric Ischemia (3)

1. Etiology/Pathogenesis

a. Acute Mesenteric Artery Embolism.   Acute mesenteric ischemia due to emboli usually originates from the heart and commonly occurs in patients with atrial fibrillation. The emboli may be from a mural thrombus in a patient with a recent myocardial infarction, from a prosthetic/rheumatic heart valve, or from atheromatous plaques dislodged by cardiovascular instrumentation. The emboli usually lodges in the superior mesenteric artery, owing to its oblique takeoff from the aorta, just distal to the origin. Many patients have a history of previous peripheral emboli.

b. Acute Mesenteric Artery Thrombosis.   Acute mesenteric ischemia due to thrombosis usually occurs in the setting of a low-flow state on the basis of diffuse atherosclerotic narrowing of the mesenteric vasculature, or in various hypercoagulable states. The occlusion usually occurs at the origin of the SMA. Acute ischemia may be superimposed on chronic mesenteric ischemia (intestinal angina). There may be a history of postprandial pain and weight loss, and a history of systemic vascular insufficiency such as angina, transient cerebral ischemic attacks, or calf claudication.

c. Nonocclusive Mesenteric Ischemia.   This clinical entity occurs when splanchnic vasoconstriction overrides the normal autoregulatory blood flow in response to shock or any other forms of severe physiologic stress resulting in a low-flow state. It may also be caused by various vasoconstrictive drugs— e.g., digitalis, vasopressin, alpha-receptor agonists, beta-receptor antagonists.

d. Acute Mesenteric venous thrombosis.   Although the underlying etiology is thought to be unknown, in as many as half the cases, various causes have been identified. Acute thrombosis of mesenteric veins causes significant hyperemia and edema of the bowel wall with significant sequestration of dark, bloody fluid. This process, if prolonged after the acute onset, will result in secondary arterial occlusion of the bowel. With the advent of ultrasonography, CT scan, and MRI, more cases of mesenteric venous thrombosis are diagnosed accurately (4–6). Based on its low incidence, most cases formerly thought to be mesenteric venous thrombosis are now thought to be nonocclusive mesenteric ischemia.

2. Patients at Risk

a. Acute Mesenteric Artery Embolism.   These are patients with chronic aterial fibrillation, recent myocardial infarction, or recent cardioversion, and elderly patients with systemic atherosclerotic vascular disease.

b. Acute Mesenteric Artery Thrombosis. These include elderly patients with systemic atherosclerotic vascular disease, congestive heart failure, recent myocardial infarction, hypercoagulable states (polycythemia vera, dehydration, carcinoma, oral contraceptives), vasculitis (e.g., SLE), trauma, and aortic dissection.

c. Nonocclusive mesenteric ischemia. These include shock, dehydration, dialysis patients, congestive heart failure, acute myocardial infarction, pericardial tamponade, major cardiac/intraabdominal surgery (cardiopulmonary bypass), and patients on vasoconstrictive drugs.

d. Acute Mesenteric Venous Thrombosis. These are patients with hypercoagulable states (antithrombin III deficiency, protein C,S deficiency, polycythemia vera, oral contraceptive pills, carcinoma), portal hypertension, Budd-Chiari syndrome, intraperitoneal irritation (appendicitis, IBD, diverticulitis, etc.), bowel obstruction (especially strangulation obstruction), and trauma.

3. Clinical Manifestations

Almost all patients with acute mesenteric ischemia have acute abdominal pain that *in its early stages is out of proportion to the physical findings.* Despite the patient complaining of excruciating abdominal pain, the abdomen is soft, flat, nontender. The pain may be colicky and the bowel sounds hyperactive initially, due to the hypermotility of early ischemic bowel. Eventually the pain will be continuous and bowel sounds will be hypoactive as ischemia progresses. Vomiting and bloody diarrhea may be associated, although the diarrhea usually occurs several hours later. Sudden presentation is characteristic of embolism; other forms present with a more gradual, insidious onset, although there is a considerable overlap. Less commonly *acute mesenteric ischemia may present without pain,* manifesting as abdominal distension and/or GI bleeding. This is especially true for nonocclusive mesenteric ischemia. It is at this stage that acute mesenteric ischemia should be detected, when bowel necrosis is limited to the mucosa and has not progressed to a transmural infarct. By the time the patient develops evidence of peritonitis (rebound tenderness, guarding), indicating the presence of irreversible transmural infarction, the mortality rate may approach the range of 50–90%. Colonic ischemia, which classically is left-sided due to the "watershed areas," may not be distinguishable clinically. If there is doubt, the diagnostic workup and management should follow that of acute mesenteric ischemia until proven otherwise, since acute mesenteric ischemia carries a dismal prognosis if there is delay. A high index of suspicion, with special note on the risk profile for the patient, cannot be overemphasized.

4. Diagnosis

As mentioned above, it is of paramount importance to diagnose mesenteric ischemia before intestinal infarction has occurred (manifested by peritonitis), due to the high mortality rate at this stage (50–90%). Therefore it is important to identify the patients at risk (maintain a high index of suspicion in the appropriate clinical setting—i.e., unexplained abdominal pain, abdominal distension, gastrointestinal bleeding), diagnose early ischemia efficiently, excluding other intraabdominal processes, and medically manage the patient so as to make the surgical intervention (i.e., embolectomy, bowel resection, vascular reconstruction) optimal.

The initial investigation should be aimed at ruling out other causes of abdominal pain and peritonitis. A upright and supine plain film of the abdomen should be obtained. This is helpful in ruling out a perforation or bowel obstruction. Bowel wall thickening, "thumbprinting," and especially pneumatosis intestinalis (air within the bowel wall) are helpful to support the diagnosis. However, these are late findings indicative of intestinal infarction. In early ischemia the plain radiographs may be normal. Thus, *a normal plain radiograph does not exclude acute mesenteric ischemia*. In acute mesenteric venous thrombosis, plain radiographs may demonstrate fluid-filled, dilated loops of bowel due to more prominent sequestration of fluid, when compared to arterial occlusion. Barium enemas are seldomly indicated in small bowel ischemia (7).

Early in the course of intestinal ischemia, laboratory findings are not helpful. Most patients with acute mesenteric ischemia will have leukocytosis and metabolic acidosis. To date, no useful laboratory marker has been identified for early intestinal ischemia (8).

The mainstay of diagnosis for the acute mesenteric ischemic syndromes is *selective mesenteric angiography* (9,10). Patients suspected of having such a syndrome should undergo an angiogram. In the patient in shock, however, resuscitative measures to correct low cardiac output, hypotension, and hypovolemia should be undertaken first. The angiogram not only confirms the diagnosis but can be used to infuse vasodilators such as papaverine to treat the vasospasm associated with ischemic injury and that seen in the perioperative period, and can aid the surgeon prior to a therapeutic surgical intervention. The angiogram may be hard to interpret, especially in the patient with preexisting but asymptomatic atherosclerotic lesions, sometimes with a total occlusion of a major splanchnic artery.

The expected angiographic findings for each entity are as follows:

1. In SMA occlusion due to embolus: The most common "positive" finding is the occlusion of the superior mesenteric artery just proximal to the origin of the middle colic artery (Fig. 2).

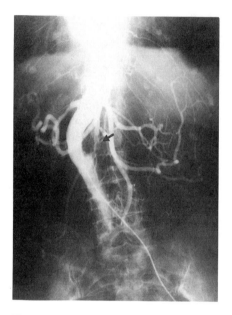

Figure 2 Mesenteric angiogram showing proximal SMA occlusion/embolus (cut-off). (Radiograph courtesy of Marlene Rackson, M.D.)

2. In SMA occlusion due to thrombosis: occlusion of the proximal portion of the superior mesenteric artery.
3. In nonocclusive mesenteric ischemia: Visible spasm of the macroscopic vessel and/or a loss of the normal arterial blush of the bowel microvessels.
4. In acute mesenteric venous thrombosis: Loss of venous flow from the bowel wall. With large sequestration of fluid in the bowel lumen as ischemia progresses, interpretation may be difficult.

An abdominal CT scan has been advocated as part of the diagnostic workup, as well as MRI, ultrasonography combined with Doppler to investigate splanchnic blood flow. However, arteriography remains the gold standard. An abdominal CT scan may be helpful to evaluate for retroperitoneal inflammation if the clinical picture is hard to distinguish from pancreatitis, or to demonstrate thrombus in the superior mesenteric vein and/or portal vein to support the diagnosis of acute mesenteric venous thrombosis. If the clinical features are suggestive of acute mesenteric venous thrombosis, especially if there is a history of deep-vein thrombosis or an inherited hypercoagulable state, a contrast-enhanced abdominal CT scan is advocated as the initial diagnostic test prior to the angiogram.

5. Treatment

a. Medical Management. The initial step in medical management is to treat the underlying and precipitating causes of acute mesenteric ischemia such as congestive heart failure, arrhythmias (atrial fibrillation), hypovolemia, and severe anemia. Before sending the patient for a diagnostic angiogram, these resuscitative measures must be undertaken; otherwise, treatment aimed at increasing intestinal blood flow will be useless. Shock must also be treated prior to the angiogram. (It should be noted that in patients in shock, selective intraarterial vasodilator therapy may result in further decrease in blood pressure.)

After the diagnosis has been established by the angiogram, intraarterial infusion of papaverine or tolazoline through an angiographically placed catheter placed in the superior mesenteric artery is recommended for all forms of acute mesenteric ischemia. This is because mesenteric vasospasm/vasoconstriction complicates ischemic injury regardless of etiology (embolism, thrombosis, nonocclusive hypoperfusion, venous occlusion). Thus, intraarterial vasodilator therapy is indicated in the patient who is scheduled for a surgical intervention, even the patient who has developed peritonitis. Optimizing intestinal blood flow is important to the surgeon when assessing bowel viability.

Papaverine, a nonselective smooth-muscle relaxant, is initially administered through a superior mesenteric artery catheter as a bolus injection of 25 mg over 20 minutes. A repeat angiogram is obtained to assess therapeutic efficacy (Fig. 3). Then papaverine is continuously infused at 30 to 60 mg/hr, and is usually continued for 12 to 24 hours with careful attention to clinical improvement/deterioration of the gastrointestinal tract (i.e., bowel sounds, abdominal distention, pain). It may be continued for a few more days if necessary. Although recommended, the efficacy of papaverine has not been fully evaluated in clinical trials, owing to difficulty in randomization of treatment.

Other supportive measures include nasogastric suction, supplemental oxygen, avoidance of vasoconstrictor agents, and antibiotics. The role of antibiotics is not clear, but they are indicated in the face of peritonitis.

The use of anticoagulants and thrombolytics is controversial in acute mesenteric ischemia. Possible use of thrombolytics has been suggested in acute mesenteric artery thrombosis, but is not recommended. The use of heparin has been advocated in acute mesenteric venous thrombosis postoperatively, and warfarin on a long-term basis. Otherwise they are not recommended in the immediate postoperative period (delayed use

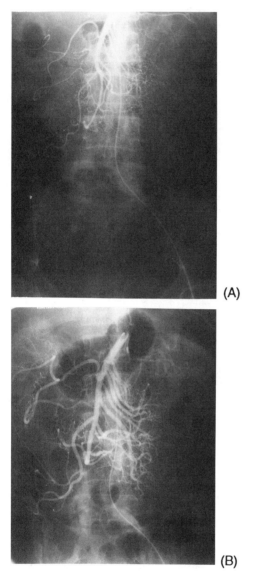

(A)

(B)

Figure 3   (A) Nonocclusive mesenteric ischemia (vasospasm). (B) Same patient S/P papaverine infusion (now a normal study). (Radiographs courtesy of Marlene Rackson, M.D.)

postoperatively has been suggested to prevent late thrombosis following embolectomy or vascular reconstruction).

   b.   *Surgical Management.*   After a diagnosis of *acute mesenteric embolism/thrombosis* is established angiographically, prompt laparotomy is usually indicated after preoperative vasodilator therapy. In mild cases of *acute mesenteric venous thrombosis*, a trial with heparin or thrombolytic therapy may be tried. However, if there is evidence of progressive intestinal infarction (peritonitis), immediate surgery is indicated. In *nonocclusive mesenteric ischemia*, surgery plays a secondary role. It is indicated only when bowel viability needs to be evaluated, with possible resection of necrotic bowel. The mainstay of treatment in nonocclusive mesenteric ischemia is correction of the underlying disorder, supportive measures (as above), and intraarterial vasodilator therapy. The high mortality rate (as high as 90%) is largely due to the severity of the underlying illness, and aggressive surgical intervention has not been traditionally undertaken.

   The role of surgery is embolectomy, thrombectomy, reconstruction of the mesenteric vasculature (i.e., bypass grafting), evaluation of the viability of the bowel, and resection of necrotic bowel. Intraarterial papaverine infusion and improving cardiac output will optimize the perfusion to the ischemic bowel so as to accurately assess bowel viability. Subjective criteria used to assess bowel viability in the initial laparotomy are bowel wall color, presence of peristalsis, and the presence of palpable mesenteric pulses. One of the difficult problems for the surgeon is that bowel viability is hard to determine until blood flow is restored to the ischemic segment. This is why many surgeons advocate a planned second-look laparotomy 24–48 hours later to reassess segments of bowel with questionable viability. There may be progression of necrosis, and a clearer demarcation between necrotic and viable bowel. There is no conclusive evidence that a planned second-look laparotomy affects mortality from acute mesenteric ischemia. Several objective methods have been investigated, including fluorescence staining, laser Doppler flowmetry, surface oximetry, and intramural pH monitoring. The fluorescence pattern of the bowel wall under Wood's lamp (3600 nm) illumination following the intravenous injection of 1 g sodium fluorescein has proven to be significantly more sensitive and specific for the rapid and convenient discrimination of viable from nonviable ischemic intestine than any other method. In controlled laboratory studies, the fluorescein technique at initial laparotomy is superior to clinical judgment at a second-look laparotomy 24 hours later (11,12).

V. CHRONIC MESENTERIC ISCHEMIA
(INTESTINAL ANGINA)

A. Etiology/Pathogenesis

1. *Chronic Mesenteric Ischemia (Intestinal Angina)*

This is an uncommon cause (5%) of intestinal ischemia and is almost always caused by chronic mesenteric atherosclerosis. It is the gastrointestinal equivalent of angina pectoris, and calf claudication in which intestinal blood flow is insufficient to meet the increased postprandial tissue demands for oxygen. Thus, it manifests as intermittent postprandial pain. The full-blown syndrome is rarely encountered due to the vast collateral circulation in the gut. When true intestinal angina occurs, it is usually the result of severe atherosclerotic narrowing of a major splanchnic artery superimposed on chronic occlusion of one or two of the remaining major arteries.

2. *Subacute and Chronic Mesenteric Venous Thrombosis*

This has an insidious onset. There may not be true intestinal ischemia in the face of subacute/chronic mesenteric venous occlusion. Subacute and chronic mesenteric venous thrombosis is a clinical entity which manifests as nonspecific abdominal pain that develops over weeks to months. Intestinal infarction rarely occurs in this category, whereas acute mesenteric venous thrombosis may lead to infarction or perforation, necessitating surgical resection.

B. Patients at Risk

1. *Chronic Mesenteric Ischemia*

This occurs when there is diffuse peripheral arterial disease (i.e., diabetes, smoker, hypercholesterolemia), especially in the middle-aged or elderly patient.

2. *Subacute and Chronic Mesenteric Venous Thrombosis*

Risk factors for this are the same as for acute mesenteric venous thrombosis.

C. Clinical Manifestations

1. *Chronic Mesenteric Ischemia*

The characteristic clinical presentation of this syndrome is postprandial pain, weight loss, and fear of eating. The abdominal pain is crampy in nature and usually occurs within 30 minutes after food intake. It slowly resolves over the next few hours. Avoidance of food and malabsorption may lead to constipation and diarrhea, respectively. Physical examination may show significant weight loss in advanced cases.

2. Subacute and Chronic Mesenteric Venous Thrombosis

This usually presents with nonspecific abdominal pain over weeks to months, and chronic mesenteric venous thrombosis is usually asymptomatic. If chronic mesenteric venous thrombosis involves the portal vein, complications of portal hypertension may be seen. They may present with gastrointestinal bleeding from esophageal varices, or with splenomegaly.

D. Diagnosis

1. Chronic Mesenteric Ischemia

Because the presentation of chronic mesenteric ischemia is insidious, and most patients do not have the typical presentation, diagnosis may be delayed due to the potential risks of selective mesenteric angiography (i.e., acute tubular necrosis, cholesterol emobli). Although the diagnosis requires an angiogram showing severe narrowing of multiple splanchnic vessels, it must be emphasized that the corresponding clinical picture of postprandial pain and significant weight loss is necessary to warrant treatment which is surgical revascularization. Other diagnostic modalities, such as barium enema, abdominal CT scan, and duplex Doppler ultrasound, are nonspecific and not helpful.

2. Subacute and Chronic Mesenteric Venous Thrombosis

These conditions are usually diagnosed when arteriograms are done to search for other intraabdominal processes. In chronic mesenteric venous thrombosis, where gastrointestinal bleeding is usually the only manifestation, the diagnostic workup is aimed at searching for the source of bleeding.

E. Treatment

1. Chronic Mesenteric Ischemia (13)

Treatment for chronic mesenteric ischemia is surgical revascularization; there is no effective medical therapy. Once the diagnosis is established by excluding other etiologies for the patient's pain and weight loss, surgery is undertaken to alleviate the pain and to prevent a superimposed acute mesenteric ischemia that may progress to intestinal infarction. Three surgical approaches have been advocated: end arterectomy, bypass grafting, and reimplantation of distal mesenteric vessels into nondiseased aortic segments. The preferred approach is bypass grafting of the superior mesenteric artery with either autogenous saphenous vein or prosthetic material. Angioplasty has been attempted but has not been successful in most circumstances.

2. Subacute and Chronic Mesenteric Venous Thrombosis

Since subacute mesenteric venous thrombosis presents with nonspecific abdominal pain and chronic mesenteric venous thrombosis presents with gastrointestinal bleeding (or no symptoms), treatment is aimed at controlling the bleeding. Asymptomatic chronic mesenteric venous thrombosis requires no treatment.

VI. FOCAL SEGMENTAL ISCHEMIA OF THE SMALL BOWEL

A. Etiology/Pathogenesis

This clinical entity of ischemic bowel disease involves nonocclusive hypoperfusion and/or intramural arterial occlusion of the small bowel, and usually results in nongangernous small-bowel ischemia due to adequate collateral circulation. However, the clinical course is variable depending on the etiology and severity of the infarct. The causes of focal segmental ischemia of the small bowel include strangulated hernias, vasculitis (i.e., SLE), coagulopathies (i.e., polycythemia vera), blunt abdominal trauma, radiation, oral contraceptives, and atheromatous emboli.

B. Patients at Risk

Risk factors for the acute mesenteric ischemia syndromes also pose risk for focal segmental ischemia. In addition, blunt abdominal trauma and radiation are possible etiologies for focal segmental ischemia of the small bowel.

C. Clinical Manifestations

The clinical patterns are variable and can present as any one of the below.

1. Acute Enteritis With Frank Peritonitis

The presentation mimics acute appendicitis, and physical examination reveals an acute abdomen with fever, tachycardia, *continuous* abdominal pain, involuntary guarding, and rebound tenderness.

2. Chronic Enteritis With Recurrent Abdominal Pain

The presentation may be clinically and radiographically indistinguishable from Crohn's enteritis.

3. Bowel Obstruction

This is the most common pattern. The patient may present with chronic diarrhea due to malabsorption caused by bacterial overgrowth in the dilated loop proximal to the stricture.

D. Diagnosis

Initial diagnostic studies should include a plain abdominal radiograph, barium studies of the small bowel. Laboratory studies will show leukocytosis, hyperkalemia, hyperphosphatemia, or metabolic acidosis, but these are nonspecific. In the patient who presents with acute enteritis, it is crucial to rule out strangulation obstruction from simple obstruction, since the presence of strangulated nonviable bowel doubles the mortality rate associated with small-bowel obstruction (5–10%). Earlier prospective studies showed that a clinician's clinical judgment, based on all available clinical and laboratory information and a personal knowledge of the patient, was no better than pure chance in making the discrimination between early strangulation and simple obstruction (15).

E. Treatment

In patients presenting with acute enteritis, since the mortality rate of small-bowel obstruction increases dramatically with the presence of bowel necrosis, prompt laparotomy, reduction of any strangulated segment, and resection of nonviable bowel provide the best clinical outcome. In the chronic enteritis and obstructive patterns, unless there is complete spontaneous resolution, treatment is surgical resection of the involved segment. Not uncommonly, the diagnosis is made on the resected segment.

VII. COLONIC ISCHEMIA (16)

A. Etiology/Pathogenesis

Colonic ischemia is the most common form of intestinal ischemia, comprising 50–60% of cases. It was first described by Boley and co-workers in 1963, and has been increasingly recognized with the advent of aortic aneurysm surgery. There is a wide spectrum of clinical manifestations including transient colitis, chronic ulcerating colitis, stricture formation, gangrene, and fulminant colitis. It is convenient to classify this entity into *gangrenous* and *nongangrenous* ischemic colitis. This is because these two entities have different etiologies and clinical courses, and are managed differently.

1. *Gangrenous Ischemic Colitis*

Although nongangrenous (nonocclusive hypoperfusion, intramural arterial occlusion) ischemic colitis can slowly progress to transmural intestinal necrosis, the vast majority of gangrenous ischemic colitis develops via the same pathogenetic mechanisms that cause small-intestinal transmural necrosis—acute mesenteric embolism/thrombosis and acute mesenteric venous thrombosis. One subgroup of patients that may develop this clinical entity are those with involvement of the ascending colon, usually occurring as a result of extensive involvement of the small bowel (superior mesenteric artery embolism/thrombosis, nonocclusive mesenteric ischemia) (17,18).

2. Nongangrenous Ischemic Colitis

As mentioned above, most colonic ischemia (85–90%) falls into this category. Noniatrogenic colonic ischemia rarely occurs from abrupt cessation of major arterial/venous blood flow, but rather occurs as a result of nonocclusive hypoperfusion from local low flow states and/or local vasoconstriction, probably mediated by the renin-angiotensin mechanism (19). Although more than 90% of patients with noniatrogenic, nongangrenous ischemic colitis are middle-aged to elderly, there is a distinct category of colonic ischemia affecting the young for which certain risk factors are identified (see Patients at Risk, below).

There are several factors that contribute to the vulnerability of the colon to nonocclusive ischemia:

1. The colon receives less blood than the small intestine (the celiac artery and superior mesenteric artery receive twice as much blood flow as the inferior mesenteric artery).
2. The colon has a less well developed collateral circulation, thus predisposing certain areas to ischemic injury, notably the splenic flexure and the rectosigmoid area (the so-called watershed areas).
3. With ongoing motor activity of the colon, increased intraluminal pressure in patients with diverticular disease, constipation, colonic malignancies, etc. results in decreased blood flow in the intestinal wall.

The ischemic injury is usually segmental and demonstrates mucosal edema, ulceration, and stenosis pathologically. A minority of patients may progress to develop strictures.

B. Patients at Risk

1. Gangrenous Colonic Ischemia

The risk is the same as for acute mesenteric ischemia (see above).

2. Nongangrenous Colonic Ischemia

a. Iatrogenic. Iatrogenic injury of the inferior mesenteric artery during aortic surgery (3–7% in elective aortic surgery, as high as 60% in ruptured aortic aneurysm (20)), barium enema, colonoscopy.

b. Noniatrogenic—Middle-aged to Elderly. Ischemic heart disease, diffuse peripheral arterial disease, diabetes prior colon pathology (diverticular disease, chronic constipation, colon cancer, etc.), severely ill patients (at risk for low flow states jeopardizing colonic blood flow; i.e., sepsis, congestive heart failure, hemorrhage, arrhythmias, etc.), vasoconstricting medications (digitalis, ergot, vasopressin, NSAIDs, etc.).

c. *Noniatrogenic—Young.* Connective tissue disorders (vasculitis; i.e., SLE), coagulopathies (i.e., polycythemia vera, thrombocytosis), sickle cell disease, cocaine abuse, marathon runners, medications (oral contraceptives, vasopressin, gold, danazol, psychotropic drugs, etc.).

C. Clinical Manifestations

1. Gangrenous Colonic Ischemia

A minority of patients (10–15%) will present as an abdominal catastrophe, with the initial presentation and clinical course resembling acute mesenteric ischemia. Patients will be gravely ill with peritoneal signs.

2. Nongangrenous Colonic Ischemia

The majority of patients will present with a sudden onset of mild to moderate crampy, left upper or lower abdominal pain, nausea, vomiting, and an urge to defecate with diarrhea, hematochezia, or melena within 24 hours. Rectal bleeding is not massive. Physical examination reveals low grade, tachycardia, localized mild to moderate abdominal tenderness without peritoneal signs. Most patients are not gravely ill. Occasionally, patients will present with clinically severe colitis with fever, chills, bloody diarrhea, abdominal distension, diminished bowel sounds, indicative of intramural necrosis. Commonly, the precipitating event of colonic ischemia cannot be identified, especially in the elderly. The early clinical presentation is similar to many other processes (i.e., acute infectious colitis, pseudomembranous colitis, Crohn's colitis, ulcerative colitis, etc.), so that the differentiation is possible only by excluding infection and demonstrating classic radiographic findings ("thumbprinting") (Fig. 4) or colonoscopic findings of *segmental* mucosal or submucosal hemorrhage, mucosal gangrene, hemosiderin, *findings which are not absolutely specific* for ischemic colitis.

The subsequent progression of nongangrenous colonic ischemia may follow one of four patterns:

a. *Mild Disease With Spontaneous Resolution Within 24–48 Hours.* The majority of patients follow this course with complete resolution in 2–3 weeks.

b. *Severe Disease Followed by Ongoing, Recurrent Chronic Colitis.* Pathologically and clinically, it may be indistinguishable from IBD.

c. *Severe Disease That Heals With Stricture Formation.* Pathologically, this indicates intramural necrosis without further progression.

d. *Severe Disease That Progresses to Gangrenous Colonic Ischemia.* Compared to patients with initial presentations of gangrenous colonic ischemia with peritonitis, the progression of nongangrenous to gangrenous

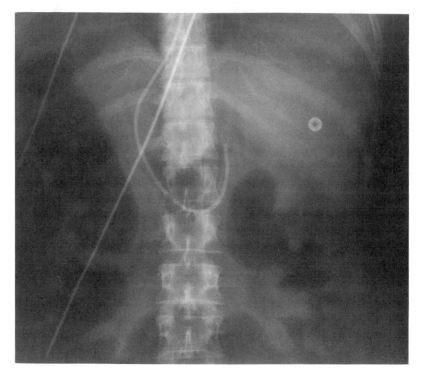

Figure 4 "Thumbprinting" on a plain abdominal radiograph. Ascending and descending colon. (Radiography courtesy of Natalie Strutynsky, M.D.)

colonic ischemia progresses over several days and may be detected only by careful follow-up roentgenographic and endoscopic examinations.

Uncommonly, it may present after a long subclinical course, with constipation and abdominal pain from strictures. There are probably many cases of colonic ischemia that go undetected or misdiagnosed, since mild cases resolve spontaneously before patients seek medical attention.

D. Diagnosis

1. Gangrenous Colonic Ischemia

As in acute mesenteric ischemia, rapid diagnosis with mesenteric angiography with preoperative papaverine therapy prior to laparotomy is the key to successful outcome. This aggressive approach for colonic ischemia should always be kept in mind when the right colon is affected and when the clinical presentation does not clearly distinguish between colonic ischemia and acute mesenteric ischemia.

Involvement of the ascending colon represents widespread involvement of the superior mesenteric artery/vein, and untreated acute mesenteric ischemia becomes rapidly irreversible. One example is when the plain abdominal radiograph does not reveal the characteristic "thumbprinting" pattern of colonic ischemia that is representative of submucosal edema and hemorrhage (it is important that the initial investigation be carried out within the first 24 hours of the onset of disease, since symptoms subside rapidly and typical radiographic findings tend to disappear rapidly). In this circumstance, a gentle air enema can be performed in an attempt to visualize "thumbprinting" against the column of air. If the thumbprinting can be seen in the classical locations (splenic flexure; descending colon), a more conservative management, as outlined below, should be taken. However, if thumbprinting cannot be observed, or thumbprinting is seen in the ascending colon only, mesenteric angiography is indicated to rule our acute mesenteric ischemia.

2. Nongangrenous Colonic Ischemia

If colonic ischemia is suspected, the initial diagnostic study should be a plain abdominal radiograph which may demonstrate "thumbprinting" against air-filled segments of the colon. This should be done within the first 24–48 hours from the onset of symptoms, since thumbprinting may disappear following clinical resolution. Thumbprinting is caused by intramural hemorrhage and submucosal edema, but is not specific and can be seen in other forms of colitis. Characteristically the involvement is segmental, with the most commonly involved segments being the splenic flexure and the recto-sigmoid areas ("watershed areas").

Mesenteric angiography is not indicated in colonic ischemia except in the two instances outlined in the previous paragraph, and can often be misleading. If there is no peritonitis and the abdominal radiograph is unremarkable, the next step is either colonoscopy or barium enema combined with flexible sigmoidoscopy. A barium enema will detect thumbprinting better, and an endoscopy will detect hemorrhagic nodules, which represents submucosal hemorrhage. Either test should be done with minimal air insufflation, because distension of the colon with air will further decrease intramural blood flow and will increase the risk of perforation. Colonoscopy is preferable to barium enema because early inspection with mucosal biopsies can differentiate between thumbprinting caused by submucosal hemorrhage and that caused by submucosal edema due to other forms of colitis (21).

Mucosal *hemosiderin*, which is indicative of previous bleeding, is typical but is not specific for ischemic colitis. Once again, these diagnostic studies should be done early in the course of disease. Thereafter the mucosa will become necrotic with ulcerations, making it especially difficult to define the etiology.

Not uncommonly, there are times when it is extremely difficult to differentiate between IBD and ischemic colitis. Poor response to steroids, segmental involvement, and no recurrence after resection of the involved segment are factors favoring ischemic colitis.

E. Treatment

The key to treatment is accurate diagnosis with special attention to exclude infectious forms of colitis (i.e., bacterial, amoebic dysentery), to exclude inflammatory bowel disease, and to exclude obstructive lesions of the colon (colon cancer, diverticular disease, fecal impaction, volvulus, strictures).

Since clinical outcome cannot be predicted based on early clinical presentation, frequent follow-up examinations are necessary. If there is no evidence of progression the patient should be treated conservatively. Administration of parenteral fluids with careful monitoring of volume status, hemoglobin, and electrolytes; nothing by mouth; administration of broad-spectrum antibiotics; optimizing cardiac function; and withdrawal of vasoconstrictive medications are important. Nutritional support is initially not necessary except in undernourished patients.

Antidiarrheal, antispasmodic, analgesic medications are contraindicated in ischemic colitis. They may precipitate toxic megacolon or colonic pseudo-obstruction. Blood transfusions are only necessary in severely anemic patients with ischemic heart disease.

No specific medical therapy is indicated for mild self-limiting disease. The role of steroids, sulfasalazine, 5-ASA, metronidazole, and immunosuppressives in chronic ischemic colitis is controversial. Controlled studies have not been done. The same can be said about the role of vasodilators (papaverine, ACE inhibitors). The setting in which sulfasalazine, 5-ASA, and steroids (usually enemas) are considered is when the patient has long-standing chronic colitis.

In gangrenous colonic ischemia from major vascular obstruction, early mesenteric angiography with preoperative papaverine followed by prompt laparotomy is indicated. This surgical approach is the same as with acute mesenteric ischemia. Whenever possible, surgery should not be delayed until the patient develops peritonitis.

In nongangrenous colonic ischemia, there are certain indications for surgical management: 1. Uncontrollable hemorrhage (rare). 2. Patients who go on to develop gangrenous colonic ischemia over the next few days (persistent fevers, increased abdominal tenderness, guarding, toxic megacolon). 3. Ongoing clinical deterioration with persistent diarrhea and rectal bleeding, as well as endoscopic evidence of disease progression. 4. Recurrent fevers, leukocytosis, and septicemia in otherwise asymptomatic patients due to nonhealing segmental colitis. 5. Patients who present with obstructive symptoms due to stricture formation from ischemic colitis (usually presenting within 6 months within onset of disease) who fail colonoscopic dilatations.

Asymptomatic ischemic strictures should be left alone and treatment should be undertaken on an elective basis. Early emergency surgery carries a high mortality rate.

Mesenteric ischemia remains one of the few gastrointestinal emergencies that require prompt recognition and treatment to minimize morbidity and mortality. The diversity of its presentation and clinical course makes it extremely difficult but challenging for the internist to suspect this clinical syndrome. A better understanding of its pathophysiology is important to improve outcome.

REFERENCES

1. Patel A, Kaleya R, Sammartano R, et al. Pathophysiology of mesenteric ischemia. Surg Clin North Am 1992; 72:31–41.
2. Reinus J, Brandt LJ, Boley SJ, et al. Ischemic disease of the bowel. Gastr Clin North Am 1990; 19:319–343.
3. Kaleya R, Sammartano R, Boley SJ, et al. Aggressive approach to acute mesenteric ischemia. Surg Clin North Am 1992; 72:157–182.
4. Boley SJ, Kaleya R, Brandt LJ, et al. Mesenteric venous thrombosis. Surg Clin North Am 1992; 72:183–201.
5. Matos C, Gansbeke V, Zaleman M, et al. Mesenteric venous thrombosis: early CT and ultrasound diagnosis and conservative management. Gastr Radio 1986; 11:322.
6. Al Karawai, Quaiz M, Clark D, et al. Mesenteric vein thrombosis; noninvasive diagnosis and follow-up (US & MRI) and non-invasive therapy by streptokinase and anticoagulants. Hepato-gastroenterol 1990; 37:507.
7. Wolf EL, Sprayregen S, Bakal CW, et al. Radiology in intestinal ischemia: plain film, contrast, and other imaging studies. Surg Clin North Am 1992; 72:107–141.
8. Thompson J, Bragg L, West W, et al. Serum enzyme levels during intestinal ischemia. Ann Surg 1990; 211:369–373.
9. Bakal CW, Sprayregen S, Wolf EL, et al. Radiology in intestinal ischemia: angiographic diagnosis and management. Surg Clin North Am 1992; 72:125.
10. Morano J, Harrison B, et al. Mesenteric ischemia: angiographic diagnosis and intervention. Clin Imaging 1991; 15:91–98.
11. Bulkley G, Zuidema G, Hamilton S, et al. Intraoperative determination of small intestinal viability following ischemic injury: a prospective, controlled

trial of two adjuvant methods (Doppler and fluorescein) compared with standard clinical judgment. Ann Surg 1981; 193:628–637.

12. Stolar CJ, Randolph JG, et al. Evaluation of ischemic bowel with a fluorescent technique. J Pediatr Surg 1987; 13:221.

13. Cunningham C, Reilly L, Rapp J, et al. Chronic visceral ischemia: Three decades of progress. Ann Surg 1991; 214:276–288.

14. Connolly JE, Kwann JH, et al. Management of chronic visceral ischemia. Surg Clin North Am 1982; 62:345.

15. Sarr MG, Buckley GB, Zuidema GD, et al. Preoperative recognition of intestinal strangulation obstruction. Am J Surg 1983; 145:176.

16. Brandt LJ, Boley SJ, et al. Colonic ischemia. Surg Clin North Am 1992; 72:203–229.

17. Sakai L, Keltner R, Kaminski D, et al. Spontaneous and shock-associated ischemic colitis. Am J Surg 1980; 140:755.

18. Guttormson NL, Bubrick MP, et al. Mortality from ischemic colitis. Dis Col Rect 1983; 26:449.

19. Bailey RW, Bulkley GB, Hamilton SR, et al. Pathogenesis of nonocclusive ischemic colitis. Ann Surg 1986; 203:590.

20. Hagihara PF, Ernst CB, Griffen WB Jr, et al. Incidence of ischemic colitis following abdominal aortic reconstruction. Surg Gynecol Obstet 1979; 149:571.

21. Scowcroft CW, Sanowski RA, Kozarek RA, et al. Colonoscopy in ischemic colitis. Gastrointest Endosc 1981; 27:156.

10

Inflammatory Bowel Disease

Arthur E. Lindner
New York University School of Medicine, New York, New York

I. INTRODUCTION

In current medical literature the term inflammatory bowel disease (IBD) means *nonspecific* inflammatory bowel disease and refers to two entities: ulcerative colitis and Crohn's disease. Both are of unknown etiology.

Ulcerative colitis is by far the older of the two diseases. Its origins have been lost amid diagnostic confusion with the infectious diarrheas, but it is possible that the disease existed in antiquity (1). The name ulcerative colitis was used by Sir Samuel Wilks, a British physician, in a letter published in 1859 in a London medical journal, reporting his testimony at a court trial (2). In this letter he described autopsy findings now considered characteristic of ulcerative colitis. In 1875 Wilks and Moxon (3) published a classic description of ulcerative colitis, and modern considerations of the disease date from this time.

Crohn's disease has a much shorter clinical history. Case reports suggestive, in retrospect, of Crohn's disease have been found in the literature of the early 1900s (4). The general recognition of Crohn's disease can be dated quite precisely to 1932, when Crohn, Ginzburg, and Oppenheimer published their description of the illness and its pathology (5).

Both ulcerative colitis and Crohn's disease occur in the elderly. This chapter will first consider IBD in general and then turn to the special considerations that must be given to management in an older population.

II. ULCERATIVE COLITIS

Characteristic findings in patients with ulcerative colitis are abdominal cramps, diarrhea with blood and mucus in the stool, and sometimes

155

fever (6). At times constipation, rather than diarrhea, may occur. In many patients the onset is insidious, with vague abdominal complaints and gradual change in the frequency and character of the stools. In others the onset is abrupt, and abdominal pain, bloody diarrhea, and fever all become rapidly more severe over a period of days or weeks. In a few patients the inception is explosive, with high fever, systemic toxicity, severe diarrhea, and electrolyte depletion or hemorrhage. Gross blood in the stool is typical and may precede the onset of diarrhea. Perianal fistulas and chronic anal disease are unusual in patients with ulcerative colitis.

Extracolonic manifestations may occur during the course of ulcerative colitis. These include iritis, spondylitis, peripheral arthritis, erythema nodosum, pyoderma gangrenosum, and a variety of liver abnormalities including pericholangitis, sclerosing cholangitis, and bile duct carcinoma. Some of these entities have qualities of autoimmune phenomena and give support to the concept that immune mechanisms participate in the clinical manifestations of ulcerative colitis. Spondylitis, when it occurs in association with colitis, follows a course unrelated to the severity or activity of the bowel disease. There is a striking association of spondylitis and, to a lesser extent, of iritis, with the tissue histocompatibility antigen HLA-B27. It appears that the B27 antigen is useful in distinguishing the arthropathies of IBD and identifies a subgroup of patients at risk for development of spondylitis and iritis, but not peripheral arthritis.

As a rule, ulcerative colitis involves the rectum, even when the rest of the colon is spared. Thus sigmoidoscopy can be expected to provide positive diagnostic findings of granularity, friability, and ulceration with blood and exudate in the lumen. Toxic dilatation of the colon and free perforation into the peritoneal cavity are dread complications of ulcerative colitis.

Carcinoma of the colon is a not infrequent sequel to chronic ulcerative colitis. The risk of cancer is related to the duration of the colitis and to the linear extent of disease in the colon (patients with universal colitis are more likely to develop cancer than those with proctosigmoiditis). The risk, however, is not related to the severity or activity of the ulcerative disease. Patients with mild colitis and those in remission—patients who would not come to colectomy for severity of their symptoms—still bear a potentially malignant colonic mucosa and must be followed carefully for possible development of cancer.

Patients with ulcerative colitis are monitored by periodic clinical and laboratory examination and by colonoscopy or barium enema. Colectomy is recommended at the first suspicion of carcinoma. Unfortunately, cancer in ulcerative colitis tends to be multicentric, atypical in its early appearance and rapidly metastasizing, so the prospects for early diagnosis and effective treatment are limited. Efforts have been made to identify a "precancer" on rectal or colonoscopic biopsy. These premalignant changes, identified by skilled pathologists, reflect a dysplasia that appears to be associated with development of colon cancer and, when confirmed and severe in degree, are an indication for colectomy.

The course of ulcerative colitis is variable. In some patients with mild disease, the clinical and sigmoidoscopic findings subside. In most, however, the disease becomes chronic, with periodic exacerbations and remissions. Medical treatment includes dietary manipulation, antispasmodics, antidiarrheal agents, oral iron and blood transfusions for anemia, sulfasalazine and its 5-ASA (mesalamine) derivatives, corticosteroids, and immunosuppressive agents. All these are useful in managing symptoms, and perhaps in inducing remissions, but the pattern of clinical exacerbations tends to persist despite treatment.

Newer methods of therapy now in clinical studies include use of intravenous cyclosporine, a potent immunosuppressive agent, in patients with severe ulcerative colitis refractory to steroid therapy. Retention enemas of budesonide, a poorly absorbed steroid, and of short-chain fatty acids, which are believed to provide nutrients for colorectal mucosal cells, are undergoing trials in patients with proctitis or proctosigmoiditis.

The indications for surgical intervention in ulcerative colitis include hemorrhage, colon carcinoma or severe dysplasia, toxic dilatation of the colon, and intractability of the illness to medical treatment. The best established surgical treatment of ulcerative colitis is a total colectomy and ileostomy, a procedure that cures the disease. In appropriate subjects, an ileoanal anastomosis can be constructed following total colectomy to obviate the need for an external ileostomy.

Although most patients do well with the ileoanal procedure, some develop an inflammatory disease of the pouch which has been termed "pouchitis." The cause of pouchitis is not well understood, but the condition usually responds to broad-spectrum antibiotics. Elderly patients are less likely to tolerate either the rigors of anastomotic surgery itself or the complication of pouchitis if it occurs, so ileostomy and colectomy are often a better choice in this age group.

III. CROHN'S DISEASE

Ulcerative colitis involves only the colon, except for a superficial involvement of the terminal ileum that sometimes occurs when the entire colon is diseased. This involvement has been called "backwash ileitis," and the small-bowel changes appear to play no important role in the course or management of ulcerative colitis.

Crohn's disease, in contrast, can involve any area of the intestinal tract (7). Rare reports of possible esophageal involvement can be found, but there are many cases involving the stomach, either alone or with the disease in the intestine. Most often the small intestine, especially the terminal ileum, is diseased, either alone or in association with disease in the colon. Colonic Crohn's disease tends to be predominantly right-sided in distribution, and often spares the rectum.

Although Crohn's disease may occur at any age, most commonly the onset is in the second or third decade of life. The clinical course usually begins with diarrhea, abdominal cramps, low-grade fever, anemia, anorexia, and weight loss. The onset is often insidious, and in early stages there may be only a gradual increase in symptoms. At times symptoms may be low-grade or so intermittent that the patient does not seek medical attention or appropriate diagnostic studies are not done for months or years. Occasionally the onset is acute and the patient presents with what seems to be acute appendicitis. At surgical exploration on these occasions, however, the small bowel is chronically inflamed, so it seems likely that what appeared to be "acute ileitis" is really an acute exacerbation of a previously quiescent chronic disease.

A characteristic finding on physical examination is the presence of a tender abdominal mass, usually in the right lower quadrant. The mass represents chronically inflamed bowel, thickened mesentery, enlarged lymph nodes, and sometimes an intraabdominal abscess.

Partial bowel obstruction and stricture formation are common in Crohn's disease, but complete obstruction is unusual even in severe disease. For this reason, obstruction may be a cause of disabling symptoms but it is rarely a cause of surgical emergency. Spasm and edema may cause obstruction, which can be relieved by bowel intubation and medical supportive measures.

Free perforation of the bowel into the peritoneal cavity is rare. On the other hand, small, sealed-off perforations of the bowel are not only common but are quite characteristic of the disease. These small perforations represent extensions of inflammatory disease through the bowel wall to the serosa and out into the mesentery. The leakage is slow, the perforation is small, and the leak becomes sealed off. Regional lymph nodes become enlarged. Such small, sealed-off perforations are the basis of the fistulas that are so common in Crohn's disease. Fistulas may extend from one loop of small bowel to another, from small bowel to colon, or from bowel to vagina, bladder, or the abdominal wall.

Perianal fistulas and abscesses are common features of the illness. It is especially interesting that perianal fistulas may be the first clinical finding in Crohn's disease and may antedate the other clinical features by many months or even years.

Microscopic bleeding is common in Crohn's disease, and iron deficiency is one cause of the anemia that occurs in this disease. Stools are often positive for occult blood. Gross blood in the stools is uncommon, however, and when it does occur it is usually only an occasional episode and not a regular feature of the course as it is in ulcerative colitis.

Extraintestinal findings, such as peripheral arthritis, anklyosing spondylitis, iritis, erythema nodosum, and pyoderma gangrenosum all occur in patients with Crohn's disease. In patients with disease of the terminal ileum or with resection of this segment of bowel, gallstones and oxalate renal calculi present with increased frequency.

In most patients Crohn's disease follows a chronic course with low-grade disability. The inflammatory process does not appear to spread anatomically, either proximally or distally, in the absence of surgery, although the inflammation may worsen within its area. The failure of the inflammation to spread under medical treatment is remarkable, for the disease is notorious for its tendency to spread and to recur after surgery. Disease recurs in most of the patients who are operated upon, usually within the first 2 years after surgery. As a rule, the disease recurs just proximal to the old diseased area, at the site of anastomosis, but sometimes the recurrence is quite distant, and skip lesions may develop. Carcinoma of the bowel does occur in patients with Crohn's disease, but the risk is less than in those with uclerative colitis, and the requirement for surveillance less demanding. A "cure" of Crohn's disease, either medically or surgically, is unusual, but prolonged remissions may occur.

The goal of medical treatment in Crohn's disease is to induce a remission or, failing this, to provide symptomatic and supportive treatment so that the patient can function in everyday life despite the activity of a chronic illness. Medical treatment includes dietary manipulation, antispasmodics, antidiarrheal agents, and iron preparations. Sulfasalazine and its 5-ASA (mesalamine) derivatives appear useful in colonic disease but are of equivocal benefit in more proximal involvement. Antibiotics are essential in management of suppurative complications associated with abscesses and fistulas and are sometimes used as well in long-term management of the underlying bowel disease, presumably by reducing infection within the bowel wall. Corticosteroids and the immunosuppressive agents azathioprine and 6-mercaptopurine play important roles in the management of Crohn's disease.

Sulfasalazine is useful in colonic Crohn's disease, as it is in ulcerative colitis, but since it remains largely inactive until metabolized by colonic bacteria, it is less helpful in small-bowel disease. The active moiety of sulfasalazine, 5-amino salicylate (mesalamine), is now available in several forms which are biologically accessible to the small-bowel mucosa as well as to the colon. These drugs provide effective treatment in Crohn's disease of both small bowel and colon.

Clinical investigations have shown a possible use for parenteral methotrexate, a folate inhibitor that interferes with DNA synthesis, in treatment of active Crohn's disease, particularly in reducing corticosteroid dosage.

Surgery is indicated for treatment of the complications of Crohn's disease. These include obstruction, fistulas that are symptomatic or causing disability, abdominal masses and abscesses, and the rare complications of perforation or hemorrhage. Intermittent partial obstruction or infection with abscess formation are usually the complications that require surgery. "Intractability" to medical treatment, without development of complications, is a difficult surgical indication to define. It includes patients who, despite good medical management, simply don't do well: they have frequent disability with diarrhea, abdominal pain, and fever. In this group one must consider treating the diseased bowel surgically. Because the risk of recurrent disease is high, many physicians prefer to treat even severe Crohn's disease medically as long as possible and reserve surgery for the time when complications occur or the clinical course is deteriorating.

The early operations for Crohn's disease were bypass procedures in which the diseased loops of bowel were simply excluded from continuity with the fecal stream. More recent surgical techniques emphasize resection of the diseased bowel with an end-to-end anastomosis. When the rectum is involved, colectomy and ileostomy are usually performed. Patients with Crohn's colitis are poor candidates for the ileoanal anastomosis that is utilized in ulcerative colitis because Crohn's disease is associated with the risk of recurrent inflammation.

IV. PREVALENCE AND INCIDENCE OF IBD IN THE ELDERLY

Statistics on the prevalence of IBD in older populations are difficult to compare because authors use different definitions of "elderly." The age of 60 has often been used as the time of entry into the age group called the "elderly population" (8).

IBD may present for the first time in an elderly person, or a subject may develop IBD at an earlier age and then continue to carry the illness into old age. In 1990, Grimm and Friedman (9) reviewed the available epidemiologic surveys in the literature and concluded that the proportion of all patients with ulcerative colitis who develop their disease after age 60 averages about 12% (range 8–20%), with more men than women in the group. The proportion of patients who develop Crohn's disease after age

60 averages about 16% (range 7–26%), with more women than men in some studies but nearly equal distribution in others.

A large European study in 1988 by Softley et al. (10) demonstrated similar gender differences between ulcerative colitis and Crohn's disease in the elderly. They report a preponderance of males with ulcerative colitis (61% to 39%) and of females with Crohn's disease (68% to 32%).

Thus it is not at all uncommon for IBD to present for the first time in elderly subjects. In the reports surveyed for the 1990 review, as in most studies, ulcerative colitis is up to three times more common than Crohn's disease in the elderly population.

For many years investigators have observed a bimodality in the incidence of IBD, a phenomenon well discussed by Mendeloff and Calkins (11). The mode of incidence for both ulcerative colitis and Crohn's disease in both sexes is between the ages of 15 and 25 years. Then there occurs a second mode about age 60–70 years in many but not all series of cases. When ischemic colitis was described in 1963, it was suspected that misdiagnosis of this common entity had been responsible for the second peak of IBD (12). During the past decades, however, ischemic colitis has become well recognized and carefully diagnosed, but the second-peak phenomenon persists. The reason is not clear, but there is a significant incidence of IBD in the elderly.

V. LINEAR EXTENT OF DISEASE IN THE ELDERLY

In its pattern of distribution of disease within the bowel, ulcerative colitis may involve the rectum alone (proctitis), the rectum and sigmoid (proctosigmoiditis), the rectum and left colon to about the splenic flexure, or the entire colon (universal colitis). The disease may sometimes be observed to spread proximally, starting in the rectum and ultimately reaching the cecum on subsequent examinations. In Crohn's disease the most common involvement is of the terminal ileum, or the ileum and the right colon, with sparing of the rectum; it is possible for any or all of the intestine to be involved in Crohn's disease.

Although any of these patterns of distribution may be found in the elderly patient with IBD, just as in the younger subject, some differences in the distribution of disease in the elderly have been noted. There is a tendency for ulcerative colitis to be less extensive, with more proctitis and proctosigmoiditis and less universal disease (9,10). In older patients, Crohn's disease tends to involve the colon, especially on the left side (9,10), with less small-bowel disease (8).

Thus, although there are many exceptions, a profile emerges of IBD in the elderly in which ulcerative colitis tends to be distal in distribution, rather than universal, and Crohn's disease tends to involve the colon rather than the small bowel and to emphasize involvement of the left side of the colon.

VI. DIAGNOSTIC EVALUATION

Because IBD is of unknown cause, its diagnosis requires exclusion of the other diseases that cause similar symptoms, physical findings, and laboratory abnormalities. After history and physical examination, a rigid or flexible sigmoidoscopy will demonstrate the status of anus, rectum, and sigmoid. A rigid sigmoidoscopy can be performed safely even in patients who are acutely ill, thus providing valuable immediate information about the distal bowel. Ultimately evaluation of the colon requires colonoscopy or barium enema. Of the two modalities, colonoscopy is generally preferred today because it permits direct visualization of the mucosa and allows biopsy for histological assessment. A small-bowel X-ray examination is the best method to evaluate the small intestine. Computerized tomography of the abdomen is not usually required for diagnosis or management of IBD, but it can be helpful in detecting extraintestinal masses and in evaluating thickness of the bowel wall.

Microbiological studies of the stool are essential and should include search for ova and parasites, enteric pathogens including *Campylobacter* and *Yersinia enterocolitica*, and for the toxin of *Clostridium difficile*, the agent responsible for pseudomembranous colitis.

VII. DIFFERENTIAL DIAGNOSIS

The diagnosis of ulcerative colitis and Crohn's disease in older patients requires acknowledgment that IBD is indeed part of the spectrum of gastro-intestinal illness in the elderly. But there must also be an awareness of even more common gastrointestinal illnesses that afflict the older age group and can cause confusion in diagnosis (13). The two most confounding problems may be ischemic colitis and colonic diverticular disease.

Ischemic colitis, now that it is well recognized, is actually fairly easy to distinguish from IBD. It characteristically presents as an acute episode of abdominal pain and bleeding and then follows a rapid progression of findings—as visualized by barium enema or CT scan—from a stage of inflammatory edema, thumbprinting of the mucosa, segmental disease, spasm, irritability, and increased secretions, all leading to complete resolution or to stenosis. This sequence rarely requires more than 6 weeks.

Diverticulitis of the colon can easily be confused with Crohn's disease. In the elderly, Crohn's disease tends to involve the colon, especially on the left side. This is also the part of the bowel that commonly develops diverticula, so Crohn's disease and diverticular disease are not only problems in differential diagnosis but they may coexist. Diverticular disease affects one-third of Americans over the age of 60 years (14).

In Crohn's disease of the colon the involved segment tends to be long—usually 10 cm or longer—whereas in diverticulitis the segment is often short, perhaps 3–6 cm in length. Unfortunately, of course, there are exceptions to these guidelines of length.

When Crohn's disease develops in a segment of bowel that contains diverticula (this will usually be the sigmoid colon), the transverse fissures of the IBD penetrate easily through the mucosa of the diverticula, causing diverticulitis. It is apparent that differential diagnosis will be difficult in this situation, but the transverse fissures and the marked mucosal edema of Crohn's disease help distinguish this entity from conventional diverticulitis, and of course other characteristics of Crohn's disease, such as extraintestinal manifestations or anal disease, may be present and helpful.

The *infectious diarrheas* often present with blood in the stool and a worsening diarrhea. Not only are intestinal infections a problem in differential diagnosis, but they may also occur in a patient who already has IBD. Multiple stool examinations and cultures are warranted. Sources of infection in elderly people include foreign travel and infectious foods or materials from nursing homes or senior citizen centers. Among the organisms to seek are *Campylobacter*, the toxigenic *E. coli* of travelers' diarrhea, *Salmonella*, *Shigella*, *Yersinia enterocolitica*, *Giardia lamblia*, and *Endameba histolytica.*

Toxin-producing *E. coli* of the serotype 0157:H7 has recently been identified as a cause of colitis (15). The disease is often acquired after eating inadequately cooked beef or unpasteurized milk. Illness can be severe, with abdominal pain and tenderness, hematochezia, and a tendency for the findings to be right-sided in the colon, so sigmoidoscopy may be normal. Stool cultures are normal unless the specific serotype is sought.

Clostridium difficile spreads among hospitalized patients and can be endemic in nursing homes. The toxin of *C. difficile* tends to be active following antibiotic therapy and may cause simple antibiotic-associated diarrhea or the much more serious pseudomembranous colitis. Diagnosis is made by the identification of *C. difficile* toxin in the stool or by visualization of the pseudomembranes on endoscopy.

Cathartic colon (16) is an unusual condition that merits consideration in the elderly patient. Prolonged use of cathartics, especially those containing cascara, may lead to changes in the radiological appearance of the colon that are difficult to distinguish from ulcerative colitis. The right side of the colon shows the more extensive alterations, with absent or diminished haustral markings, bizarre contractions, and inconstant areas of narrowing.

The correct diagnosis can be made by history and by colonoscopy and biopsy.

The nonsteroidal antiinflammatory drugs (NSAIDs) used so frequently by the elderly for management of arthritic complaints have been found to produce nonspecific ulceration of the small-intestinal mucosa. Such ulcerations are less common than the long-recognized drug-induced ulcers of the stomach and duodenum, but they can be serious in their manifestations (17).

In the Western world, *intestinal tuberculosis* is uncommon, but it is important that tuberculosis be considered in patients who seem to have Crohn's disease of the distal ileum and proximal colon. The chest X-ray may fail to demonstrate tuberculosis, and diagnosis is suggested by a positive PPD test and the individual circumstances of the case.

Carcinoma of the colon or small bowel, especially in its scirrhous or linitis plastica form, may suggest Crohn's disease. In carcinoma, however, nodularity is prominent and the inflammatory mucosal alterations of IBD are not seen. *Lymphoma of small bowel or colon or multiple carcinoids of the small bowel* may resemble Crohn's disease. Laparotomy may be required for diagnosis.

Radiation injury of the small bowel or the colon, especially following treatment for cancer of the prostate or female genital tract, can be associated with diarrhea and bleeding as long as months to years after the course of treatment. Diagnosis is aided by history and by the presence of prominent submucosal telangiectases on endoscopy.

VIII. MANAGEMENT OF IBD IN THE ELDERLY

Reviews of the recent literature (9,13,18), as well as the experience of contemporary gastroenterologists, indicate that both ulcerative colitis and Crohn's disease exist as important entities in the geriatric population. The course and the prognosis for the elderly subject do not differ in major responses and goals from those in younger people. The basic treatment modalities for the elderly are those outlined earlier in this chapter for the management of IBD.

The general considerations that are of particular importance in treating IBD in the elderly are these:

1. Older patients tend to have concurrent unrelated diseases, especially heart disease, and these other conditions may require modifications in medications or treatment programs.
2. Older patients tend to have serious or even incapacitating arthritic complaints and so they are often treated with NSAIDs. Because these drugs may have deleterious effects on the small bowel and

colon, they should be avoided when possible or used judiciously when they must be employed.

3. Some drug effects in the elderly merit special attention and may require alterations in treatment of IBD. Sulfasalazine and its related drugs are well tolerated, but they block the absorption of folic acid (19), so folate supplements are indicated. Immunosuppressive agents are also well tolerated. Metronidazole interferes with warfarin metabolism, and this effect must be considered in patients receiving anticoagulant therapy. Corticosteroids are a particular problem for the elderly because steroid complications seem correlated with age. In particular, the effects on bone calcium can be severe, leading to vertebral compression and bone fractures. Corticosteroids should be avoided if possible, and if required they should be used for short periods and in the lowest possible doses.

4. The risk of intestinal cancer increases with age. Although our concerns are mainly with ulcerative colitis, there is also increased risk of cancer of the small bowel and colon in patients with Crohn's disease. No particular management seems practical to try to forestall development of cancer in the elderly, but the surveillance principles established in younger people should be maintained.

5. When surgery is required for IBD in the elderly it can usually be performed with appropriate attention to concurrent illnesses. Elderly patients with ulcerative colitis generally tolerate ileostomy well, but they are less successful candidates for the stresses and adjustments of the ileoanal anastomosis.

REFERENCES

1. Goligher JC, DeDombal FT, Watts JM, et al. Ulcerative Colitis. Baltimore: Williams and Wilkins, 1965:1–3.
2. Wilks S. The morbid appearance of the intestine of Miss Banks. Med Times Gaz (Lond) 1859; 2:264.
3. Wilks S, Moxon W. Lectures on Pathological Anatomy. 2d ed. London: Churchill, 1875:408, 672.
4. Marshak RH, Lindner AE. Chronic inflammatory disease of the colon: historical perspective. In: Berkowitz ZT, Kirsner JB, Lindner AE, et al., eds. Ulcerative and Granulomatous Colitis. Springfield, Ill: Charles C. Thomas, 1993:xvii–xxii.
5. Crohn BB, Ginzburg L, Oppenheimer GD. Regional ileitis: a pathological and clinical entity. JAMA 1932; 99:1323–1328.
6. Lindner AE. Ulcerative colitis. In: Marshak RH, Lindner AE, Maklansky D, eds. Radiology of the Colon. Philadelphia: W.B. Saunders, 1980:64–66.

7. Lindner AE. Regional enteritis. In: Marshak RH, Lindner AE, eds. Radiology of the Small Intestine. 2d ed. Philadelphia: W.B. Saunders, 1976:179–231.
8. Woolrich A. Inflammatory bowel disease in older age. In: Korelitz BI, Sohn N, eds. Inflammatory Bowel Disease. St. Louis: Mosby, 1992:24.
9. Grimm IS, Friedman LS. Inflammatory bowel disease in the elderly. Gastro Clin North Am 1990; 19:361–389.
10. Softley A, Myren J, Clamp SE, et al. Inflammatory bowel disease in the elderly patient. Scand J Gastro 1988; 23(suppl 144):27–30.
11. Mendeloff AI, Calkins BM. Epidemiology. In: Kirsner JB, Shorter RG, eds. Inflammatory Bowel Disease, 3rd ed. Philadelphia: Lea and Febiger, 1988:3–16.
12. Brandt LJ. Gastrointestinal Disorders of the Elderly. New York: Raven Press, 1984:299–300.
13. Lashner BA, Kirsner JB. Inflammatory bowel disease in older people. Clin Geriatr Med 1991; 7:287–299.
14. Reichel W. Clinical Aspects of Aging, 3rd ed. Baltimore: Williams and Wilkins, 1989:194.
15. Griffin AM, Olmstead LC, Petras RA. *E. coli* 0157:H7-associated colitis. Gastroenterology 1990; 99:142–149.
16. Heilbrun N. Roentgen evidence suggesting enterocolitis associated with prolonged cathartic abuse. Radiology 1943; 41:486–491.
17. Allison MC, Howatson AG, Torrance MB. Gastrointestinal damage associated with the use of nonsteroidal antiinflammatory drugs. N Engl J Med 1992; 327:749–754.
18. Fleischer DE, Grimm IS, Friedman LS. Inflammatory bowel disease in older patients. Med Clin North Am 1994; 78:1303–1319.
19. Holt PR. Gastrointestinal drugs in the elderly. Am J Gastro 1986; 81:403–411.

11

Liver Disease in the Elderly

David J. Clain
Albert Einstein College of Medicine, Bronx, and Beth Israel Medical Center, New York, New York

I. INTRODUCTION

Aging has been frequently invoked as a cause of disease. The term senile cirrhosis like senile dementia is an echo of past ignorance. We have learned that specific entities account for these disorders in the elderly just as in younger age groups. For example alcoholism and hepatitis C are major causes of cirrhosis over the age of 60. The liver does show age-related changes in structure and function, but the clinical significance is relatively small. Alterations in the handling of drugs and toxins are often mediated by factors outside the liver and may be independent of the intrinsic function of hepatocytes. We need to understand the physiology of the aging process in the liver. Even if time itself does not bring inevitable decline in clinical function or changes in the profile of disease, all cells eventually show deterioration at a subcellular level due to an accumulation of biological errors in transcription and translation. The ultimate clinical test of an older organ may be its performance after transplantation. Several studies report similar results for graft and patient survival whether young or old livers were used (1) (Fig. 1). Successful liver transplantation has been reported from donors as old as 86 years (2).

II. REGENERATION

The liver is unusual in having enormous powers of regeneration after cellular death or rejection. There is partial protection from the effect of aging by the ability to regenerate. In older livers the rate of replacement

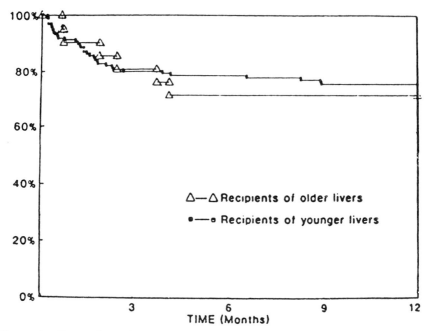

Figure 1   Comparison of survival of recipients of livers from older (> age 50) and younger donors. One-year survival was 71.4% (older donors), compared with 75.6% (younger donors). (From Ref. 1.)

of liver cells after injury is reduced, so repair is probably slower. The lifespan of an hepatocyte in the absence of injury is about one-third that of the human, which means that liver cells are replaced once or twice in a lifetime. Cell division takes place mainly in the periportal area of the lobule. Hepatocytes move slowly toward zone 3, the perivenular area, before dying. The size, shape, and function of liver cells vary with their zonal location. Gene expression and the metabolic roles of liver cells therefore change during their lifespan as they migrate transzonally along the cell plates of each lobule. The mechanism of aging in hepatocytes probably relates to accumulation of abnormal proteins due to reduced degradation by lysosomes. These abnormal proteins may interfere with metabolic functions and lead eventually to cell death (3).

III. AGING AND LIVER STRUCTURE

There are no meaningful changes in liver cell morphology with age. Hepatocytes are larger in size and smaller in number. Liver weight is decreased and exceeds the overall reduction in body weight. The interpretation of liver biopsies in aging individuals follows the same criteria as histopathologic diagnosis in younger patients. Popper described variations in a group of old and infirm subjects which include periportal proliferation of bile ductules, excess inflammatory cells, and accumulation of lipofuscin pigment in Kupffer cells. These findings were termed nonspecific reactive hepatitis and in many instances were probably the result of systemic disease (4).

IV. LIVER DYSFUNCTION WITH AGE

Changes in many biochemical pathways in the liver in older patients should be contrasted with the normal results of clinical tests of liver function. The results of animal studies may be species-specific. For example, cytochrome P450 enzymes decline with age in some strains of rat but not in others. In humans, on the other hand, the specific activities of many microsomal and other liver enzymes are constant with aging. Because of the disparity between animal and human data, the clinical relevance of experimental findings, such as quantitative changes in protein synthesis, is undetermined (3,5). The increased secretion of cholesterol into bile and the reduction in bile acid synthesis lead to a rise in lithogenic index, which may be the explanation for the higher incidence of gallstones in the elderly. In a group of people of mean age 84 years living in an institution, the prevalence of gallstones was 65% compared with 10% in the general population (6).

V. DRUGS AND THE LIVER

Pharmacokinetics and drug-induced liver diseases are two distinct but interrelated issues in the elderly. Those over 65 years old constitute 12% of the population but account for 30% of prescription drugs and 40% of nonprescription drugs. Older people not only use more drugs but also have frequent adverse reactions, may have less efficient clearance and metabolism, and are susceptible to certain hepatotoxic injuries. The practical impact of these alterations on the choice of the correct dose of drugs in the elderly has been one of the major areas of research in liver disease in aging. However, it is not established that age is an independent variable separate from associated diseases and multiple drugs. A study of "geriatric polypharmacy" recorded an average of 12 prescriptions per year in the over-65 age group compared to 5 in the 25-to-44-year-olds (4). The prevalence of drug taking is emphasized by the high incidence of adverse reactions, which is reported to be 20% or more among the elderly. Specific hepatotoxic side effects are evident from a French study in which admissions for acute hepatitis were due to medication in more than 40% of cases (8). In a survey of causes of jaundice in a geriatric setting, 20% were drug-induced (9).

There is substantial evidence that altered kinetics in the elderly are in large part due to factors extraneous to the liver. These include renal insufficiency, reduced cardiac output, diminished protein binding of drugs, and altered distribution through body compartments. There is relatively more fat than water and lean body mass, so water-soluble drugs are distributed in a smaller space. The ability of the liver to eliminate drugs and toxins is mainly dependent on two factors: *delivery* (hepatic blood flow) and *hepatocyte function* (liver mass X enzyme activity).

A major unresolved question is to what extent biochemical changes in the liver play a significant role in the handling of drugs in the aged. Drugs that are efficiently cleared by hepatocytes (high hepatic extraction ratio) are relatively unaffected by metabolic changes in the liver, but are very sensitive to liver blood flow. For example, there is a major decline in the extraction of propranolol after portacaval shunting, and heart failure may reduce by 50% the clearance of lidocaine (10). The progressive fall in hepatic blood flow with age also affects clearance of drugs and results in higher plasma level and a longer half-life of many commonly used agents (11). The clearance of drugs that are less rapidly metabolized is largely dependent on the total activity of liver enzymes. Conjugation reactions such as glucuronidation are generally unaffected, but there is a reduction in clearance of many drugs such as diazepam which are transformed by cytochrome P450-dependent oxygenases (12). There is evidence that many of these enzymes are normal in the aging human liver, and impaired hepatic metabolism may be adequately explained by a reduction in liver mass and by extrahepatic factors such as initial volume of distribution and protein binding. On the other hand, it is established that the hepatotoxicity of drugs such as INH has a biochemical component. There is significant enhancement of toxicity with age as well as by alcohol and Rifampin, which may be related to specific P450 isoenzymes (13).

In summary, the clearance of drugs by the liver cannot be predicted by age, presence of disease, or measurement of liver function tests. Consequently, there is no quantitative means of deriving a dosage regimen. There are also many extrahepatic factors. That is why all medications should be used with caution in the elderly. The standard dose may need to be reduced. Therapeutic goals should be established and dosage modified according to the patient's response. High-extraction drugs such as propranolol and lidocaine are most affected, but hepatic metabolism may be impaired and agents such as diazepam, fluraz pam, and quinidine often show higher blood levels in the elderly (14).

VI. LIVER FUNCTION TESTS

The normal range of standard liver function tests is not significantly different in the geriatric population. There is no change in the serum levels of bilirubin, aminotransferases, and alkaline phosphatase. There is a decline with age of measurements which reflect liver cell mass and blood flow such as galactose elimination and aminopyrine clearance, which are generally used for investigative rather than clinical purposes. Abnormal liver function tests may be differently interpreted in older patients because of a change in frequency of individual diseases. The principles, however, remain the same at any age. Mild abnormalities should be confirmed before embarking on costly investigations. Asymptomatic abnormalities are frequently discovered by the use of routine chemistry screens, by insurance examinations, and at the time of blood donation. Age is not the cause, and all abnormalities require evaluation. Some causes may be innocuous such as mild fatty liver or a transient reaction to drugs. Others are extrahepatic—for example, muscle injury or bone disease. Associated symptoms, signs, and test results may point to the origin or to a clear line of investigation (15).

VII. AMINOTRANSFERASES

The levels of aspartate transaminase (AST) and alanine transaminase (ALT) are primarily a guide to etiology not severity. Chronic hepatitis shows mild to moderate elevation of transaminases. When AST and ALT are more than 20× normal, the cause is usually acute hepatitis due to viruses or drugs, ischemia following low cardiac output, or acute stone obstruction of the bile duct (Table 1). Hepatic necrosis from combined abuse of alcohol and acetaminophen may lead to very high aminotransferases in excess of 2,000 IU/L. Causes of chronic hepatitis and an approach to investigation are summarized in Tables 2 and 3.

Alcoholism is common in the geriatric age group, and there is a high prevalence of chronic hepatitis C often contracted from blood transfusion

Table 1 Causes of AST or ALT More Than 20 Times Upper Limit of Normal

Drugs and toxins
Viral hepatitis
Acute stone obstruction of bile duct
Ischemia
Combined alcohol and acetaminophen

Table 2 Common Causes of Persistently
Raised AST and ALT in Elderly (2–10
times upper limit of normal)

Drug-induced liver disease
Fatty liver disease (steatohepatitis)
Alcohol
Chronic viral hepatitis (B, D, and C)
Systemic disease (heart, skeletal muscle)

(16). Chronic hepatitis C sometimes culminates in cirrhosis or even hepatocellular carcinoma, but follow-up for an average of 18 years of patients
with transfusion-related non-A, non-B hepatitis from five major prospective
trials in the United States showed no increase in mortality from all causes
and a barely significant excess of deaths related to liver disease, most of
which were attributed to alcoholism (17). Recent data from survivors in
this study, indicate that biochemical and histological morbidity is common,
but clinical changes are seldom evident at 20 years after infection. Fatty
liver (nonalcoholic steatosis) is frequently seen in older patients and rarely
progresses to fibrosis or cirrhosis. While most common in women who may
be overweight and diabetic, it is also seen in euglycemic men of normal
weight. Liver biopsy is not indicated if aminotransferases respond to simple
measures such as abstention for suspected alcoholic hepatitis or weight

Table 3 Management of Abnormal AST or ALT (elevated 2–10
times upper limit of normal)

1. Check previous results *or* repeat to confirm
2. Exclude systemic disease, eg, heart or skeletal
3. Repeat AST or ALT after withdrawing drugs and/or alcohol
4. Laboratory tests
   a. Hepatitis
   b. Serum iron, TIBC, ferritin
   c. Antinuclear antibody
      Anti-smooth-muscle antibody
   d. Alpha-1 antitrypsin
5. Sonogram for fat or cirrhosis
6. If steatohepatitis is suspected:
   Reduce weight and/or control glucose, *then* repeat AST or ALT.
7. Liver biopsy in selected patients

reduction and control of diabetes for steatosis. The chief indications for liver biopsy in this setting are to evaluate the histological severity of chronic hepatitis before deciding on therapy, to measure iron for the diagnosis of hemochromatosis, and to establish a cause for persistence or progression of markedly elevated AST and ALT.

VIII. ALKALINE PHOSPHATASE

Isolated elevation of alkaline phosphatase (ALP) may be seen on routine screening of an apparently healthy population. The incidence rises with age and may be higher in women. A normal gamma glutamic transpeptidase (GGTP) suggests a source outside the liver. The origin is often bone. In a study of 602 members of a health maintenance organization, 5.5% had a prior diagnosis that could have explained an abnormal ALP, and in another 3.5% active disease appeared during a 2-year follow-up. Cancer, liver disease, and Paget's were the most common findings. The other 91% developed no ALP-associated disease, and in one-fifth, liver function reverted to normal (18). Similar findings have been recorded in patients admitted to a geriatric service. Bone disease such as osteomalacia, fractures, and Paget's predominated. Hepatic ALP was most often elevated from heart failure and gallstones (15). Overall, there is uncertain significance to a lone elevation of ALP up to twice normal in elderly patients (19). Many abnormal values will resolve within months. Others have an obvious, often extrahepatic, cause. Limited studies suggest that stable values do not justify intensive evaluation. Occult disease is seldom found. If the diagnosis is not apparent when first detected, enzymes should be repeated at 3- to 4-month intervals.

A different picture emerges when ALP is more than three times increased, and especially when there was a clinical indication for the test. While a normal GGTP points to a source outside the liver, an increased value may be misleading because nonspecific elevations are caused by toxins, drugs, and many systemic illnesses. Abnormal aminotransferases and bilirubin are generally reliable in confirming a hepatobiliary cause for raised ALP. The combination of history, physical findings, and an imaging study will frequently be diagnostic. The crucial point of decision in the algorithm of elevated hepatic ALP is whether ultrasound shows dilated bile ducts. Dilatation indicates obstruction of a major duct most often due to tumor, especially carcinoma of the head of the pancreas, gallstones, or benign stricture from chronic pancreatitis or cholecystectomy. Nondilated ducts with a high ALP and a normal or slightly elevated bilirubin may be due to an extrahepatic cause, but intrahepatic cholestasis or infiltrative diseases of the parenchyma are more likely. These include primary biliary cirrhosis, hepatic malignancy, drug toxicity, hepatic cirrhosis, granulomatous hepatitis, and lymphoma.

In the presence of persistent jaundice above 7 or 8 mg/dl, however, the absence of duct dilatation virtually excludes major bile duct obstruction. Notable exceptions to this rule are stones in the common bile duct when jaundice is moderate and fluctuating and, less often, primary sclerosing cholangitis in which fibrosis may prevent dilatation.

IX. VIRAL HEPATITIS

There is little accurate information about the contribution of viruses A, B, C, and D to the occurrence of acute hepatitis in elderly patients. Hepatitis C predominates, and hepatitis B is the next most frequent. There are many ethnic, geographic, and socioeconomic factors that influence the incidence of these infections. Figure 2 shows the marked difference between the prevalence of antibodies to hepatitis A (anti-HAV) and B (anti-HBs) in middle-class whites, middle-class blacks, and Chinese in various age groups

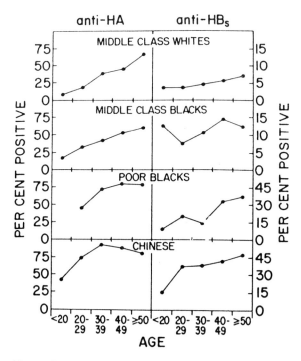

Figure 2 Percentage prevalence of hepatitis A antibodies (anti-HA) and hepatitis B surface antibodies (anti-HBs) according to age in four populations in greater New York. (From Szmuness et al. (20), with permission.)

in New York City (20). In the white and black populations the prevalence of anti-HAV was 2–4 times higher in those over age 50 than in those under 20. These data suggest a cohort of older patients who were exposed decades before when hepatitis A was more prevalent rather than a cumulative incidence with age (21). Therefore, older patients in New York City are less susceptible to hepatitis A, and this accords with general clinical experience in the United States. Improved living conditions have changed this pattern of antibodies in children, and in due course may modify the incidence of hepatitis A in the elderly.

Several studies suggesting greater severity and poor prognosis were published before serological testing became available (22). There are anecdotal descriptions of subacute hepatic necrosis with a prolonged, often fatal outcome, especially in postmenopausal women. Fulminant disease is more frequent in adults, and an even higher mortality is expected in an older population with frequent comorbid conditions such as heart and lung disease and diabetes. An adverse outcome has been attributed to the frequency of hepatitis C in the elderly, but in the Sentinel Counties study of non-A, non-B hepatitis there was a subset of mainly elderly patients with no viral markers who ran a rather mild course (23).

Chronic hepatitis is common in older patients because at least 50% of hepatitis C infections are persistent. Hepatitis C is an important cause of cirrhosis and end-stage liver disease. The tendency to chronicity of hepatitis C is inherent to the virus and is seen at all ages. This contrasts with hepatitis B infection, in which immune competence is important for viral clearance. Impairment of immunity in the very young and the very old leads to a higher incidence of chronic hepatitis. An outbreak of hepatitis B in a nursing facility resulted in a chronic carrier rate of 59% (24). There is a poor response to hepatitis B vaccine in the elderly for similar reasons (25).

The main purpose of treating asymptomatic chronic infection with HBV and HCV with alpha-interferon are to avoid the development of cirrhosis and primary hepatocellular carcinoma (PHC). The effect of age on therapy has not been studied, but there is sound evidence that mortality in hepatitis C does not increase within 18 years of infection (17). Treatment is therefore not justified in elderly patients with a limited life expectancy and a recent onset of chronic hepatitis or mild histological changes. Iron overload increases with age, and may reduce the efficacy of treatment with alpha-interferon in chronic hepatitis C. Venesection will leach out liver iron and may improve the response to treatment. Both HBV and HCV appear to have an important role in the etiology of PHC. The incidence of the two viruses varies with age; in a Korean study the ratio of HBV/HCV was 29.7 before age 50 and 0.9 over 60 years in PHC (26).

X. DIFFERENTIAL DIAGNOSIS OF ACUTE HEPATITIS
A. Ischemia

Ischemic hepatitis may simulate the clinical picture of acute viral hepatitis. There may be anorexia and fatigue (27). Physical examination shows a tender, enlarged liver and often jaundice. Aminotransferases are strikingly elevated. Underlying heart disease is common, and persons of any age may be affected. The clinical picture and pattern of liver function tests due to ischemia vary with the relative contribution of right heart failure, low cardiac output, and hypoxemia (28). Shock liver is an acute ischemic event due to hypotension often associated with myocardial infarction or arrhythmia. AST and ALT may be very high, often in the 1,000s, and the rise and fall are rapid, within a few days, which is quite unlike the profile of enzymes in viral infection. Absence of hepatitis A IgM and hepatitis B core IgM will also help exclude viral hepatitis. Hepatitis C antibodies are usually present at the onset of symptomatic infection. Many patients with ischemic hepatitis never have a drop in blood pressure, and in some cases, with extremely low output and marked hepatic venous hypertension, the laboratory profile is similar to that of viral hepatitis. Liver histology will show zone 3 (perivenular) ischemic necrosis in contrast to zone 1 (periportal) inflammation in viral hepatitis, but liver biopsies are rarely required for diagnosis. The mortality may exceed 50% because liver ischemia signals a profound circulatory disorder.

B. Drugs and Toxins

Hepatic drug reactions are common in the elderly and are responsible for more than 40% of acute hepatitis (9). The clinical and laboratory features may be identical to the pattern in viral hepatitis. A detailed history of medications and toxins is essential. Viral serology is useful in diagnosis, but chronic carriers of HBV and HCV are not immune to the effects of drugs and toxins. In allergic reactions to drugs, presence of rash, fever, and eosinophilia may be valuable etiologic features. Liver biopsy may not be helpful because hepatotoxic damage, as is seen for example with INH and carbon tetrachloride, often cannot be distinguished from viral. While alcoholic hepatitis presents a distinctive clinical and laboratory profile, the combination of alcohol and acetaminophen may cause acute necrosis with very high AST and ALT, which can be mistaken for viral hepatitis.

C. Common Duct Stones

Three patterns of abnormal liver function tests may be associated with choledocholithiasis. Most frequently, there is intermittent obstruction of the common duct with fluctuating ALP, bilirubin, and aminotransferases. Larger stones may impact with gradually increasing ALP and jaundice typical of cholestasis (Table 4). A third profile which resembles acute hepatitis shows a sudden marked elevation of AST and ALT caused by passage of a small stone through the papilla. Pain is variable. Transient jaundice may be present. The aminotransferases usually fall rapidly, but values occasionally remain elevated for many days.

XI. AUTOIMMUNE HEPATITIS

Autoimmune hepatitis was originally described in young women, but is now known to occur in males and females of any age. Autoimmune hepatitis is occasionally seen in the elderly, but viruses and drugs are much more frequent causes of chronic hepatitis. There are no special clinical features in the geriatric group, but treatment with corticosteroids should be used with special caution. Prednisone causes a high incidence of serious complications including pain and fractures due to osteopenia, diabetes, sodium retention, and hypertension. In asymptomatic, elderly patients with moderate, stable elevation of liver enzymes and normal synthetic function, corticosteroids should be withheld because there is a high ratio of risk to benefit. Symptomatic patients with florid clinical features do need therapy. Azathioprine can be used to minimize the steroid dosage. Prednisone is usually started at a

Table 4 Common Causes of Cholestasis

Intrahepatic[a]
    Drug-induced
    Viral hepatitis
    Alcoholic hepatitis
    Right heart failure
    Primary biliary cirrhosis
    Systemic sepsis
Large bile duct obstruction
    Carcinoma of the pancreas
    Gallstones in common duct[b]
    Bile duct tumor
    Stricture of common duct
    Chronic pancreatitis
    Primary sclerosing cholangitis[b]

---

[a] Bile ducts not dilated.
[b] May be undilated bile ducts.

dose of 30 mg daily and reduced gradually over several weeks to 15 mg or less, guided by the response of symptoms and laboratory findings.

XII. ALCOHOLIC LIVER DISEASE

Medicare patients with alcohol as the primary reason for admission cost the taxpayers $233,543,500 in 1989. Twenty-one percent of 33,039 elderly patients had cirrhosis, fatty liver, or other alcoholic-related damage. These figures underestimate the problem because they do not reflect admissions in which alcohol was a secondary diagnosis, and because VA hospitals, where alcoholism is not uncommon, were excluded. Chronic liver disease and its complications are much more frequent in elderly drinkers than young drinkers. The age-specific incidence of cirrhosis in white men living in the urban areas of Baltimore is highest in the seventh decade (29). Several studies show a 1-year mortality as high as 50% from alcoholic liver disease in patients over 60 years of age. The consequences of dependent drinking in the elderly are seldom obvious. Alcoholism with or without liver disease frequently masquerades as falling, dizziness, insomnia, muscle pains, malnutrition, hypothermia, or general medical problems unrelated to ethanol. The potential for rehabilitation of older over-users of alcohol is better if they started drinking later, due to social factors such as depression and loneliness and if these can be successfully addressed (30).

XIII. PRIMARY BILIARY CIRRHOSIS

Primary biliary cirrhosis (PBC) is a chronic cholestatic disease due to destruction of intrahepatic bile ducts by an immunological process. There is predictable progression to cirrhosis and liver failure. Ninety percent of patients are women between the ages of 40 and 59. About 5% are in their 60s and 70s, but younger asymptomatic patients often survive more than 10 years into this age range. PBC should always be considered in the differential diagnosis of cirrhosis or cholestatic syndromes in the elderly (Table 4). Medical therapies are beginning to influence prognosis. Colchicine is safe but marginally effective. Ursodiol improves liver function tests and histology and slows clinical progression. Methotrexate has toxic side effects, which limits its current use to clinical trials (31). Treatment is mainly directed at controlling pruritus and preventing osteopenia, which is especially common in older patients. Vitamin D should be given to patients with chronic cholestasis, jaundice, and low levels of 25-(OH)D to prevent bone pain and fractures. PBC is the second most common indication for liver transplantation. Prognostic models based on clinical data determine the best time for operation (32). Age is an important criterion independent of serum bilirubin, albumin, prothrombin time, and edema. Patients should be referred to a transplant center when serum bilirubin reaches 150 μmol/L, because the best results are achieved when prognosis is relatively good at the time of transplantation.

XIV. CIRRHOSIS

Decompensated liver disease in elderly patients may not present with frank features, such as portal hypertensive ascites, variceal bleeding, and hepatic encephalopathy, but rather may appear more obscurely with loss of weight, muscular atrophy, edema, anemia, osteoporosis, or change in mental status. Hepatic encephalopathy may be subtle, and may be confused with other causes of the organic mental syndrome. Cirrhosis is often far advanced when first diagnosed late in life. The causes of cirrhosis in persons over 60 years of age vary with geography, economic status, and social customs. Chronic hepatitis C and alcohol use are most common in the United States. Hepatitis B and D, PBC, and sclerosing cholangitis are also frequently seen. No etiology is evident in many cases. Less common are drug-induced chronic hepatitis, autoimmune hepatitis, hemochromatosis, and, rarely alpha-1 antitrypsin deficiency. Older cirrhotics are in general treated like younger cirrhotics. There are some exceptions. Vasopressin is risky in patients with cardiovascular disease because arrhythmias, angina, and myocardial infarction may be induced. Portal systemic shunts for bleeding, whether created surgically or by insertion of a transjugular intrahepatic stent, result in an unacceptable incidence of encephalopathy.

Body iron stores in hemochromatosis increase with age. The diagnosis is usually made in middle-aged men and can be confused with alcoholic cirrhosis. Older patients tend to have more severe liver disease. Hemochromatosis is 10 times as common in men as in women, and female patients with overt disease usually present many years postmenopausal. Hepatomegaly and diabetes are common. Recognition is vital because prognosis may be improved by removal of iron through venesection.

Primary hepatocellular carcinoma (PHC) is a frequent complication of cirrhosis caused by chronic viral hepatitis, alcohol, and hemochromatosis. The peak incidence varies with geography and underlying cause. PHC is the commonest solid tumor reported from Asia and sub-Saharan Africa, and commonly presents between age 30 and 50 in chronic carriers of hepatitis B or C. The tumor ranks only 22nd in the United States and appears at a later age. The carcinomas have often grown to a large size and may be multicentric when first seen. Older patients seldom have operable tumors. Transplantation may be indicated for PHCs that are small and not multicentric, but there is a high incidence of recurrence in the allograft.

XV. LIVER TRANSPLANTATION

Orthotopic liver transplantation (OLT) is an established treatment of severe chronic liver disease with survival rates that approach 80% at 1 year. Improved results have been achieved by enhanced preservation of donor livers, better surgical techniques, and the introduction of cyclosporine for immunosuppression. Outcome is dependent on many factors in patient selection. Evaluation of risk includes serum bilirubin, prothrombin time, encephalopathy, ascites, and nutritional status. However, no evidence has emerged to support the use of age alone as a criterion for selection.

The preference for younger patients in the early years of liver transplantation largely excluded candidates over 55 years, but as experience has broadened, excellent results have been achieved with survival in patients over 60 years equal to survival at younger ages (33). Observations at several centers suggest, however, that elderly transplant patients who are in a high-risk category with severely decompensated liver disease do less well than their younger counterparts (34). Some of these comparisons were made with historical controls. One center reported data on 202 consecutive liver transplant patients who were classified into four groups according to age and UNOS (United Network for Organ Sharing) status (Fig. 3) (35). Hepatitis C

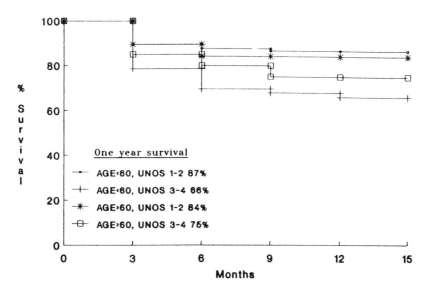

Figure 3 Comparison of percentage survival in months according to age and UNOS status of recipients after liver transplantation. (From Emre et al. (35), with permission.)

cirrhosis, primary biliary cirrhosis, sclerosing cholangitis, and alcoholic liver disease were the commonest etiologies. Many patients had pretransplant renal failure, gastrointestinal bleeding, encephalopathy, and diabetes. The main conclusion was that selected patients over age 60 can be transplanted with overall 1-year graft and patient survival rates equal to those achieved in younger patients even when stratified to an adverse pretransplant medical status.

A "bonus" for elderly transplant recipients is that the impairment of immune function accompanying older age reduces the incidence of allograft rejection, and may also allow lower dosage of immunosuppressive drugs with reduced side effects such as infection, cataracts, and osteoporosis. The shortage of donor organs is unfavorable to the choice of elderly recipients whose long-term life expectancy even after successful transplantation will be less than in younger patients. Selection of older patients requires careful exclusion of cancer, serious heart disease, and serious lung disease.

These excellent results have not only made OLT readily available to patients in their 60s and 70s, but Medicare has also broadened its criteria for reimbursement. The best results are achieved by anticipating severe decline in status and transplanting earlier in the course of advanced liver disease, especially in the elderly, in whom deterioration is often unpredictable.

REFERENCES

1. Wall WJ, Mimeault R, Grant D, Bloch M. The use of older liver donors for hepatic transplantation. Transplantation 1990; 49:377–381.
2. Wall W, Grant D, Roy A, Asfar S, Bloch M. Elderly liver donor (letter). Lancet 1993; 341:121.
3. Dice JF, Goff SA. Aging and the liver. In Arias IM, Jakoby WB, Popper H, Schachter D Shafritz DA, eds. The Liver: Biology and Pathobiology. 2d ed. New York: Raven Press 1988:1245–1257.
4. Popper H. Aging and the liver. In: Popper H, Schaffner F, eds. Progress in Liver Disease. Vol VII. Orlando Fla: Grune & Stratton, 1986:659–683.
5. Butler JA, Heydari AR, Richardson A. Analysis of effect of age on synthesis of specific proteins by hepatocytes. J Cell Physiol 1989; 141:400–409.
6. Ratner J, Lisbona A, Rosenbloom M, Szabolesci S Tupaz T. The prevalence of gallstone disease in very old institutionalized persons. JAMA 1991; 265:902–903.
7. Williams L, Rush DR. Geriatric polypharmacy. Hosp Prac (Off) 1989; 21:109–112.
8. Benhamou JP. Drug induced hepatitis: clinical aspects. In: Fillastre JP, ed. Hepatotoxicity of Drugs. Rouen, France: University of Rouen, 1986:23–30.
9. Eastwood HOH. Causes of jaundice in the elderly; a survey of diagnosis and investigation. Geront Clin 1971; 13:69–71.

10. Castleden CM, George CF. The effect of aging on the hepatic clearance of propranolol. Br J Clin Pharmacol 1979; 7:49–54.
11. Wynne HA, Cope LH, Mutch E, Rawlins MD, Woodhouse KW, James OFW. The effects of age upon liver volume and apparent blood flow in healthy man. Hepatology 1989; 9:297–301.
12. Klotz U, Avant GR, Hoyumpa A, Schenker S, Wilkinson CR. The effects of age and liver disease on the disposition and elimination of diazepam in adult man. J Clin Invest 1975; 55:347–359.
13. Lewis JH, Zimmerman HJ. Drug induced liver disease. Med Clin North Am 1989; 73:775–792.
14. Vestal RE. Drug use in the elderly. A review of problems and special considerations. Drugs 1978; 16:358–382.
15. Lubin JR, Coles JA, Millward BA, Croker JR. Value of profiling liver function in the elderly. Postgrad Med 1983; 59:763–766.
16. Katkov WN, Friedman LS, Cody H. Elevated serum alanine aminotransferase levels in blood donors: the contribution of hepatitis C virus. Ann Intern Med 1991; 115:882–884.
17. Seeff LB, Buskell-Bales Z, Wright EC, et al. Long term mortality after transfusion-associated non-A, non-B hepatitis. N Engl J Med 1992; 327:1906–1911.
18. Rubenstein LV, Ward NC, Greenfield S. In pursuit of abnormal serum alkaline phosphatase: a clinical dilemma. J Gen Intern Med 1986; 1:38–43.
19. Lieberman D, Phillips D. Isolated elevation of alkaline phosphatase: significance in hospitalized patients. J Clin Gastroenterol 1990; 12:415–419.
20. Szmuness W, Dienstag JL, Purcell RH, Harley EJ, Stevens CE, Wong DC. Distribution of antibody to hepatitis A antigen in urban and adult populations. N Engl J Med 1976; 295:755–759.
21. Gust ID, Lehman NI, Lucas CR. Relationship between prevalence of antibody to hepatitis A antigen and age: a cohort effect? J Infect Dis 1978; 138:425–426.
22. Goodson JD, Taylor PA, Campion EW, Richter JM, Wands J. The clinical course of acute hepatitis in the elderly patient. Arch Intern Med 1982; 142:1485–1488.
23. Alter MJ, Margolis HS, Krawczynski K, et al. The natural history of community-acquired hepatitis C in the United States. N Engl J Med 1992; 327:1899–1905.
24. Kondo Y, Tsukada K, Takeuchi I, et al. High carrier rate after hepatitis B virus infection in the elderly. Hepatology 1993, 18:768–774.
25. Denis F, Mounier M, Hessel L, et al. Hepatitis B vaccination in the elderly. J Infect Dis 1984; 149:1019.
26. Lee HS, Han CJ, Kim CV. Predominant etiologic association of hepatitis C virus with hepatocellular carcinoma compared with hepatitis B virus in elderly patients in a hepatitis B endemic area. Cancer 1993; 72:2564–2567.
27. Bynum TE, Boitnott JK, Maddrey WC. Ischemic hepatitis. Dig Dis Sci 1979; 24:129–134.
28. Cohen JA, Kaplan MM. Left sided heart failure presenting as hepatitis. Gastroenterology 1978; 74:583–587.

29. Garagliano CF, Lilienfeld AM, Mendeloff AL. Incidence rates of liver cirrhosis and related diseases in Baltimore and selected areas of the United States. J Chron Dis 1979; 32:543–554.
30. Dunne FJ, Schipperheijn JAM. Alcohol and the elderly. (Editorial.) BMJ 1989; 298:1660–1661.
31. Poupon RE, Poupon R, Balkau B, UDCA-PBC Study Group. Ursodiol for the long term treatment of primary biliary cirrhosis. N Engl J Med 1994; 330:1342–1347.
32. Neuberger JM. Predicting the prognosis of primary biliary cirrhosis. Gut 1989; 30:1519–1522.
33. Pirsch JD, Kalayoglu M, D'Alessandro AM, et al. Orthotopic liver transplantation in patients 60 years of age and older. Transplantation 1991; 51:431–433.
34. Castaldo P, Langnas A, Stratta RJ, Wood RP, Shaw BW. Liver transplantation in patients over 60 years of age. Gastroenterology 1991; 100:A717.
35. Emre S, Mor E, Schwartz ME, et al. Liver transplantation in patients beyond 60. Transplant Proc 1993; 25:1075–1076.

12

Biliary Disease in the Elderly

Franklin E. Kasmin
Beth Israel Medical Center, New York, New York

Jerome H. Siegel
Beth Israel Medical Center, New York, and Albert Einstein College of Medicine, Bronx, New York

I. INTRODUCTION

Diseases of the biliary tract have become an important entity affecting the elderly. Older patients are more predisposed to developing certain complications resulting from benign or malignant disease affecting the biliary tree ostensibly because of the time requirements for these conditions to develop. Also, biliary tract diseases often present in an atypical manner in the elderly. Additionally, the application of therapeutic options must take into consideration the general physical condition of the older patient, and preexisting or comorbid processes.

The diagnostic challenge confronting the gastroenterologist is first establishing a correct diagnosis despite misleading clues. The treatment plan must take into account the natural history of the disease, the likelihood of disease-related complications, and the risks of the various treatment modalities available.

II. ANATOMIC CONSIDERATIONS

Although the morphology of the biliary tree is not greatly altered during the aging process, there are some important differences to be noted. First, a gradual narrowing of the distal common bile duct has been reported. This change occurs as a result of the development of fibrous tissue located in the periampullary bile duct. However, this occurrence is not necessarily associated with a dilatation of the proximal biliary tree (1,2). Secondly, there is an increased incidence of periampullary diverticula found in the elderly, indicating that these diverticula are, for the most part, acquired changes related to aging (3). Both of these anatomic changes could conceivably play a role in the development of common bile duct stones, a condition seen with increased frequency in the aged.

The gallbladder may become more distensible with age. However, early studies of emptying in the elderly do not demonstrate an appreciable loss of gallbladder emptying (4). It is likely that the gallbladder does not undergo important physical change over time regarding pathophysiologic function or its propensity for disease.

III. GALLSTONES AND DISEASES OF THE GALLBLADDER

Gallstone disease is one of the most common indications for surgery in people over the age of 60. Since an important factor in the development of gallstones is time, it is not unusual that the elderly have a high incidence of cholelithiasis. Autopsy studies indicate that up to 33% of people over the age of 70 have gallstones, most of them asymptomatic (5–7). However, with increasing age, there is an increased likelihood that asymptomatic stones may become more clinically important, and the elderly have an increased rate of complications of gallstone disease, including pancreatitis, cholangitis, and gallbladder carcinoma.

The clinical presentation of stone disease in the elderly usually follows one of several courses. Certainly, it is not unusual that biliary colic worsens in patients who have aged into the seventh decade or beyond. In most surgical series, half the elderly patients presented with chronic cholecystitis and cholelithiasis (5,8,9). Most of these patients are treated electively.

Alternatively, cholecystectomy may be necessary because of complications of gallstone disease. Approximately 30% of elderly patients who undergo cholecystectomy do have acute cholecystitis. In addition, choledocholithiasis is found in 10–20% of elderly patients undergoing cholecystectomy (8,9). If cholecystectomy is performed as an emergency in an elderly patient, the incidence of common duct stones rises to 50%. (10) Gangrenous cholecystitis occurs in 5–10% of elderly patients with cholecystitis (8,11,12). Bacterial cultures of the bile are positive in a high proportion of elderly patients undergoing both elective and emergent cholecystectomy (12).

Acalculous cholecystitis is a recognized condition occurring more frequently in the elderly. This special condition represents an ischemic inflammation of the gallbladder wall, which can rapidly progress to necrosis and perforation if left untreated (13). Its particular importance in older patients is its association with vascular insufficiency of the gut, a condition often related to cardiovascular disease and atherosclerosis, both of which occur more frequently with advanced age.

Torsion of the gallbladder can present as biliary colic, simulating acute cholecystitis (14). A loose serosal attachment between the gallbladder and the liver allows the gallbladder to twist, either around the axis of the cystic duct or across the common bile duct, causing intermittent obstruction of those structures. However, this uncommon condition does not appear to occur more frequently in the elderly population.

An important point should be made regarding the clinical presentation of stone disease in the aged. The diagnosis of this condition is often obscured by a relative paucity of symptoms. For reasons that are unclear, elderly patients tend to complain less of pain during attacks of colic or cholecystitis, and frequently present with fewer positive findings on physical exam. Coexisting medical conditions occur with increased frequency in the elderly. Two of these conditions, diabetes and dementia, may obscure clinical signs and symptoms, making the evaluation of gallbladder disease more difficult. Furthermore, aging is associated with deficiencies which affect a normal immune response, limiting the patient's ability to respond to an inflammatory response. To emphasize this, one report of six octogenarians showed that changes in these patients' mental status or progressive physical feebleness were the only presenting signs of serious biliary tract disease (15). A high index of suspicion is helpful when evaluating an elderly patient who presents with few phsyical findings. A delay in diagnosis can easily lead to rapid deterioration of the patient's condition such as perforation of a gangrenous gallbladder or sepsis from cholangitis.

A. Diagnosis

The diagnosis of cholelithiasis, cholecystitis, and stone-related disease of the biliary tree is based on the correlation of historical, physical, and biochemical evidence. The diagnosis is supported by the prudent use of invasive and noninvasive imaging.

The clinical history of right upper quadrant colic, fatty food intolerance, and, in the case of acute cholecystitis, fever, and malaise may be elicited. While pain is often present, its absence in the elderly by no means rules out gallbladder disease. A positive "Murphy's" sign is elicited when the tender gallbladder fundus rises toward the anterior abdominal wall during deep inspiration and is struck by the examiner's fingers.

Blood work should include liver chemistries, white blood count, and serum amylase levels. During most attacks of acute cholecystitis, liver chemistries are either normal or slightly elevated due to contiguous hepatic inflammation. The white blood count is often elevated to between 15,000 and 20,000 cells/dl. Marked elevations of the liver chemistries or the presence of a high serum amylase may indicate the presence of choledocholithiasis.

The ultrasound examination of the upper abdomen remains the best imaging study when considering cholelithiasis and associated disease of the biliary tree (Fig. 1). The echogenicity of gallstones makes them visible to sonography, even when they are radiolucent. Sonography is inexpensive, noninvasive, usually portable, and rapidly performed. It provides accurate information regarding intrahepatic and extrahepatic duct dilatation as well as the status of the gallbladder wall.

Nuclear scans are useful in assessing the function of the gallbladder (16,17). Radioisotopes such as HIDA, DISIDA, and PIPIDA are injected intravenously, accumulated by the liver, and excreted into the biliary tree (Fig. 2).

In the correct clinical setting, the lack of uptake by the gallbladder is very specific for cystic duct obstruction and cholecystitis. The time for transit into the gallbladder can be used as a method to assess sphincter of

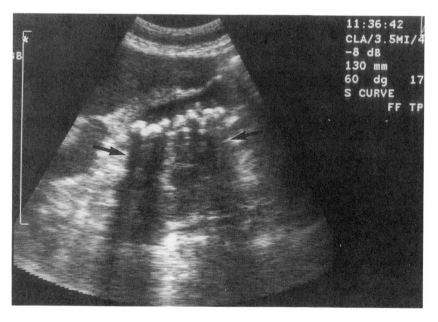

Figure 1 Sonogram showing gallbladder with acoustic "shadowing" (arrows), indicating the presence of gallstones.

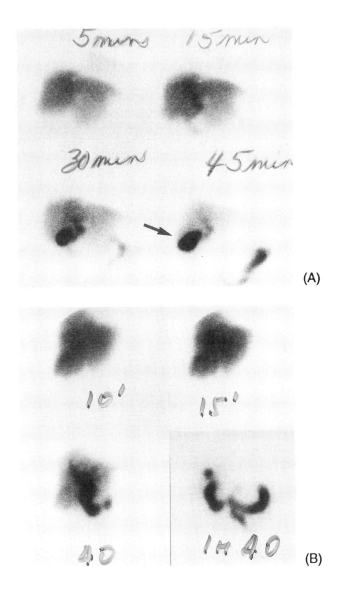

Figure 2 A. A normal HIDA scan, showing rapid uptake of radionuclide in the area of the gallbladder fossa (arrow), indicating patency of the cystic duct. B. An HIDA scan in a patient with acute cholecystitis and cystic duct obstruction. Note the absence of radionuclide in the gallbladder fossa after 1.5 hours. Isotope is seen flowing through a dilated common bile duct into the duodenum.

Oddi function or patency. computerized assessments of the emptying rates of the gallbladder following a standardized dose of a stimulant of contraction (i.e., cholecystokinin) can be used to assess functional (nonobstructive) disease of the gallbladder.

False-positive findings (the absence of gallbladder filling) can occur in a clinical setting without cholecystitis. False-positive results occur during fasting, in patients with an overfilled gallbladder, and in the patient who has had a sphincterotomy of the sphincter of Oddi. The gallbladder fails to function in patients who have undergone sphincterotomy because of the loss of the pressure in the common bile duct required to fill the gallbladder.

Computed tomography (CT) assumes a lesser role in confirming the diagnosis of cholecystitis and cholelithiasis. While the liver architecture is well seen with CT, much of the gallbladder is often lost between slices of the scan. Also, radiolucent stones may not be seen by CT. The cost of the exam and its radiation exposure are also disadvantages of this technique when compared to sonography.

Endoscopic retrograde cholangiopancreatography (ERCP) is a useful modality for performing minimally invasive cholangiography. One can diagnose choledocholithiasis pre- or postcholecystectomy, and cystic duct patency can also be determined. The great advantage of ERCP over other modalities is its therapeutic capability, which includes extraction of stones, drainage of cholangitis, and even disimpaction of an obstructing cystic duct stones.

B. Treatment

The gold standard for the treatment of cholecystitis remains cholecystectomy. Removal of the gallbladder is safe and effective in both acute and nonemergent situations and provides complete cure of the disease process. The mortality rate for elective open cholecystectomy in the general population is approximately 0.1% (18). Mortality rises in the emergent situation and when the common bile duct is explored. Laparoscopic cholecystectomy has not been responsible for a rise in the mortality rate, although the incidence of common duct injuries is greater than that reported in open cholecystectomies (19).

Cholecystectomy in the elderly is generally safe when performed in the nonemergent situation. The mortality rate for elective cholecystectomy is accepted as 3% in patients 65 years or older (7–12,20–22). However, there is a significant increase in morbidity and mortality rates when emergent cholecystectomy is performed in the elderly or when it is performed for acute cholecystitis. The mortality rate for these situations ranges from 6% to 15%, respectively, and can increase to as much as 20% or higher if common duct exploration is part of the emergent operation.

While cholecystectomy remains the gold standard of treatment for diseases of the gallbladder, several other treatment options can be considered, especially in the elderly population.

An important surgical option remains cholecystostomy. This procedure is simpler to perform than cholecystectomy and is generally reserved for patients too ill to undergo the risk of a more extensive procedure. In some series, however, cholecystostomy is associated with a higher mortality than cholecystectomy, but that may be because the less extensive procedure was performed on the most ill patients (23).

Medical dissolution therapy is available for the management of cholelithiasis. Ursodiol and chenodeoxycholic acid taken orally are agents for the treatment of cholesterol stones provided the load is not great (24). Cessation of oral treatment often leads to stone recurrence, and some advocates of bile acid dissolution therapy incorporate a chronic therapy protocol to prevent recurrence. Direct dissolution of gallbladder stones is available in some centers. The drug MTBE (methyl tert-butyl ether) is instilled into the gallbladder via a percutaneous route and is very effective in dissolving cholesterol stones (25).

Extracorporeal shockwave lithotripsy (ESWL) provided by transabdominal electrohydraulic shock waves has gained popularity in Europe but is not generally available in the U.S. (26). ESWL was under investigation in several centers in the U.S. It was never approved by the Food and Drug Administration and was withdrawn from use. The protocol limited the size and number of stones to be fragmented.

Endoscopic therapy for cholecystitis is controversial. Several reports of transpapillary stenting for the treatment of both acute and chronic cholecystitis have been published (27,28). In addition, endoscopic catheter manipulation and injection of the cystic duct with disimpaction of cystic duct stones have been reported to be useful in relieving the symptoms of acute cholecystitis (27). These therapies would be recommended only in patients who are too ill to undergo cholecystectomy. A more definitive role for ERCP in cholecystitis awaits further study.

IV. CHOLEDOCHOLITHIASIS

Common duct stones are an important complicating factor of gallstone disease in the elderly population. The incidence of choledocholithiasis is approximately 5% at the time of cholecystectomy in the general population, but as mentioned this figure rises to 10–20% in the aged.

There are several predisposing factors affecting the elderly that account for the development of common duct stones. One factor is thought to be due to changes of the sphincter anatomy, as described above, which leads to sphincter dysfunction. Another factor is the higher incidence of periampullary diverticula in the elderly which compress the distal common bile duct and promote stasis. Finally, time must play a role; the presence of gallbladder stones over a period of many years in the elderly population allows for more time for passage of stones into the common duct.

Common duct stones often present atypically in the elderly. Symptoms include painless jaundice, malaise, and loss of appetite. Asymptomatic elevations of liver functions (cholestasis) or the incidental radiologic findings on imaging studies alert the clinician to bile duct pathology. Clinical features of choledocholithiasis include right upper quadrant colic, cholangitis, and pancreatitis. While it is difficult to separate the symptoms of gallbladder colic from those of colic due to choledocholithiasis, it is certain that many older patients undergo cholecystectomy (with removal of common duct stones) for symptoms that were due mostly to the duct stones. It is important to remember that complications of gallstone disease, such as cholangitis, biliary colic, or gallstone pancreatitis, can present in the absence of cholecystitis.

Cholangitis occurs when a stone impacts, at least temporarily, in the ampulla or distal bile duct, allowing for the development of bacterial infection. Increased pressure in the biliary tree allows for the translocation of bacteria from the bile ductules into the bloodstream, producing bacteremia and sepsis. At times, frank suppuration of the bile will occur, and liver abscesses may develop. Common bacterial pathogens are *Escherichia coli*, *Klebsiella pneumoniae*, and *Enterococcus*. The mortality from untreated cholangitis approaches 100%. The mainstays of therapy are hydration, antibiotics, and decompression of the bile duct. Elderly patients tolerate cholangitis and survive this insult provided they tolerate definitive therapy for decompression of the common duct.

Gallstone pancreatitis occurs when a stone migrates into or passes the ampulla of Vater. While it is not clear what role obstruction of the pancreatic duct plays in this condition, a longer-than-usual "common channel" between the distal common bile duct and the distal pancreatic duct seems to be frequently present in patients who develop gallstone pancreatitis.

Gallstone pancreatitis presents with abdominal pain occurring over a 12- 48-hour period and is frequently associated with nausea and vomiting. Supportive care usually is responsible for resolution of this syndrome. It is thought that the resolution of symptoms occurs when the stone disimpacts, either during its passage into the duodenum, or as it becomes dislodged and floats back up into the duct. In patients who have normalized their liver functions after an episode of gallstone pancreatitis, up to 85% will have no evidence of persistent common bile duct stones at the time of cholangiography. When symptoms and signs of pancreatitis persist or worsen, a continuing stone impaction is suspected. With this scenario, clinical deterioration is evident, and specific treatment is directed at the stone. The morbidity and mortality rates in elderly patients in this situation are high, and standard surgical therapy is risky (29,30). For this reason early investigation is recommended (31).

A. Diagnosis

Serum liver chemistries are the mainstay for confirming the presence of choledocholithiasis. Elevations of any of the serum liver enzymes or elevation of the serum bilirubin or amylase should raise suspicion of duct stones. It should be noted that stones can present with minimal or marked elevations of one or several serum markers. As discussed previously, some elderly patients have choledocholithiasis with normal serum liver chemistries, but this is atypical.

Sonography is recommended as the first-line diagnostic imaging study for evaluating the biliary tree. Important clues to the presence of choledocholithiasis include common bile duct dilatation to greater than 8 mm in diameter (or greater than 11 mm postcholecystectomy), visualization of echogenic defects in the duct, or the presence of pancreatitis. The absence of these findings, however, does not rule out duct stones, and in the proper clinical setting, a cholangiogram is essential.

ERCP is an important technique for confirming the presence of common duct stones, as not only is the technique an excellent method for opacifying the bile duct, but it also allows for immediate treatment of the disease process (Fig. 3). The disadvantage of ERCP is that it is invasive, and a level of expertise is a prerequisite which may not be available at all centers.

B. Treatment

The management of choledocholithiasis can be endoscopic, surgical, or radiologic. A fourth modality, extracorporeal lithotripsy, available only in Europe or in some research centers in U.S. and Canada, may be useful for large stones when combined with ERCP.

The endoscopic method for removing common duct stones is efficacious, cost-effective, and associated with a low morbidity and mortality (32–34). ERCP, usually combined with sphincterotomy, is successful in approximately 85–95% of reported series. The procedure, which usually takes about 1 hour, is performed under intravenous, conscious sedation. It is associated with a 1–2% incidence of serious complications and a mortality rate of less than 1%, even in the elderly (35). Interestingly, a recent study demonstrated that therapeutic ERCP in patients 90 years of age or older had a lower

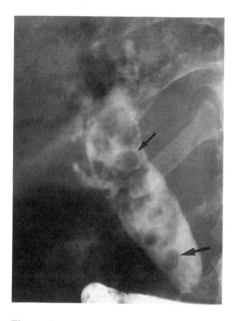

Figure 3   An ERCP film showing multiple gallstones (arrows) in a dilated common bile duct.

complication rate than that quoted in studies looking at all age groups combined (36).

Very large stones can be treated with either mechanical, electrohydraulic, or laser lithotripsy, all accomplished through the endoscope (Fig. 4). In patients in whom stone extraction is incomplete, an indwelling bile duct stent can prevent occlusion of the biliary orifice (37,38). In the latter group of patients, repeat attempts at stone extraction can be made after a variable interval. Ursodiol may be taken orally on a daily basis between procedures to soften the stone material. In some medically frail patients, recurrent or prolonged stent therapy alone is a viable option (37). Failure of ERCP can be due to inability to cannulate the common bile duct, inability to reach the biliary orifice in patients with a Roux-Y anastomosis or with a hepatico-jejunostomy, or failure to approach the stone within the duct because of a biliary stricture. The procedure's success depends on the skill of the endoscopist.

Open cholecystectomy with common bile duct exploration is the time-honored approach to common bile duct stones. This procedure is effective and relatively safe, although the morbidity and mortality associated with this operation are greater than for simple cholecystectomy. In the elderly

Lithotripsy technique

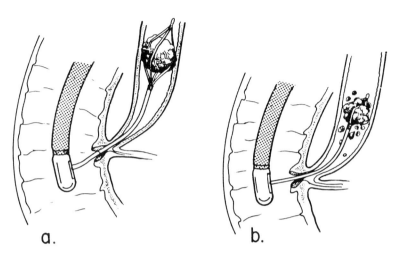

Figure 4 A diagram of the technique of mechanical lithotripsy, in which a basket (a), ensnaring a large stone, is forcefully withdrawn into a coil sheath in order to crush the stone (b).

population, nonemergent common duct exploration carries a mortality of 4%. In emergent situations, the mortality ranges from 5% to 20% or higher (8–12).

Failure of open bile duct exploration may occur because of strictures of the biliary tree, numerous intrahepatic stones, or very large bile duct stones. In these situations, intraoperative choledochoscopy, sometimes incorporating lithotripsy, may be utilized to achieve success. At times, a T-tube is left in place to allow for later attempts at percutaneous stone extraction. Alternatively, a choledocho- or hepaticoenterostomy is performed to allow passage of retained stones.

Percutaneous bile duct stone extraction via the transhepatic approach is performed using baskets or lithotripters. External drains or internal stents can also be placed to temporize an acute situation. The radiologic approach is generally reserved for situations where endoscopy is unsuccessful or unavailable, but simple percutaneous drainage may be a first-line therapy in patients who are particularly unstable.

Cholangitis due to bile duct stones presents a particular problem. Severe cholangitis due to an occluded biliary tree accounts for rapid deterioration and is often fatal. Emergent drainage is imperative, even in the oldest and sickest patients (39–41).

Surgical drainage for severe acute cholangitis is associated with morbidity and mortality rates of up to 66% and 33%, respectively (42–45). Broad-spectrum antibiotic therapy is utilized immediately in an attempt to reverse the septic state prior to surgery. However, a subgroup of patients will remain unsalvageable by any technique, including surgery, because of progressive sepsis and irreversible consequences. For this reason, less invasive forms of drainage should be performed at the time of presentation of cholangitis, even in the sickest patients.

Percutaneous transhepatic drainage can be performed emergently with excellent response (46–49). This procedure provides time for recuperation prior to the performance of a definitive endoscopic or surgical procedure, or it may be a prelude to further radiologic therapy. The disadvantages to the percutaneous approach are the necessity for subsequent therapy and the associated complications of an indwelling tube such as hemorrhage and sepsis.

Endoscopic drainage by ERCP has been shown to be the safest method for dealing with acute cholangitis (50–56). ERCP can be performed in patients who are gravely ill, even at the bedside in the intensive care unit. The immediate goal of therapy is to decompress the biliary tree internally, either by sphincterotomy and stone extraction, or by simply placing a transpapillary stent. Purulent material is usually seen draining into the duodenum after a successful procedure, and the rapidity of clinical improvement, from moribund to becoming alert and responsive, may be measured in minutes. The advantage of endoscopy is its safety compared to other techniques (Table 1). Also, endoscopy often provides definitive therapy. In elderly patients in whom cholangitis is present in the absence of cholecystitis, cholecystectomy can be avoided. This minimally invasive approach is well tolerated. In a large group of patients followed longitudinally, only 8% of patients ultimately required cholecystectomy (57).

V. BILIARY NEOPLASMS

Neoplastic lesions arising from the biliary tree and pancreas are a frequent cause of biliary problems in the elderly. While some benign tumors are occasionally found, the clinician is usually correct in assuming that most newly discovered strictures of the biliary tree in the aged are malignant. The management of these lesions has changed over the last 15 years, ostensibly because of improvement in imaging techniques, allowing for dramatic improvements in staging.

Table 1 Therapy of Acute Cholangitis: 30-Day Mortality

Reference	Surgical	Radiologic	Endoscopic
Welch (42)	40%		
Saharia (43)	14%		
Lygidakis (44)	20%		
Thompson (45)	9%		
Gould (46)		29%	
Kadir (47)		17%	
Pessa (48)		5%	
Kinoshita (49)		14%	
Vallon (50)			7%
Neoptolemos (51)			5%
Leung (52)			5%
Gogel (53)			8%
Siegel (54)			7%
Lai (55)	33% (66%)[a]		10% (34%)[a]

[a] Mortality (morbidity).

A. Bile Duct Cancer

Adenocarcinoma arising from the bile ducts is an unusual form of cancer. Early reports estimated the incidence to be 500 cases per year in the United States, but this is probably an underestimation because of the limitations of antemortem diagnosis. Bile duct cancer is common in parts of China and Thailand, and is attributed to infestation with liver flukes such as *Clonorchis sinensis.* Other predisposing conditions include primary sclerosing cholangitis and previous exposure to thorium compounds, most notably Thorotrast, a radiologic contrast agent used until the 1950s. Cystic lesions of the biliary tree such as choledochal cysts and those due to Caroli's disease are precursor lesions.

The peak incidence by age of bile duct cancer is in the 60s and 70s. In most patients in the United States, no predisposing factor will be found. The tumor is generally slow-growing, spreading along the serosal plains of the biliary tree and its associated vasculature. While obstructive jaundice, with or without pain, is the usual clinical presentation of bile duct tumors, progressive cholestasis without jaundice occurring over several months is not uncommon (58,59).

Carcinomas arising within the liver are known as cholangiocarcinomas and often present in advanced stages. Lesions located at the bifurcation of the bile duct are called Klatskin tumors (Fig. 5), presenting more commonly as obstructive jaundice. Lesions located in the distal bile duct, known simply as bile duct adenocarcinoma, also present with obstructive jaundice, and are difficult to differentiate from pancreatic or periampullary carcinoma.

B. Gallbladder Carcinoma

Carcinoma of the gallbladder, a disease that peaks in incidence in the 50s and 60s, also affects the elderly (60). The major predisposing factor for this type of cancer is the presence of gallstones. Most patients have a history of several years of mild right upper quadrant pain by the time the diagnosis of gallbladder cancer is confirmed. It is unclear whether the pain experienced in this situation is related to the development of the cancer or to chronic cholecystitis. Many patients, however, ultimately seek medical attention because of a change in the character or severity of their symptoms.

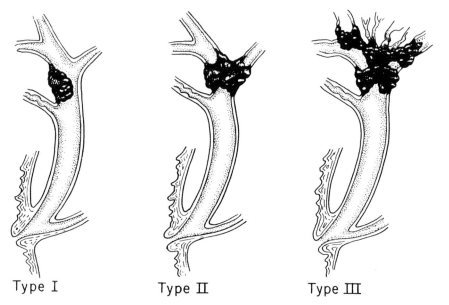

Type I   Type II   Type III

Figure 5 Anatomic drawing of the three stages of Klatskin tumors: type I disease involves the common hepatic duct, type II disease involves the entire bifurcation, and type III disease involves the bifurcation as well as secondary branches of the right and left hepatic ducts.

In most affected persons, gallbladder carcinoma becomes extremely aggressive by the time the diagnosis is made. While it is thought that the lesion grows insidiously for years prior to presentation, there is little chance for effective therapy by the time the diagnosis is confirmed. The mean survival of gallbladder carcinoma is about 6 months, and surgery offers a less than 5% cure rate in most instances. Most gallbladder carcinomas that are resected for cure have been discovered incidentally at the time of cholecystectomy for cholecystitis (60).

C. Pancreatic Cancer

The most common malignant stricture of the biliary tree is pancreatic carcinoma. This disease has a peak incidence in the age range of 50 to 60 years, and there is a male predominance (61,62). Recent data associate this lesion with chronic pancreatitis (63) and cigarette smoking (62), but there is little else known to predispose one to this disease. Because the distal one-third of the bile duct courses through the head of the pancreas, lesions in this region produce obstructive jaundice because of extrinsic compression. The bile duct is obstructed by the mass effect of the tumor or to local pancreatitis caused by the cancer. This cancer spreads along the local tissue planes and by invading the portal blood supply. Duodenal obstruction is not uncommon, again, because of the tumor invasion or mass effect. The resectability and cure rates for pancreatic cancer are extremeley low, and most patients die within 6 months of diagnosis.

D. Ampullary Carcinoma

This unusual form of adenocarcinoma produces a biliary stricture or obstruction by invasion of the distal choledochus. It is relatively slow-growing and spreads along local tissue planes. The peak age incidence is in the 60s and 70s, while the epidemiology of this lesion is thought to be similar to that of colon cancer (64). Periampullary cancer presents as obstructive jaundice, and the lesion is usually obvious endoscopically. Since pancreatic cancers can invade the duodenum and appear endoscopically as an ampullary mass, it is important to differentiate the two if possible. Ampullary carcinoma, even with local spread, responds favorably to resection, with a 5-year survival rate of up to 30%.

E. Other Malignant Neoplasms

Mucoepidermoid carcinoma, cystadenocarcinomas, and primary biliary carcinoids are all rare. Metastatic lesions to the lymph nodes of the porta hepatis are not unusual in patients with colon or breast cancer. These strictures are present similar to a nonoperable primary malignancy of the proximal biliary tree and carry a poor prognosis.

F. Benign Biliary Neoplasms

Benign tumors of the bile duct are rare. Adenomas arising from bile duct epithelium occur both intra- and extrahepatically. These lesions produce obstructive jaundice if located in the extrahepatic biliary tree. Intrahepatic lesions are usually discovered incidentally. Adenomas of the wall of the gallbladder are not unusual and are usually discovered incidentally either during sonography or at the time of cholecystectomy. Other lesions such as papillomas and myoblastomas can involve the intrahepatic and extrahepatic biliary tree, but these lesions are also quite rate.

G. Diagnosis

Computed tomography and ERCP are the two most frequently used modalities for evaluating neoplasias affecting the biliary tree. CT scans provide the best evaluations of the pancreatic parenchyma and associated vasculature. CT scans visualize the liver and are specific for determining the presence of metastatic disease and lymph node metastases. Though the scan may or may not demonstrate the presence of a hilar mass lesion, it can easily assess the caliber of the intrahepatic biliary system.

ERCP is invaluable as both a diagnostic and a therapeutic modality in these disease states (Fig. 6). The location, length, and quality (smooth vs. irregular) of a biliary stricture is assessed, and the ampulla and pancreatic duct are examined simultaneously. Tissue can be obtained by advancing cytology brushes through strictures, and biopsies of both ampullary and intraductal lesions can be performed (65,66).

Often, a diagnosis of malignancy is suspected but brushings at the time of endoscopy fail to provide a tissue diagnosis. In these instances, percutaneous biopsy under CT guidance is considered. If an experienced cytologist examines the cells after each pass of the needle, the yield can be as high as 60–70% (67,68). Serum markers for malignancy such as CA 19-9 (pancreas) and CEA (biliary adenocarcinoma) are also helpful in confirming a suspicion of malignancy if the serum levels of these are markedly elevated.

Transabdominal sonography is useful in the diagnosis of neoplastic lesions of the pancreas and biliary tree, but it lacks the sensitivity of CT. Endoscopic ultrasound, however, may play an important role in the staging of these lesions since real-time, high-resolution images of the mesenteric vasculature and local lymph nodes can be obtained.

H. Treatment

Treatment of malignant lesions arising from or involving the bilitary tree must take into account several factors. First, the general physical condition

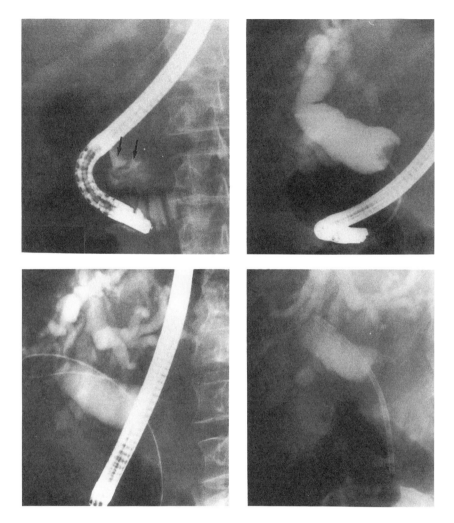

Figure 6   The "double-duct sign" of pancreatic cancer, in which the tumor causes obstruction to both the bile duct and the pancreatic duct (arrows).

of the patient may place restrictions on proposed therapies. Second, the aggressiveness, nature, and stage of the disease must be a consideration in determining the respective roles of palliation and resection. Finally, the relative risks and benefits of each treatment must be considered.

Because jaundice is often the presenting symptom of these lesions, palliation of biliary obstruction becomes a primary goal since most malignancies that affect the biliary tree are incurable. Jaundice can be treated surgically by either bypass or resection, or nonsurgically by stenting or percutaneous drainage. Since these tumors are not particularly responsive to chemotherapy or radiation therapy, only resection holds the possibility of long-term survival.

Surgical therapy can be considered as either palliative or curative. For lesions involving the distal bile duct and ampullary area, such as pancreatic cancer affecting the head of the pancreas, distal bile duct carcinoma, and ampullary carcinoma, surgical resection via pancreaticoduodenectomy (Whipple procedure) may be attempted for cure. Resection of more proximal bile duct carcinomas and disease at the bifurcation usually entails en-bloc resection of the affected areas, and a significant hepatectomy is sometimes necessary. Resection of gallbladder carcinoma is possible if the disease is limited to the gallbladder and involves a simple cholecystectomy. Palliative surgical therapy addresses jaundice by creating a choledochoenterostomy in the case of distal lesions or the performance of an hepaticoenterostomy for proximal obstructions. A gastrojejunostomy is performed for apparent or impending gastric outlet obstruction.

The success of resection for malignant lesions depends on the type of tumor treated. For cancer of the head of the pancreas, proximal cholangiocarcinomas, and gallbladder carcinoma, there is, at best, a 5% 5-year survival rate. As mentioned, ampullary carcinoma has a 5-year survival rate of 20–30%, even when locally invasive disease is present. Unfortunately, the latter tumor is the most uncommon of the malignant diseases listed. Survival rates vary from study to study depending on the selection of patients regarding their general medical fitness, age, and extent of disease. The elderly tend to be underrepresented in these studies, and thus a realistic survival rate for this group following surgery is difficult to ascertain.

Morbidity following extensive or radical operations is not uncommon and includes anastomotic leaks, gastrointestinal dysmotility, and medical complications such as pneumonia, thromboembolic phenomena, and cardiac events. These complications occur more frequently in the elderly, but they are related more to the patient's general medical fitness level than to age per se. In a recent report, the mortality rate for pancreaticoduodenectomy performed in the elderly was 9% (69).

Palliation is often best accomplished during ERCP by placing a biliary endoprosthesis (stent), which allows for the drainage of bile into the duodenum (Fig. 7). The advantages of endoscopic therapy include its low morbidity and mortality rate (70), a shortened length of stay and recovery period compared to surgery, and its lower initial costs. However, there are some drawbacks to endoscopic stenting. Stents become clogged by a mix of bacterial (biofilm) and stone debris and require replacement if the patient

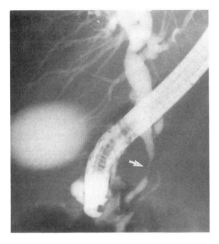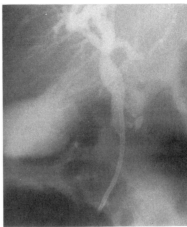

Figure 7 A malignant biliary stricture (arrow) palliated by the endoscopic insertion of a stent.

"outlives" the stent. Complicated tumors of the hilum can be difficult to stent, and incomplete therapy often leads to cholangitis. Finally, reliably successful endoscopic therapy may not be available in many centers due to lack of expertise.

The major difficulty of endoscopic therapy, stent clogging, has been addressed through the search for improved stent designs. Due to improved flow, a larger-caliber stent appears to be best, and 11.5-Fr plastic stents last a mean of 4–6 months. The newest development is the expandable stainless-steel mesh stent (WallStent) which reaches 36 Fr in greatest diameter (71). WallStents are not removable and are prone to ingrowth of tumor through the steel lattice. However, WallStents are particularly useful in hilar tumors because of their mesh design which allows drainage through its side mesh as well as through the proximal end of the stent, and avoids the early complication of cholangitis (72).

Percutaneous approaches to palliation allow drainage both externally and internally. Percutaneous drainage tends to be a quick procedure requiring a brief period of recuperation. Its limitations include: 1. a higher rate of infectious complications when compared to the other palliative modalities, and 2. the need for highly skilled radiologists. External drainage leads to resolution of jaundice, but, because bile is diverted from the digestive tract, intestinal absorption is affected and essential nutrients are lost.

Chemotherapy offers little to most patients with malignant biliary strictures. High-dose combination chemotherapy may lead to a significant response in about 10–30% of patients with pancreatic, bile duct, or gallbladder adenocarcinoma. These therapeutic regimens include 5-fluorouracil and may include a combination of mitomycin-C and/or streptozotocin (73). Adjuvant radiotherapy has not been proven to change outcomes significantly. Local, high-dose irradiation (brachytherapy) using an iridium wire placed within the bile duct by ERCP or PTC is technically possible; further experience is needed to accurately assess its value (73).

Our approach to the treatment of malignant strictures is one of "palliation until proven resectable" (Fig. 8). Most patients undergo an ERCP and stent placement to relieve jaundice, which immediately restores a sense of well-being and improves the patient's nutritional status. In patients who are found to have unresectable disease at the time of diagosis or who are medically frail, a permanent mesh stent should be considered. Supportive care is provided, and ERCP is repeated when the stent clogs.

In patients in whom resection is possible and desirable, further staging for resectability is incorporated into the workup and evaluation. Mesenteric angiography and endoscopic ultrasound are performed for more accurate staging. In patients who appear resectable, laparoscopy is performed prior to laparotomy to ensure that no small metastatic lesions have been overlooked. Even with the best staging and selection of patients for resection, the 5-year survival for these tumors does not generally exceed 10% (75–77). Again, the exception is ampullary carcinoma, and, though unusual, more liberal staging guidelines for resection are employed because of a better response to surgery.

Regardless of the disease, some young patients or very healthy elderly patients with malignant biliary strictures do outlive an endoscopic stent and thus require multiple stent changes. Palliative bypass may be indicated in these patients to avoid repeated hospitalizations and the costs of multiple ERCPs, and to eliminate the emotional problems associated with impending mortality.

VI. NONNEOPLASTIC STRICTURES

Nonneoplastic strictures of the biliary tree are either iatrogenic or acquired. Iatrogenic strictures are usually caused by operative injury at the time of biliary tract surgery. Acquired strictures include external compression due to inflammatory conditions such as chronic stone disease, pancreatitis, reactive lymphadenopathy, or sclerosing cholangitis.

A. Duct Injuries

Postoperative strictures usually occur in the mid to proximal common bile duct or in the common hepatic duct. These strictures, which are generally

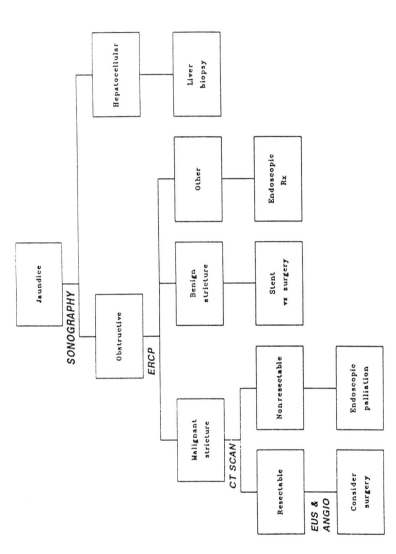

Figure 8 Evaluation and treatment of obstructive jaundice.

postischemic and fibrous, result from either direct duct injury or injury to the ductal blood supply. Occasionally, a surgical staple is actually seen on the duct.

The presentation of strictures varies. If the duct is occluded by a misplaced staple, jaundice occurs soon after surgery. In the event of ischemic injury due to damage to the periductal blood supply, cholestasis and/or cholangitis can occur weeks or months postoperatively.

ERCP is the procedure of choice for the treatment of strictures (78–80). Following confirmation of the stricture through cholangiography, hydrostatic dilating balloons are introduced through the stricture. A large-caliber stent is placed to maintain the effects of the dilatation and the integrity of the lumen. The stent is usually left in place 6 weeks or more before removal (Fig. 9). In cases where endoscopic therapy fails, either because of a technically unsuccessful procedure or due to recoil of the stricture following several dilatations, surgical bypass is considered. Surgical anastomoses themselves may stricture, but, if technically possible, dilatation of surgical anastomoses is also effective (81).

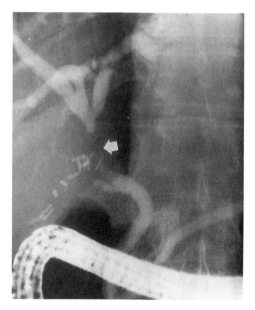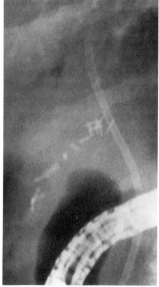

Figure 9   A postoperative stricture (arrow) is seen in association with surgical clips. Following balloon dilatation, an endoprosthesis was placed.

B. External Compression

Chronic relapsing pancreatitis can produce compression of the distal common bile duct and, ultimately, jaundice, if there is significant disease strategically located where the bile duct traverses the head of the pancreas. Similarly, lymph nodes in the porta hepatis can enlarge to compress the common hepatic duct. A special type of inflammation, caused by an impacted gallstone in the neck of the gallbladder, produces obstructive jaundice near the insertion of the cystic duct. This phenomenon is known as Mirrizzi's syndrome.

Endoscopic decompression of these conditions is recommended and includes stent placement for relief of jaundice. However, there is often recurrence of these strictures after a stent is removed because of the persistence of the extrinsic disease. Definitive surgical bypass is often needed.

C. Cholangitides

Longstanding cholangitis, either infectious or idiopathic, leads to strictures of the biliary tree.

Infectious cholangitis and strictures are most often seen in the Far East and are referred to as Oriental cholangitis. Chronic parasitic infestation of the biliary tree leads to stasis of bacterial byproducts, the formation of "brown" stones, chronic inflammation, scarring, and strictures. These strictures are occasionally treated with ERCP, but, often, the disease is so extensive that biliary bypass and even partial hepatectomy are required.

Primary sclerosing cholangitis (PSC) often causes stricturing of the extrahepatic biliary tree. Presentation of this disease in the elderly is unusual, as the mean age of first manifestation is 39 years (82). PSC is associated with ulcerative colitis in 70% of cases. The strictures and cholestasis associated with PSC are amenable to endoscopic stent therapy, but this approach remains investigational (83). Other therapies under evaluation include the use of ursodeoxycholic acid, cyclosporine, and methotrexate.

VII. SUMMARY

Disorders of the biliary tree remain an important cause of morbidity and mortality in the elderly. Symptomatology in these disorders can be atypical or absent, even in the presence of severe disease. Appropriate diagnostic evaluation must be performed with a high index of suspicion. Therapeutic intervention must take into account the natural history of the disease processes, the risks of therapy, and the general medical condition of the patient.

Alternatives to standard surgical therapies, such as ERCP, may provide optimum results with reduced morbidity in the appropriate setting.

REFERENCES

1. Boyden EA. The anatomy of the choledochoduodenal junction in man. Surg Gynecol Obstet 1957; 104:641.
2. Nakada I. Changes in morphology of the distal common bile duct associated with aging. Gastroenterol Jpn 1981; 16:54.
3. Eggert A, Teichmann W, Wittmann DH. The pathologic implication of duodenal diverticula. Surg Gynecol Obstet 1982; 154:62.
4. Boyden EA, Grantham SA Jr, Evacuation of the gall bladder in old age. Surg Gynecol Obstet 1936; 62:34.
5. Amberg JR, Zboralske FF. Gallstones after 70. Requiescat in pace. Geriatrics 1965; 20:539.
6. Gracie WA, Ransohoff DF. The natural history of silent gallstones. The innocent gallstone is not a myth. N Engl J Med 1982; 307:798.
7. McSherry CK, Ferstenberg H, Calhoun WF, et al. The natural history of diagnosed gallstone disease in symptomatic and asymptomatic patients. Ann Surg 1985; 202:59.
8. Pigott JP, Williams GB. Cholecystectomy in the elderly. Am J Surg 1988; 155:408.
9. Harness JK, Strodel WE, Talsma SE. Symptomatic biliary disease in the elderly patient. Am Surg 1986; 52:442.
10. Krarup T, Sonderstrup J, Kruse-Blinkenberg HO, Schmidt A. Surgery for gallstones in old age: do no operate too late? Acta Chir Scand 1982; 148:263.
11. Houghton PWJ, Jenkinson LR, Donaldson LA. Cholecystectomy in the elderly: a prospective study. Br J Surg 1985; 72:220.
12. Margiotta SJ Jr, Willis IH, Wallack MK. Cholecystectomy in the elderly. Am Surg 1988; 54:34.
13. Glenn F, Becker CG. Acute acalculous cholecystitis. An increasing entity. Ann Surg 1982; 195:131.
14. Wetstein L, Attkiss M, Aufses AH. Acute torsion of the gallbladder: review of the literature and report of a case. Am Surg 1976; 42:138.
15. Cobden I, Venables CW, Lendrum R, James OFW. Gallstones presenting as mental and physical debility in the elderly. Lancet 1984; 1:1062.
16. Ralls PW, Colletti PM, Halls JM, Siemsen JK. Prospective evaluation of ^{99m}Tc-IDA cholescintigraphy and gray-scale ultrasound in the diagnosis of acute cholecystitis. Radiology 1982; 144:369.
17. Eikman EA, Cameron JL, Colman M, et al. A test for patency of the cystic duct in acute cholecystitis. Ann Intern Med 1975; 82:318.
18. McSherry CK, Glenn F. The incidence and causes of death following surgery for nonmalignant biliary tract disease. Ann Surg 1980; 191:271.
19. NIH Consensus Development Panel on Gallstones and Laparoscopic Cholecystectomy. Gallstones and laparoscopic cholecystectomy. JAMA 1993; 269:1018.

20. Glenn F. Hays DM. The age factor in the mortality rate of patients undergoing surgery of the biliary tract. Surg Gynecol Obstet 1955; 100:11.
21. Glenn F, Surgical management of acute cholecystitis in patients 65 years of age and older. Ann Surg 1981; 193:56.
22. Hosking MP, Warner MA, Lobdell CM, et al. Outcomes of surgery in patients 90 years of age and older. JAMA 1989; 261:1909.
23. Glenn F. Cholecystectomy in the high risk patient with biliary tract disease. Ann Surg 1977; 185:185.
24. Fromm H. Gallstone dissolution therapy—current status and future prospects. Gastroenterology 1986; 90:1560.
25. Thistle JL, May GR, Bender CE, et al. Dissolution therapy of cholesterol gallstones by methyl tert-butyl ether administered by percutaneous trans-hepatic catheter. N Engl J Med 1989; 320:633.
26. Ferrucci JT. Gallstone ESWL—the first 175 patients. Am J Radiol 1988; 150:1231.
27. Siegal JH, Kasmin FE, Cohen SA. Endoscopic retrograde cholangiopancrea-tography treatment of cholecystitis: possible? yes; practical?? Diag Ther Endosc 1994; 1:51.
28. Tamada K, Seki H, Sato K, et al. Efficacy of endoscopic retrograde cholecys-toendoprosthesis for cholecystitis. Endoscopy 1991; 23:2.
29. Kelly TR, Wagner DS. Gallstone pancreatitis: a prospective randomized trial of the timing of surgery. Surgery 1988; 104:600.
30. Neoptolemos JP, Carr-Locke DL, London NJ, et al. Controlled trial of urgent endoscopic retrograde cholangiopancreatography and endoscopic sphinctero-tomy versus conservative treatment for acute pancreatitis due to gallstones. Lancet 1988; 2:979.
31. Fan ST, Lai ECS, Mok FPT, et al. Early treatment of acute biliary pancreatitis by endoscopic papillotomy. N Engl J Med 1993; 328:228.
32. Cotton PB, Chapman M, Whiteside CG, et al. Duodenoscopic papillotomy and gallstone removal. Br J Surg 1976; 63:709.
33. Davidson BR, Neoptolemos JP, Carr-Locke DL. Endoscopic sphincterotomy for common bile duct calculi in patients with gallbladder in-situ considered unfit for surgery. Gut 1988; 29:114.
34. Neoptolemos JP, Carr-Locke DL, Leese T, Janes D. Acute cholangitis in association with acute pancreatitis: incidence, clinical features and outcome in relation to ERCP and endoscopic sphincterotomy. Br J Surg 1987; 74:1103.
35. Gandolfi L, Rossi A, Vaira D, et al. Endoscopic retrograde cholangiopancrea-tography in the elderly. Acta Gastro Belg 1986; 49:602.
36. Kasmin FE, Fenig DM, Cohen SA, Siegel JH. Biliary endoscopy in nonagenari-ans—"ERCP in the nineties." Gastrointest Endosc 1995; 41(4):A423.
37. Siegel JH, Yatto RP. Biliary endoprostheses for the management of retained common bile duct stones. Am J Gastroenterol 1984; 79:50.
38. Rustgi AK, Schapiro RH. Biliary stents for common bile duct stones. Gastro Endosc Clin North Am 1991; 1:79.
39. Andrew DJ, Johnson SE. Acute suppurative cholangitis, a medical and surgical emergency. Am J gastroenterol 1970; 54:141.

40. Hinchey EJ, Couper CE. Acute obstructive suppurative cholangitis. Am J Surg 1969; 117:62.
41. Reynolds BM, Dargan EL. Acute obstructive cholangitis: A distinct clinical syndrome. Ann Surg 1959; 150:299.
42. Welch JP, Donaldson GA. The urgency of diagnosis and surgical treatment of acute suppurative cholangitis. Am J Surg 1976; 131:527.
43. Saharia PC, Cameron JL. Clinical management of acute cholangitis. Surg Gynecol Obstet 1976; 142:362.
44. Lygidakis NJ. Acute suppurative cholangitis: comparison of internal and external biliary drainage. Am J Surg 1982; 143:304.
45. Thompson JE, Tompkins RK, Longmire WP. Factors in management of acute cholangitis. Am Surg 1982; 195:137.
46. Gould RJ, Vogelzang RL, Nieman HL, et al. Percutaneous biliary drainage as an initial therapy in sepsis of the biliary tract. Surg Gynecol Obstet 1985; 160:523.
47. Kadir S, Boassiri A, Barth KH, et al. Percutaneous biliary drainage in the management of biliary sepsis. AJR 1982; 138:25.
48. Pessa ME, Hawkins IF, Vogel SB. The treatment of acute cholangitis: percutaneous transhepatic drainage before definitive therapy. Ann Surg 1987; 205:389.
49. Kinoshita H, Hiroshashi K, Igawa S, et al. Cholangitis. World J Surg 1984; 8:963.
50. Vallon AG, Shovron PJ, Cotton PB. Duodenoscopic treatment of acute cholangitis. Gut 1982; 23:A915.
51. Neoptolemos JP, Carr-Locke DL, Fossard DP. Prospective randomized study of pre-operative sphincterotomy versus surgery alone for common bile duct stones. Br Med J 1987; 294:470.
52. Leung JWC, Chung SCS, Sung JY, et al. Urgent endoscopic drainage for acute suppurative cholangitis. Lancet 1989; 1:1307.
53. Gogel K, Runyon BA, Volpicelli NA, et al. Acute suppurative obstructive cholangitis duct stones: treatment by urgent endoscopic sphincterotomy. Gastrointest Endosc 1987; 33:210.
54. Siegel JH, Rodriguez R, Cohen SA, et al. Endoscopic management of cholangitis: critical review of an alternative technique and report of a large series. Am J Gastroenterol 1994; 89:1142.
55. Lai ECS, Mok FPT, Tan ESY, et al. Endoscopic biliary drainage for severe acute cholangitis. N Engl J Med 1992; 326:1582.
56. Leese T, Neoptolemos JP, Baker AR, Carr-Locke DL. Management of acute cholangitis and the impact of endoscopic sphincterotomy. Br J Surg 1986; 73:988.
57. Siegel JH, Safrany L, Ben-Zvi JS, et al. Duodenoscopic sphincterotomy in patients with gallbladders in-situ: report of a series of 1272 patients. Am J Gastroenterol 1988; 83:1255.
58. Kuwayti K, Baggenstoss AH, Stauffer MH, Priestley JI. Carcinoma of the major intrahepatic and extrahepatic bile ducts exclusive of the papilla of vater. Surg Gynecol Obstet 1957; 104:357.
59. Klatskin G. Adenocarcinoma of the hepatic duct at its bifurcation within the porta hepatis. Am J Med 1965; 38:241.

60. Perpetuo M, Valdivieso M, Heilburn LK, et al. Natural history of gallbladder cancer. Cancer 1978; 42:330.
61. Gold EB, Gordis L, Diener MD, et al. Diet and other risk factors for cancer of the pancreas. Cancer 1985; 55:460.
62. Gordis L, Gold EB. Epidemiology of pancreatic cancer. World J Surg 1984; 8:808.
63. Lowenfels AB, Maisonneuve P, Cavallini G, et al. Pancreatitis and the risk of pancreatic carcinoma. N Engl J Med 1993; 328:1433.
64. Wilson JM, Melvin DB, Gray GF, Thorbjarnarson B. Primary malignancies of the small bowel: a report of 96 cases and a review of the literature. Ann Surg 1974; 180:175.
65. Foutch PG, Kerr DM, Harlan JR, et al. Endoscopic retrograde wire-guided brush cytology for diagnosis of patients with malignant obstruction of the bile duct. Am J Gastroenterol 1990; 85:791.
66. Gagnon P, Ponchon T, Labadie M, et al. Value of endobiliary brushing cytology and biopsies of bile duct stenosis. Gastrointest Endosc 1990; 36:A200.
67. Ferrucci JF Jr, Wittenberg J. CT biopsy of abdominal tumors: aids for lesion localization. Radiology 1978; 129:739.
68. Yeh H. Percutaneous fine needle aspiration biopsy of intraabdominal lesions with ultrasound guidance. Am J Gastroenterol 1981; 75:148.
69. Levi J, Stollman N, Barkin JS, et al. Pancreaticoduodenectomy in the elderly. Am J Gastroenterol 1994; 89:A133.
70. Siegel JH, Snady H. The significance of endoscopically placed prostheses in the management of biliary obstruction due to carcinoma of the pancreas: results of non-operative decompression in 277 patients. Am J Gastroenterol 1986; 81:634.
71. Huibregtse K, Cheung J, Coene PPLO, et al. Endoscopic placement of expandable mesh stents for biliary strictures—a preliminary experience with 33 patients. Endoscopy 1989; 21:280.
72. Kasmin FE, Aviles L, Cohen SA, Siegel JH. Comparison of early complications of Wallstent placement vs. plastic stent placement for malignancy. Am J Gastroenterol 1993; 88:A1534.
73. Mallinson C. Cytotoxic chemotherapy in pancreatic exocrine cancer. In: Cancer of the Bile Ducts and pancreas. Philadelphia: W.B. Saunders Co., 1989.
74. Urban MS, Siegel JH, Pavlou W, et al. Treatment of malignant biliary obstruction with a high-dose rate remote afterloading device using a 10 F nasobiliary tube. Gastrointest Endosc 1990; 36:292.
75. Carter DC. Surgery for pancreatic cancer. Br Med J 1980; 280:744.
76. Tompkins RK, Saunders K, Roslyn JJ, Longmire WP. Changing patterns in diagnosis and management of bile duct cancer. Ann Surg 1990; 211:614.
77. Lai ECS, Tompkins RK, Roslyn JJ, Mann, LL. Proximal bile duct cancer—quality of survival. Ann Surg 1987; 205:111.
78. Berkelhammer C, Kortan P, Haber G. Endoscopic biliary prosthesis as treatment for benign post-operative bile duct stricture. Gastrointest Endosc 1989; 35:95.

79. Davids PHP, Tanka AKF, Rauws EAJ, et al. Benign biliary strictures; surgery or endoscopy? Ann Surg 1993; 217:237.

80. Johnson KG, Geenen JE, Venu RP, et al. Endoscopic treatment of biliary strictures and sclerosing cholangitis: a larger series and recommendations for treatment. Gastrointest Endosc 1991; 37:38.

81. Teplick SK, Wolferth CC Jr, Hayes MF Jr, et al. Balloon dilatation of benign post-surgical biliary-enteric anastomosis strictures. Gastrointest Radiol 1982; 7:307.

82. Wiesner RH, Grambsch PM, Dickson ER, et al. Primary sclerosing cholangitis: natural history prognostic factors and survival analysis. Hepatology 1989; 10:430.

83. Gaing AA, Geders JM, Cohen SA, Siegel JH. Endoscopic management of primary sclerosing cholangitis: review and report of an open series. Am J Gastroenterol 1993; 88:2000.

13

Pancreatic Disease in the Elderly

Seth A. Cohen
Beth Israel Medical Center, New York, New York

I. ALTERATIONS OF THE PANCREAS WITH AGING

The pancreas is an unobtrusive gland about 12–24 cm in length which lies in the retroperitoneum with its head encompassed by the C-loop of the duodenum. In adults, the average weight of the gland is 60 g. It is made up of multiple acinar units in which the exocrine cells surround the microscopic ducts. This ductal system coalesces into the main pancreatic duct. When stimulated the exocrine cells secrete digestive enzymes, bicarbonate, and water.

The weight of the pancreas decreases after age 70 from an average weight of 60 g to 40 g or less at age 85. Macroscopically, this loss of mass correlates with atrophy of the gland. Atrophy of the parenchyma is accompanied by symmetrical ductal dilatation in the head and body of the main pancreatic duct as measured by pancreatography (1,2). It is estimated that the main pancreatic duct dilates 8% per decade (2). Pancreatic duct stones may increase in frequency in the elderly (3). Histologically, patchy areas of parenchymal fibrosis and adipose infiltration are found as the pancreas ages. Ductal dilatation, with scant lymphocytic infiltration, rare areas of ductal metaplasia, and evidence of arteriolar sclerosis may be seen. Some authors have postulated that some of these age-related changes may occur on an ischemic basis (4).

It is difficult to demonstrate a decline in pancreatic exocrine function with age. The secretory response of volume and bicarbonate output is unchanged (5); however, enzymatic output declines linearly with age and is more pronounced after age 65 (4). Due to the excessive amount of baseline enzyme secretion, these declines are not clinically significant.

II. ACUTE PANCREATITIS

Acute pancreatitis develops in the elderly just as it does in the younger population. Alcohol is a much less common cause in older patients, as the mean age of the first attack of alcohol-related pancreatitis is 37 years. The most common cause of acute pancreatitis in the geriatric population is gallstone pancreatitis, and, like biliary calculus disease, it has a slight female preponderance. Other causes include structural lesions such as ampullary tumors, periampullary diverticula, and carcinoma of the pancreas (6). Less commonly, patients with chronic pancreatitis will present with acute pancreatitis. Ischemia or emboli are rare causes of acute pancreatitis in the older population (7). Hypercalcemia can also lead to acute pancreatitis. Hyperlipidemia and heredity pancreatitis should not present for the first time in an older person. Medications are often suspected of causing pancreatitis, but this is difficult to prove clinically. A definite association has been established for thiazides, 6-mercaptopurine, sulfonamides, estrogens, valproic acid, and L-asparaginase (8). The list of medications probably associated with pancreatitis is much larger. Postoperative pancreatitis may occur following laparotomy due manipulation, and can also occur after cardiac bypass surgery related to the calcium infusion (9).

A. Clinical Presentation and Diagnosis

In a fit, elderly person the presentation of pancreatitis is similar to other adult patients: acute onset of sharp burning epigastric pain radiating to the back associated with nausea, vomiting, and ileus. The patient is restless but often finds relief sitting upright. On physical examination, there is evidence of peritoneal irritation with direct tenderness and guarding, localized rebound tenderness, diminished bowel sounds, and mild distension. It is important to note that in the older, less physiologically fit geriatric population, the presentation may be muted. The pain may be less localized, and if muscle tone is poorly developed, the signs of local peritoneal inflammation may be masked or absent. Lethargy and increased confusion with evidence of systemic inflammation may be the only presenting signs. Extravasation of fluid into the extravascular space ("third spacing") is important early in all severe pancreatitis, and evidence of hypovolemia may be present.

Diagnosis depends heavily upon laboratory results and noninvasive imaging. Serum amylase and lipase levels are most helpful in establishing the diagnosis of pancreatitis. It is postulated that elevated serum amylase levels are the result of increased permeability due to the inflammation of pancreatitis. It should be remembered that the differential diagnosis of abdominal pain and elevated amylase includes biliary tract disease, complicated peptic ulcer disease, intestinal obstruction, intestinal ischemia, and peritonitis. Modest elevations of serum amylase are nonspecific and are dependent on renal function. Elevations of greater than four times normal, in the appropriate clinical setting, however, is specific for pancreatitis. Levels of amylase >1,000 units are generally more suggestive of gallstone pancreatitis.

Gallstone pancreatitis has traditionally been diagnosed when a patient has an otherwise unexplained attack of pancreatitis in the presence of cholelithiasis. As would be expected, based on the hypothesis that it is caused by migrating gallstones, patients who develop gallstone pancreatitis tend to have small, multiple gallbladder stones, have wider cystic ducts, and are more likely to have a common pancreaticobiliary channel at the ampulla compared to controls (10). Clinically, there is often a rapid rise and fall in hepatic transaminases with a mild elevation of alkaline phosphatase which is specific for gallstone pancreatitis.

Up to 30% of patients will have "idiopathic" pancreatitis. Recently, interest has returned to microscopic bile analysis for crystals. As many as 60–70% of patients with "idiopathic" pancreatitis have either calcium bilirubinate or cholesterol monohydrate crystals on microscopic analysis. The presence of calcium bilirubinate crystals corresponds to sludge in the gallbladder on sonography (11).

Noninvasive imaging has become central to the diagnosis and management of acute abdominal conditions. It is especially helpful in older patients in whom the presentation may be atypical and in whom the history may not be reliable (12). Ultrasonography is readily available, quick, and comparatively inexpensive; however, the pancreas is often obscured by overlying bowel gas. Computed abdominal tomography (CT scanning) provides excellent images of the pancreas and surrounding organs, and is very important in diagnosing and assessing the severity of pancreatitis. It requires ionizing radiation, however, and is more expensive than ultrasonography.

B. Assessing Severity

Acute pancreatitis can range from a mild attack lasting a single day to a fulminant attack with multiorgan failure and death. The mortality of pancreatitis increases with age (13). One of the important goals in caring for older patients is to identify those at high risk for serious disease. The best-known clinical system to grade severity of pancreatitis is Ranson's Criteria (which notably includes age greater than 55 years old as an independent risk factor). A newer classification is Acute Physiology and Chronic Healthy Inquiry (APACHE II) (14). APACHE II has the advantage of being able to stratify severity immediately, compared to Ranson's Criteria, which requires 48 hours of observation, and is more accurate. CT scanning also provides a radiologic system for assessing severity (15).

The stages of pancreatitis of increasing severity are interstitial edematous pancreatitis and necrotic pancreatitis. Necrotic pancreatitis can remain sterile or it can become secondarily infected (infected necrosis). Overall mortality for acute pancreatitis approaches 20%. Mortality is directly related to the number of complications (16). Complications are likely in patients with sterile necrosis, and even more so in infected necrosis. "Dynamic" CT scanning with rapid bolus of IV contrast is essential in distinguishing between severe interstitial pancreatitis and necrosis in patients who are severely ill. The importance of this distinction is that in the absence of necrosis most patients will recover without developing complications.

Fatal attacks are four times more likely in people over 60 years (13). Much of this is because of comorbidities. In one study from the United Kingdom in no less than 35% of the fatal cases of pancreatitis, the diagnosis was made only at autopsy (13). This indicates a need to maintain a clinical suspicion of pancreatitis in severely ill, older patients. The mortality of recurrent attacks of pancreatitis, mostly from untreated gallstone disease, was not significantly lower than that of the initial attack.

C. Treatment

Supportive care, and prompt recognition and treatment of complications are the goals of treatment. This includes adequate hydration, supplemental oxygen if required, analgesia, placement of a nasogastric tube if the patient has persistent vomiting, and prophylaxis for gastrointestinal bleeding with IV H_2 receptor antagonists. Potential complications include shock, respiratory failure, renal failure, pancreatic abscess, coagulopathy, and GI bleeding.

Patients who are at risk for severe pancreatitis should be treated in an intensive care unit, with careful attention to intravascular volume and respiratory status. Patients with severe pancreatitis can easily sequester 6–10 L of fluid in the first several days. In patients with renal or cardiovascular impairment, fluid status should be monitored by central venous pressure or Swan-Ganz catheter.

Gallstone pancreatitis represents a special case of pancreatitis because there is a potentially reversible cause. A gallstone may be lodged in the distal common bile duct or impacted at the papilla of Vater. Common bile duct stones are found in 30–60% of patients who die of gallstone pancreatitis. It is very important to assess the patient with one of the clinical systems. Management depends on whether the patient is predicted to have a mild or severe attack. Patients predicted to have a mild attack will have a good outcome regardless of treatment or intervention, and only require supportive care. Whereas in elderly patients with predicted severe pancreatitis complications occur in up to 60%, and they have an 18% mortality rate. These patients, with severe gallstone pancreatitis, will benefit from urgent endoscopic intervention. Urgent ERCP reduces complications, hospital stay, and mortality compared to supportive care, (17) whereas early surgery in severe gallstone pancreatitis has been shown to have a prohibitive mortality (18).

The natural history of gallstone pancreatitis is one of recurrent attacks unless the gallbladder is removed. Therefore, after resolution of an attack, an early cholecystectomy, during the index hospitalization, is recommended in patients who are good surgical risks. There is evidence that endoscopic sphincterotomy alone, without cholecystectomy, prevents recurrent attacks of gallstone pancreatitis by ablating the common channel (11,19). This is an alternative in patients unfit for surgery.

Pseudocysts can complicate either acute or chronic pancreatitis. They are encapsulated collections of pancreatic secretions that have leaked out of the ductal system. The cysts will grow until they equalize pressure with either the gland or the duct. Pseudocysts, by definition, have a fibrous nonepithelial lining. Most cysts communicate with the pancreatic duct. In order to avoid confusion with true pancreatic cysts, which can be neoplastic, the patient should have history compatible with either acute or chronic pancreatitis (20). Most acute pseudocysts resolve and do not require intervention unless they become infected or otherwise complicated.

Survival in patients with pancreatic infection is related to early diagnosis and operative drainage. CT-guided aspiration for Gram's stain and culture permits an earlier diagnosis of infected pancreatic necrosis than previously believed, usually within 14 days of the initial attack (21). Aspiration should be considered in toxic patients selected with fever, leukocytosis, abdominal pain, tachycardia, or altered sensoria, known to have an inflammatory mass on CT scan (21). These criteria identify only 5% of all patients with pancreatitis, but 60% of those tested have infection. CT-guided aspiration has replaced laparotomy as the initial diagnostic test. Patients with infected pancreatic necrosis or abscess require surgical drainage and appropriate antibiotics.

III. CHRONIC PANCREATITIS

Chronic pancreatitis is morphologically defined as an irreversible, irregular sclerosis of the gland with destruction of the exocrine parenchyma and

Table 1 Classifications of Chronic Pancreatitis

Etiologic: alcoholic, idiopathic, obstructive, tropical, miscellaneous, hereditary
Morphologic: calcific, noncalcific
Clinical: latent, painful, exocrine insufficiency, painless

ductal distortion. Clinically it is associated with recurrent or persistent abdominal pain often accompanied by signs of pancreatic exocrine insufficiency. There are multiple classifications of chronic pancreatitis. No single one is universally accepted (Table 1).

A. Etiology

In Western countries alcohol abuse is the leading cause of chronic pancreatitis, responsible for about 70% of cases (22). Alcoholic chronic pancreatitis (ACP), however, is not a common problem among older patients because the mean age of onset is 37 years ($\pm$10 years), and it rarely develops after age 60. ACP usually "burns out" after a mean of 10 years, and the majority of patients do not live beyond age 70 (23). Chronic pancreatitis can also develop due to obstruction of the main pancreatic duct at the level of the ampulla or upstream due to benign stenosis, anatomic abnormalities, and tumors. Other, rare causes include hyperparathyroidism and primary idiopathic inflammatory pancreatitis (4).

Many older patients with newly diagnosed chronic pancreatitis fall into the idiopathic category. A second peak in the incidence of idiopathic chronic pancreatitis occurs at age 65 years. Some authorities have suggested that "idiopathic senile chronic pancreatitis" be recognized as a distinct clinical entity (22). Generally, these are men, 65 years old or older, who present with some combination of steatorrhea, diabetes, weight loss, pancreatic calcification, and abdominal pain, with or without hyperamylasemia. Other authorities do not recognize this as an distinct entity (4).

B. Presentation

Most patients with chronic pancreatitis present with abdominal pain, weight loss, maldigestion, or diabetes (24). Those who develop chronic pancreatitis in the geriatric age group are more likely to have "painless" disease compared to younger patients. In those who do experience pain, they complain of dull epigastric pain radiating to the back, exacerbated by eating, often associated with nausea and vomiting. Pain may be episodic, lasting several days, or constant. The cause of pain in chronic pancreatitis is not understood but is presumed to be related to inflammation of the gland, perineural inflammation, and/or increased pressures in the gland and ducts due to ductal obstruction.

Other causes of pain associated with chronic pancreatitis include pseudocysts, peptic ulcer disease, and biliary strictures. Strictures of the bile duct are seen in 6–9% of patients due to external compression of the duct by the fibrotic pancreas. These patients may present with pain, weight loss, and cholestasis or jaundice.

Clinically, overt malabsorption of fat, carbohydrates, and protein occurs late in chronic pancreatitis, not until 90% of the exocrine function is lost. Steatorrhea may also occur because of deactivation of lipase when the duodenal pH falls below 4, due to inadequate pancreatic bicarbonate secretion. Patients complain of foul-smelling, greasy stools; passing oil per rectum can occur.

In patients suspected of having chronic pancreatitis who are losing weight it is important to determine whether caloric intake is adequate. A stool test for fecal fat with the patient on a high-fat diet can be performed. Patients who have persistent abdominal pain and weight loss should be evaluated for the possibility of a coexisting underlying pancreatic malignancy.

Pancreatic diabetes is a late sign of chronic pancreatitis, as destruction of the endocrine tissue occurs slowly. Many patients demonstrate glucose intolerance, but overt diabetes is less common. Complications of pancreatic diabetes are rare.

C. Diagnosis

Because many older patients who present with chronic pancreatitis do not have an appropriate clinical history, establishing the diagnosis may be clinically challenging. There are several important issues posed by the consideration of chronic pancreatitis: 1. In patients with chronic abdominal pain, is chronic pancreatitis the cause? 2. In patients with malabsorption, is it due to chronic pancreatitis? and possibly most important, 3. In older patients with abdominal pain and weight loss with an abnormal pancreas is the cause chronic pancreatitis or carcinoma? Chronic pancreatitis is a risk factor for carcinoma of the pancreas (25). This must be considered in all patients with an established diagnosis of chronic pancreatitis who have a change in symptom pattern.

In patients with the appropriate history and clinical findings demonstration of pancreatic calcifications on plain abdominal X-rays is the only test necessary to diagnose chronic pancreatitis. Pancreatic calcification is a dynamic process which may increase with time and then may spontaneously regress (26). When plain films do not demonstrate calcification, the other imaging modalities of increasing sensitivity and expense are sonography, computerized tomography, and endoscopic pancreatography. Evidence of chronic pancreatitis includes calcification and/or ductal irregularities with dilation and stricturing. In the absence of histology, endoscopic pancreatography is still considered the gold standard in diagnosing chronic pancreatitis and distinguishing it from carcinoma. Care must be taken in interpreting minor changes of ductal caliber and side branches, or even the presence of pancreatic calculi, since they may be associated with "normal" aging of the pancreas.

In patients with a morphologically normal pancreas (by CT and ERCP), but in whom there is still a suspicion of chronic pancreatitis, the secretin pancreatic function test is the most sensitive test. This test, however, is not readily available.

D. Treatment

Treatment of chronic pancreatitis is directed to the symptoms of the patient. Pain is usually the prime complaint. Medical management begins with evaluation to eliminate other treatable causes of pain such as peptic ulcer disease, pseudocysts, or bile duct strictures. Patients are placed on a low-fat diet and given pancreatic enzyme supplementation. Studies in humans have shown that a high level of pancreatic protease in the duodenum suppresses pancreatic enzyme secretion by negative feedback inhibition, leading to pain reduction in many patients (27). Nonsteroidal antiinflammatory agents or narcotic analgesics can be used. Care must be taken to avoid addiction.

Patients with recurrent attacks of acute pancreatitis or persistent pain and an obstructed dilated pancreatic duct who do not respond to medical management should undergo surgical or endoscopic decompression. Surgical drainage involves resection and pancreaticojejunostomy (distal pancreatectomy or Puestow procedure), with 50–70% of patients obtaining relief. Endoscopic sphincterotomy, pancreatic stone extraction, and pancreatic stenting with or without extracorporeal shock-wave lithotripsy (ESWAL) has been shown to be effective in selected patients (28).

Pseudocysts may complicate chronic pancreatitis, and care must be taken to avoid confusion with true pancreatic cysts. Patients with pseudocyst should have an appropriate history. The pancreatogram is generally abnormal and usually communicates with the cyst. Fluid aspirated from the cyst is high in amylase, and cellular debris should not be present. If the pseudocyst is biopsied, no epithelial lining should be present (20). Pancreatic pseudocysts, if not symptomatic, can usually be observed as long as they are not increasing in size and are under 8 cm in diameter. Symptomatic pseudocysts can be drained surgically, percutaneously, or endoscopically. Percutaneous drainage will fail to resolve the cyst if there is downstream obstruction of the pancreatic duct.

Patients with weight loss should be put on a high-calorie diet and given pancreatic enzyme supplements. Steatorrhea can be easily treated, but not abolished, with pancreatic enzyme supplementation. Addition of an H_2 receptor antagonist or proton pump inhibitor may be necessary to prevent lipase inactivation by gastric acid. With persistent weight loss, the possibility of carcinoma must always be considered.

The diabetes that accompanies chronic pancreatitis is usually mild and does not predispose the patient to acidosis. Glucose levels can usually be maintained with diet and oral hypoglycemics.

Traditionally it was recommended that patients with significant biliary strictures undergo elective biliary drainage procedures to avoid the complications of cholangitis and biliary cirrhosis, but recently other data suggest that only symptomatic patients require bypass surgery (29).

IV. CANCER OF THE PANCREAS

Cancer of the pancreas is the second leading cause of death among gastrointestinal malignancies. The incidence in the United States increased several decades ago, but is now stable. The incidence of carcinoma of the pancreas is related to age, and increases sharply after age 60. Comparative studies have shown that Western diet and environment are associated with cancer of the pancreas, but cigarette smoking, chronic pancreatitis, and diabetes are the only definitely identified risk factors. Coffee consumption has been suggested as a risk factor, but the epidemiologic data are flawed (30).

Eighty-five percent of pancreatic malignancies are adenocarcinoma arising from ductal epithelium. Biologically, it is an aggressive tumor with a high predilection to metastasize. Eighty percent of patients have metastases at the time of the initial presentation, to regional lymph nodes, the peritoneum, and the liver via the portal circulation. Two-thirds of the carcinomas develop in the head of the pancreas. Because the distal common bile duct runs through the head of the pancreas, painless, obstructive jaundice due to compression of the bile duct is one of the most common presentations of cancer of the pancreas. Other common signs and symptoms include weight loss, epigastric pain, anorexia, and weakness.

Older patients who complain of abdominal pain and/or weight loss can be a diagnostic challenge. Weight loss is a common complaint among geriatric patients, and often unsubstantiated. Traditionally these patients have been investigated for "occult malignancies," but only 10–15% have organic gastrointestinal disease (31). Although many of these patients have inadequate caloric intake that may be associated with depression or dementia, one must nevertheless maintain a clinical suspicion of carcinoma of the pancreas.

In patients who complain of abdominal pain, it is important to elicit whether the pain is longstanding, such as in the irritable bowel syndrome, or this is a new symptom. An abdominal ultrasound is the most cost-effective test to image the pancreas when there is a clinical suspicion of cancer. If a pancreatic mass is seen, an endoscopic retrograde pancreatogram is indicated. As cancer of the pancreas is of ductal origin, pancreatography is both sensitive and specific (32).

There are no serum screening tests for pancreatic cancer in asymptomatic people. In patients with a pancreatic mass, CA 19-9, a new carbohydrate antigen test, is promising and can be useful (33). Carcinoembryonic antigen (CEA), neither sensitive nor specific, is not helpful.

Surgical resection is the only chance to cure cancer of the pancreas. Therefore, resectability is always the pivotal issue in its diagnosis and treatment. Traditionally, only 10–20% of cancers in the head of the pancreas were resectable. With better diagnostic capabilities and tertiary referral, up to 30% of highly selected patients may be resected (34). This is opposed to only 8% of cancers in the body and tail of the pancreas being resectable, because these patients present at a later stage. Some surgeons believe that pancreaticoduodenectomy offers better palliation in young, fit patients with extensive local disease; whether this applies to older, less fit patients is unknown. It is important to emphasize that cancers of the ampullary area (ampulla of Vater and distal common bile duct) are resectable in 80% of patients and should be pursued more aggressively.

Preoperative evaluation to determine resectability should include CT scan with intravenous contrast, angiography, and possible endoscopic ultrasonography to rule out vascular invasion, and laparoscopy to evaluate for peritoneal and liver metastases. Exploratory laparotomy is no longer justifiable as the initial diagnostic test. No longer does the argument hold true that exploration is the only reliable method to assess resectability, and that biliary and/or intestinal by-pass (single or double bypass) is required in all nonresectable patients. Only 10–15% of patients with cancer of the pancreas develop duodenal obstruction requiring gastrojejunostomy. Also, in many older patients endoscopic or percutaneous biliary stenting is superior to surgical bypass for relief of jaundice. Patients judged suitable for pancreatic resection should be referred to specialized centers where the mortality for pancreaticoduodenectomy (Whipple's resection) should be under 5%. In less experienced hands the mortality can be several times higher.

In geriatric patients, the question of whether patients are medically fit for pancreatic resection is also very important. Generally, healthy patients in their 80s may undergo coronary bypass surgery and total joint replacements, but the demands of upper abdominal surgery can be great. Serious cardiac, pulmonary, and/or vascular diseases are relative contraindications to surgery. Patient attitude and wishes are paramount; some older patients do not want to subject themselves to major surgery. In general, resection is optimal for younger, more fit patients. Decisions concerning surgery in older patients need to be made on an individual basis.

Although a clinical diagnosis of cancer of the pancreas can be made with a high degree of certainty based on history, CT scan, ERCP, and angiography, in the absence of histologic confirmation confusion with chronic pancreatitis still occurs in a small number of patients. Many authorities recommend that a CT-guided skinny needle aspiration *not* be performed in patients with potentially resectable disease due to the fear of peritoneal seeding. Low-dose radiation prior to needle biopsy has been suggested, but not proven, to prevent this (30). Rather, patients who appear to be resectable are advised to proceed directly to surgery for resection. Obviously this needs to be discussed frankly with the patient. Endoscopic brush cytology can be obtained at the time of ERCP in many patients, and although this has a lower sensitivity, it is safe. An emerging technology is endosonographic-guided needle aspiration of pancreatic lesions.

CT-guided fine-needle aspiration for cytologic confirmation of carcinoma is appropriate in patients who are not resectable, and most physicians would recommend it. The diagnostic yield is greatly enhanced if a cytopathologist can examine the aspirate at the time of the procedure, so that if the aspirate is nondiagnostic, it can be repeated.

Several rare types of pancreatic cancer have a better prognosis than typical ductal carcinoma and need to be identified and treated appropriately. The first is cystadenocarcinoma. This typically presents as an abdominal mass in an older middle-aged women. Noninvasive imaging demonstrates a cystic structure, which should not be confused with a pseudocyst. Histologically, the cyst is lined with malignant columnar, mucus-producing epithelia. Cyst adenocarcinoma may be resectable, with a good prognosis, if diagnosed early in the disease. Once it has metastasized, the prognosis is similar to typical cancer of the pancreas. Intraductal mucin-secreting adenocarcinoma is another unusual lesion with a better prognosis (35). Patients present with pancreatitis or abdominal pain as a result of pancreatic duct obstruction by globs of mucus. Ductal dilation is evident on CT scanning. Mucus extruding from a dilated pancreatic duct is an impressive sight for the endoscopist. Surgical resection can be curative in the majority of these patients, as metastases are unusual.

V. PALLIATION

The majority of older patients with cancer of the pancreas are not candidates for surgery, either because the tumor is not resectable or because comorbidities place them at high risk for surgery. These patients need palliation. The most common problems are obstructive jaundice, pain, glucose intolerance, and weight loss.

Jaundice can lead to pruritus, a general feeling of malaise, and the risk of cholangitis. Prolonged jaundice also has a negative impact on renal and cardiac function. In unresectable disease, endoscopic placement of an internal biliary stent at the time of ERCP is the optimal method to relieve obstructive jaundice in poor-risk, older patients. Randomized controlled trials performed in England have shown that endoscopic stenting is superior to both percutaneous biliary drainage and surgical bypass (36,37). The success rate is 90–95% when performed by a skilled endoscopist. Traditionally, large-bore plastic stents 10 and 11.5 French have been placed, which provide biliary drainage with a mean patency of approximately 4 months. If the patient survives longer than that and the stent becomes occluded (many older patients die before this occurs), the patient can have the stent changed as an outpatient procedure. Since stent occlusion is the limiting factor for endoscopic stenting, new, expandable metal stents have been developed which have a mean patency of 9 months (38). If endoscopic stenting is technically unsuccessful, percutaneous transhepatic biliary drainage provides another nonsurgical alternative.

It is important to adequately treat patients' pain. Narcotics on a fixed schedule are more effective than on an "as-needed" basis. New transdermal narcotic patches supply a steady-state concentration of high-efficacy narcotic. For patients with severe pain, intravenous or subcutaneous morphine pumps are employed and may be used at home. In patients with incurable cancer there should be no fear concerning addiction to opiates. Percutaneous celiac ganglia blocks with neurolytic agents may also give relief.

Glucose intolerance and newly diagnosed diabetes mellitus occur in the majority of patients with cancer of the pancreas. The diabetes is generally mild and controlled by diet, oral hypoglycemic agents, or a low dose of insulin. Diabetes only becomes a problem if the patient needs a high-calorie supplement. Then fingersticks to monitor blood glucose and insulin may be required.

Weight loss is inexorable in patients with carcinoma of the pancreas. Most of the weight loss is related to inadequate caloric intake, but also to some degree of maldigestion. Treatment with pancreatic enzymes improves steatorrhea and azotorrhea. Anorexia is a systemic symptom and improves slightly after relief of biliary obstruction. More than 50% patients have abnormal gastric emptying in absence of duodenal obstruction; this, too, may lead to impaired food intake.

Managing the various complications that arise during palliative treatment can be as challenging as treating for potential cure. A truism that cannot be repeated too often, is that the patient with incurable malignancy needs a lot of care and should not be abandoned.

REFERENCES

1. Anand BS, Vij JC, Mac HS, et al. Effect of aging on the pancreatic ducts: a study based on the study of endoscopic retrograde pancreatography. Gastrointest Endosc 1989; 35:210–213.
2. Kreel L, Sandin B. Changes in pancreatic morphology associated with aging. Gut 1973; 14:962–970.
3. Nagai H, Ohtsubo K. Pancreatic lithiasis in the aged clinicopathology and pathogenesis. Gastroenterology 1984; 86:331–338.
4. Laugier R, Sarles H. The pancreas. Clin Gastroenterol 1985; 14:749–756.
5. Dreiling DA, Triebling AT, Koller M. The effect of age on human exocrine pancreatic secretion. Mt Sinai J Med 1985; 52:336–339.
6. Linn A, Feller ER. Pancreatic carcinoma as a cause of unexplained pancreatitis: report of 10 cases. Ann Intern Med 1990; 113:166–167.
7. Steinberg W, Tenner S. Acute pancreatitis. N Engl J Med 1994; 330:1198–1210.
8. Mallory A, Kern P. Drug-induced pancreatitis: a critical review. Gastroenterology 1980; 78:813–820.
9. Fernandez–del Castillo C, Harringer W, Warshaw AL, et al. Risk factors for pancreatic cellular injury after cardiopulmonary bypass. N Engl J Med 1991; 325:382–387.
10. Kelly TR. Gallstone pancreatitis: pathophysiology. Surgery 1976; 80:488–492.
11. Lee SP, Nicholls JF, Park HZ. Biliary sludge as a cause of acute pancreatitis. N Engl J Med 1992; 326:589–593.
12. Taourel P, Baron MP, Pradel J, et al. Acute abdomen of unknown origin: impact of CT on diagnosis and management. Gastrointest Radiol 1992; 17:287–291.
13. Corfield AP, Cooper MJ, Williamson RCN. Acute pancreatitis: a lethal disease of increasing incidence. Gut 1985; 26:724–729.
14. Larvin M, McMahon MJ. APACHE-II score for assessment and monitoring of acute pancreatitis. Lancet 1989; 2:201–205.
15. Balthazer EJ. CT diagnosis and staging of acute pancreatitis. Radiol Clin North Am 1989; 27:19–37.
16. Karimgani I, Porter KA, Langevin RE, Banks PA. Prognostic factors in sterile pancreatic necrosis. Gastroenterology 1992; 103:1636–1640.
17. Neoptolemos JP, Carr-Locke DL, London NJ, et al. Controlled trial of urgent endoscopic retrograde cholangiopancreatography and endoscopic sphinctero-tomy vs. conservative treatment for acute pancreatitis due to gallstones. Lancet 1988; 2:979–983.
18. Kelly TR, Wagner DS. Gallstone pancreatitis: a prospective randomized trial of the timing of surgery. Surgery 1988; 104:600–605.
19. Siegel JH, Veerappan A, Cohen SA, Kasmin FE. Endoscopic sphincterotomy for biliary pancreatitis: an alternative to cholecystectomy in high-risk patients. Gastrointest Endosc 1994; 40:573–575.

20. Warshaw AL, Rutledge PL. Cystic tumors mistaken for pancreatic pseudocysts. Ann Surg 1987; 205:293–298.
21. Gerzof SG, Banks PA, Robbins AH, et al. Early diagnosis of pancreatic infection by computed tomography-guided aspiration. Gastroenterology 1987; 93:1315–1320.
22. Ammann RW. Chronic pancreatitis in the elderly. Clin Gastroenterol 1990; 19:905–914.
23. Ammann RW, Akovbiantz A, Largiader F, Schueler G. Course and outcome of chronic pancreatitis. Gastroenterology 1984; 86:820–828.
24. Bank S. Chronic pancreatitis: clinical features and medical management. Am J Gastrology 1986; 81:163–167.
25. Lowenfels AB, Maisonneuve P, Cavallini G, et al. Pancreatitis and the risk of pancreatic cancer. N Engl J Med 1993; 328:1433–1437.
26. Ammann RW, Muench R, Atto R. Evolution and regression of pancreatic calcification and chronic pancreatitis. Gastroenterology 1988; 95:1018.
27. Isaksson G, Ihse I. Pain reduction by an oral pancreatic enzyme preparation in chronic pancreatitis. Dig Dis Sci 1983; 28:97–101.
28. Sherman S, Lehman GA, Hawes RH, et al. Pancreatic ductal stone: frequency of successful endoscopic removal and improvement in symptoms. Gastrointest Endosc 1991; 37:511–517.
29. Stahl TJ, O'Connor M, Ansel HJ, Vennes JA. Partial biliary obstruction caused by chronic pancreatitis. Ann Surg 1988; 207:26–32.
30. Warshaw AL, Fernandez–del Castillo C. Pancreatic carcinoma. N Engl J Med 1992; 326:455–465.
31. Morton KI, Sox HC, Krupp JR. Involuntary weight loss: diagnostic and prognostic significance. Ann Intern Med 1981; 95:568–574.
32. Moossa AR, Levin B. The diagnosis of "early" pancreatic cancer: University of Chicago experience. Cancer 1981; 47:1688–1695.
33. Steinberg W. The clinical utility of the CA 19-9 tumor-associated antigen. Am J Gastroenterol 1990; 85:350–355.
34. Warshaw AL, Gu ZY, Wittenberg J, Waltman AC. Pre-operative staging and assessment of resectability of pancreatic cancer. Arch Surg 1990; 125:230–233.
35. Rickaert F, Cremer M, Deviere J, et al. Intraductal mucin-hypersecreting neoplasms of the pancreas. Gastroenterology 1990; 101:512–519.
36. Speer AG, Cotton PB, Russell RCG, et al. Randomised trial of endoscopic vs percutaneous stent insertion in malignant obstructive jaundice. Lancet 1987; 2:57–62.
37. Smith AC, Dowsett JF, Russell RCG, et al. Randomised trial of endoscopic stenting versus surgical bypass in malignant low bileduct obstruction. Lancet 1994; 344:1655–1660.
38. Davids PHP, Groen AK, Rauws EA, et al. Randomised trial of self-expanding metal stents vs polyethylene stents for distal malignant biliary obstruction. Lancet 1992; 340:1488–1492.

14

Nutrition, Aging, and the Gastrointestinal Tract

Hillel S. Hammerman
Beth Israel Medical Center, New York, New York

I. INTRODUCTION

The purpose of this chapter is to review the relationship of age-related body changes to alterations in nutrition and the gastrointestinal tract. Aging starts with birth, but the concern here is with those who are frequently, albeit subjectively, called the elderly. In this setting, the variable rate of aging results from genetic and cumulative environmental exposures. Their effects may be minor from a health standpoint (i.e., hematologic cell counts, liver function, and wrinkles). Alternatively, they result in a slow, significant, degenerative process, usually silent under normal conditions (bone density, glomerular filtration rate, vital capacity). This decline in reserve organ function in the affected elderly increases their morbidity and mortality at times of illness and injury.

Nutrition includes the intake, absorption, and utilization of food material. These factors can be altered in the aged. There are subsets of age-related changes, alterations in nutrition, and GI tract functions, which interface in either a predominant or minor manner (Fig. 1). The following discussion is aimed at recognizing and explaining those age-associated disorders which, in total or in part, are caused by, result in, or are treatable with nutritional modifications.

Table 1 is an overview of this subject. Before discussing the individual age-related disorders, we must define the nutritional standards and deviations from them.

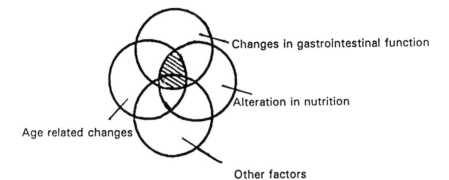

Figure 1 Relationship of age related disorders to nutritional and gastrointestinal considerations.

II. NUTRITIONAL STANDARDS AND DEFICIENCIES

A. Recommended Dietary Allowances (RDAs)

Over the centuries, proper food consumption was deemed sustenance, excess intake was gluttony, and malnutrition had the names of many diseases that are rare to the modern world. Nowadays, the same categories of nutrient intake are generally referred to as Recommended Dietary Allowances (RDAs), obesity or megadoses, and marasmus, kwashiorkor, clinical or subclinical micronutrient deficiencies, respectively.

RDAs represent estimated requirements in health to prevent nutritional deficiencies. They are not necessarily the amounts needed during illness or special situations (1). Adult RDAs change slightly with age. They are grouped in two categories: 23–50 years old, and greater than 51 years old (Table 2). Depending on the study reviewed, there are some changes for men and women over the age of 70 (2). These changes are based on known age-related variations in lean body mass, absorptive abilities, hormone effects, and other physiological functions.

In many cases, age-related disorders develop in the setting of adequate food intake. Such diseases have marginal if any etiological relation to nutrition. Nevertheless, they may cause secondary nutritional changes or, alternatively, respond in part to nutritional therapy.

B. Insufficient Nutrient Intake

In other cases disorders are fully or partially explained by nutritional deficiencies caused by decreased nutrient intake (Table 3). Although not limited to the older population, the elderly are susceptible to more of these conditions.

C. Decreased GI Tract Absorption

GI tract function is indispensable for maintaining good nutrition. Therefore, age-related changes could potentially have a serious health impact. Fortunately, due to the extensive reserve capacity present, digestion and absorption are generally preserved throughout life. There are two exceptions. The incidence of atrophic gastritis increases with age. It can result in varying degrees of malabsorption of B_{12}, B_6, folic acid, calcium, and iron. Another age-related event is decreased intestinal absorption of calcium and vitamin D. Both of these conditions are discussed later.

The older population frequently uses medications on a long-term basis. Drug-nutrient interactions can result in deficiencies which should be addressed (Table 4).

III. DISORDERS OF AGING WITH NUTRITIONAL ASSOCIATION

A. Weight Gain

Many older patients will describe their frustration about weight gain despite no perceptible increase, and often even with a documented decrease, in food intake. This phenomenon is explained by the following three points:

Although often assumed, it should be noted that for the same intake of protein, fat, and carbohydrates, there is equal absorption and utilization in all age groups. Unless there is a non-age-related specific disease entity present, young and old derive equal caloric value from the same ingested foods.

Another factor is the often considered but not usually quantitated decrease in physical activity with age. As this can represent 20% of total energy expenditures, the calories and pounds quickly add up in the sedentary (4).

The last factor to consider is less obvious and relates to age-associated changes in body composition. Between the ages of 20 and 79 there is an approximate 20–25% decline in muscle mass, and a 50% increase in fat (5). The energy needed to maintain lean body mass is three to five times greater than that required to maintain a similar amount of body fat (6). This change in body composition results in a 15–30% decrease in the basal metabolic rate. Consequently, equal or even decreased caloric intake may result in weight gain.

B. Diminished Muscle Mass

Decreased muscle mass results in an overall decrease in muscle strength. This finding is present in any age category where there is insufficient caloric

Table 1 The Association Between Changes in the Aging Body and Nutrition

Disorders of aging	Nutrition-related conditions			Other factors	Can diet change or correct disorder?
	Occurs with decreased intake	Occurs with same intake	Occurs because of decreased absorption		
Weight gain	Possible	Yes	No	↓ Activity	Yes
Decreased muscle strength	Possible	Yes	No	↓ Exercise and hormone changes	Only in the nutritionally deficient
Weight loss	Often	No	Rare		Where deficient
Osteoporosis	In calcium and vitamin D-rich foods	Yes	Partially	Hormones Genetics Exercise	2–4 × ↑ RDA VITD ~2× ↑ RDA Calcium ↑ Milk/dairy products
Immune function	Yes	Possible	Unknown	Genetics	Yes
Constipation	Yes	Possible	No	Exercise Fluid intake Muscle strength	"Fiber"

Specific nutrient-deficiency disorders				
Vit D/Ca^{++} → osteoporosis	Yes	Yes	Yes	Hormones	↑ Intake needed
B$_{12}$	Rare	Yes	Yes	Atropic gastritis; drug-induced pH changes	Yes, by maintaining RDAs
Folic acid	Rare	Yes	Yes		
B$_6$ (pyridoxine)	Yes	Rare	Yes		
Iron	Yes	Rare	Yes		
Neurocognitive changes	Possible	Rare	Yes	Multiple	Same
Vision	Possible	Possible	No	Excessive UV light exposure Smoking	Protective effect of Vit C, E, and beta carotene-rich yellow and orange fruits and vegetables
Vascular aging	Possible	Possible	Yes	Lipid metabolism Hypertension Diabetes	Maintain RDAs for B$_{12}$, folic acid, and B$_6$

Table 2 Recommended Daily Dietary Allowances for Persons Over Age 51[a]

	RDAs for Women (Men) Over 51 Years Old	Changes for Elderly[b]
Calories	1,800 (2,400) kcal	1,600 (2,050)
Protein	44 (56)g	
Vitamin A (retinol)	800 (1,000) μg RE[c]	Possible decrease
Vitamin D (calciferol)	5 μg	10 (20) μg
Vitamin E (tocopherol)	8 (10) μg	
Vitamin K (phylloquinone)	70 (140) μg	
Vitamin B_1 (thiamine)	1 (1.2) mg	
Vitamin B_2 (riboflavin)	1.2 (1.4) mg	
Vitamin B_4 (niacin)	13 (16) mg	
Vitamin B_5 (pantothenic acid)	4 (7) mg	
Vitamin B_6 (pyridoxine)	2 (2.2) mg	
Vitamin B_7 (biotin)	100 (200) μg	
Vitamin B_9 (folic acid)	400 μg	
Vitamin B_{12} (cobalamin)	3 μg	
Vitamin C (ascorbic acid)	60 mg	
Calcium	800 μg	1,000 (1,500) mg
Phosphorus	800 mg	
Magnesium	300 (350) mg	
Iron	10 mg	
Zinc	15 mg	
Iodine[(D)]	150 μg	
Copper[(D)]	2.0–3.0 mg	
Manganese[(D)]	2.0–3.0 mg	
Fluoride[(D)]	1.5–4.0 mg	
Chromium[(D)]	50–200 μg	
Selenium[(D)]	50–200 μg	
Molybdenum[(D)]	150–200 μg	

[a] In accordance with the Food and Nutrition Board Committe on Dietary Allowance: 1990[(1)].
[b] From Suter PM[(2)].
[c] Retinol equivalents.
[d] Estimated safe and adequate intake.

and protein intake. In the older population, especially after the age of 60, decreased muscle mass, and therefore lean body weight, occurs universally, even with adequate age-adjusted nutrition. In part, decreased activity results in muscle atrophy. However, other nonnutritional causes have been examined including changes in growth hormone and insulinlike hormone secre-

Table 3 Factors Contributing to Decreased Intake and Weight Loss
in the Elderly

I. Anorexia
  A. Psychological: depression, dysphoria, perceived food intolerances
  B. Neurologic: dementia, altered cognition, possible decreased CNS
    modulated feeding drive
  C. Sensory:
    1. Decreased taste and smell due to aging; medications (digoxin,
      theophylline, ACE inhibitors); dry mouth due to TCA, clonidine,
      dentures/gingival disease
    2. Restrictive diets (institutional); chronic excessive alcohol
  D. Chronic diseases
II. Social
  A. Isolation: living alone and unable to shop, prepare, or consume due to
    physical handicaps (arthritis, cardiopulmonary symptoms, impaired vision,
    stroke, tremor)
  B. Economic limitations
III. Physical limitations
  A. Difficulty chewing due to dentition or neurologic changes (after CVA)
  B. Dysphagia due to esophageal motor disorders, chronic peptic strictures,
    or neuromuscular dysphagia
  C. Food avoidance due to eating-related abdominal discomfort (gastric
    motility disorders, intestinal angina, diarrhea and/or constipation)

tion and sensitivity (7). Decreased muscle mass and increased body fat explain the often observed age associated redistribution of body weight from the extremities to the torso. Similar findings occur in hypercortisol states which are not age related. When they exist, protein-calorie deficiencies should be corrected. However, loss of muscle mass with age is more often prevented and reversed by weight-bearing exercises.

C. Weight Loss

Common is the observation of the lean, wiry older person whose "clothes hang" and he or she "is not as plump as before." Some of these visual changes occur despite good nutrition. They are secondary to normal physiological age-related loss of lean muscle mass. Although some people become thinner by purposeful dieting, others experience advanced disease-related cachexia (cardiac, pulmonary, oncologic).

There are still other patients, however, without overt underlying disease who have documented weight loss. When this exceeds 5% of the body weight over a 6–12 month period, it is considered pathological and should

Table 4 Chronically Used Drugs That May Interfere With Nutritional Status in the Elderly (Modified from Durnin and Lean [3])

	Increased levels	Decreased levels
Vitamins	None	Isoniazid (pyridoxine)
		Metformin (folate, B_{12})
		Phenothiazines (folate)
		Tricyclics (folate)
		Methotrexate (folate)
		Colchicine (B_{12})
		Cholestyramine (A, B_{12}, D_3, E_3, K)
		Tetracycline (C)
		Aspirin (C)
		Antacids, H_2-receptor blockers, omeprazole (B_{12}; B_6, folate)
		Corticosteroids (C)
		Sulfasalazine (folate)
		Anticoagulants (D_3 folate)
Minerals and electrolytes	Amiloride (K)	Thiazide/loop
	Spironolactone (K)	Diuretics (Na, K, Ca, Mg, Zn)
	Corticosteroids (Na)	Phosphates (iron)
	Phenylbutazone (Na)	Tetracycline (iron)
	Carbenoxolone (Na)	Antacids, H_2-receptor blockers, omeprazole, (Ca, iron)
		Ethanol (Fe)
		lithium (I)?
		Iron supplements (Zn)

be studied (8). The many causes include decreased intake due to social, psychological, and economic factors. In addition, one often encounters decreased absorption due to gastrointestinal tract, hormonal, or medication-related changes (Tables 3, 4).

D. Osteoporosis

Osteoporosis has become a major health issue for the geriatric population. Simply put, bone mass is proportional to bone strength and inversely proportional to the rate of fracture. Genetics, exercise, and calcium intake are the major determinants of peak bone mass that occurs in men and women by age 30–35 (9). Men usually have a higher peak mass. Over the next 40–50 years, total bone mass is diminished in women and men by approximately 40% and 25%, respectively. Women have an accelerated rate of cancellous bone loss in the 10–15 years postmenopause. Men are generally spared that loss. Later, however, both women and men have a slow age-related loss of both cancellous and cortical bone (10).

Hormone replacement therapy has been and continues to be extensively studied (11). The accelerated postmenopausal bone loss in women is primarily retardable by hormone replacement therapy. To a lesser extent, weight-bearing exercises also contribute to reverse the osteoporotic process in men and women.

Osteoporosis also occurs in the setting of age-related nutritional changes. The latter plays a partial etiological role, as well as having a therapeutic potential. Vitamin D intake is derived from skin synthesis and diet. Transformation in the liver and kidneys results in the active metabolite 1,25-dihydroxyvitamin D. This potentiates calcium absorption from the small intestine.

In the elderly, several events occur that can interfere with these steps. Compared to the young, senior citizens often have significantly less exposure to the sun, decreased ability to form previtamin D_3 after UV exposure, have low dietary vitamin D intake, and have decreased renal synthesis of 1,25-dihydroxyvitamin D (12). Much of this can be overcome by increasing the oral intake of vitamin D. However, in the nonsupplemented state, the net result is to decrease the absorption of calcium. This aggravates the tendency toward calcium deficiency in the elderly, who, by avoiding milk and dairy products, already have less than the RDA of calcium (13). Calcium losses can also result from decreased absorption in an alkaline intestinal pH present in atrophic gastritis, or through the use of antacids and H_2 receptor blockers.

Therefore the nutritional recommendations to prevent osteoporosis include sun exposure, vitamin D supplementation of 400–800 IU/day (10–20 μg) and elemental calcium supplementation of 1,000–1,500 mg/day (11). Note that the multiple types of available calcium supplements vary by elemental calcium content and the type of associated salt. They are best taken with meals and exposed to acid. Where there is medical or drug-induced achlorhydria, a pH-independent salt such as gluconate, citrate, or lactate should be used (14).

E. Immune Function

Independent of age, nutritional deficiencies are associated with immune dysfunction. Anergy and decreased total lymphocyte counts are consistent findings in malnutrition states. The improvement of immunologic responses often parallels improved nutritional status.

With aging, there exist a spectrum of immune response capabilities. Likewise, nutritional status varies from excellent to poor. Population studies have shown that these two variables parallel each other, suggesting that impaired immunity in the elderly may be due in part to associated nutritional deficiencies (15).

Zinc supplementation has been documented to improve T-cell function in delayed hypersensitivity reactions. Vitamins E, C, and B_6 have been shown to stimulate various aspects of the immune system (16). Deficiencies in these nutrients should be corrected by supplemental or dietary intake. However, specific dosages other than current RDAs have not been proven.

F. Constipation

Constipation has many meanings and is seen for different reasons in all age groups. It is sometimes considered an age-related disorder, as its incidence, or at least complaints about it, are greater in the elderly. The cause of this relationship is multifactorial and not purely based on decreased intake of fiber-rich nutrients. Other factors include decreased colonic motility, physical inactivity, and decreased abdominal muscle strength.

Among the treatment options, the recommendation for increased dietary and supplemental fiber is commonly given. From a nutrition standpoint, the fiber content of wheat bran, whole grains, and other foods should be considered. Another reason exists for discussing constipation in a chapter about nutrition: that is, severe constipation can often result in meal-associated pain, thereby impairing dietary intake and nutritional health.

In modern society, normal fiber intake is approximately 15–20 g/days. Although there is no fixed RDA, supplemental fiber intake for a total of 25–30 g/day is often advised (17).

Dietary fiber is not considered a nutrient, as it has minimal absorption and nutritional value. To some extent, it binds and partially prevents cholesterol absorption. However, it has minimal effects on intraluminal binding of protein, calcium, or trace minerals. A detailed review of its physiology and relation to gastrointestinal disorders can be found elsewhere (18).

G. Micronutrient Deficiencies

1. Overview

In general, most of the population does not analyze and choose food based on nutrient content. Rather, the nutrient intake is proportional to the amount of food consumed. For most people in our society, the total food intake approaches, equals, or exceeds most of the RDAs. We homeostatically consume calories, and therefore micronutrients, in amounts equal to our energy expenditures, thereby maintaining a steady weight.

In the elderly, a similar homeostasis often remains. There is a decrease in total calorie, and therefore micronutrient, intake proportional to diminished physical activity. Although this is healthy from a calorie and weight stand-point, the decreased micronutrient intake increases the risk of specific micronutrient deficiencies. This is additive to the multiple other causes of age-associated decreased intake and absorption. In this setting, vitamin and mineral supplementation may become necessary. The increasingly common use of vitamin supplements may therefore have a medical basis in some segments of the older population.

2. Vitamin D and Calcium

Age-related vitamin D and calcium deficiencies have been explained in the above discussion of osteoporosis.

3. B_{12} Deficiency

B_{12} deficiency can result in peripheral neuropathy, megaloblastic anemia, and cognitive and cerebellar changes. The age-related increased incidence of these conditions results from decreased dietary intake and absorption.

Atrophic gastritis results in decreased acid secretion. Its incidence in-creases with age and it is present in approximately 55% of people greater than 60 years of age (19). Intrinsic factor is still secreted (20). However, decreased acid results in impaired digestion of B_{12} from food protein. The combined lack of acid and rise in intestinal pH promotes bacterial growth, which then competes for free B_{12} (21). If atrophic gastritis is present, the RDA may be insufficient and B_{12} injections will be required.

4. Folic Acid, B_6, Calcium, Iron

A rise in intestinal pH can decrease the absorption of folic acid, B_6, calcium, and iron. Although the 0.4 mg RDA for folic acid is usually met, the elderly population frequently consumes less than the RDA for B_6. Folic acid deficiencies results in megoblastic anemia and possible central nervous system and vascular changes (2). B_6 deficiency is also related to vascular and neurological changes. Calcium intake and deficiency were previously described. Iron intake is usually adequate if there are no unusual losses. Iron deficiency results in weakness and anemia.

H. Neurocognitive Changes

Age-related central nervous system changes are multifactorial. Nutritional causes have been studied extensively (22). Vitamin deficiencies are known to cause specific neurological disorders (Table 5). Mild subclinical vitamin deficiencies of B_{12}, B_6, and folic acid may develop in the aging population and result in cognitive and peripheral nervous system changes. Folic acid,

Table 5   Neurological and Behavioral Effects of Vitamin Deficiencies

Vitamin	Presentation
Thiamin	Beri-beri, Wernicke-Korsakoff's psychosis
Niacin	Pellagra, dementia
Pantothenic acid	Myelin degeneration
Pyridoxine (B_6)	Peripheral neuropathy, convulsions
Folate	Irritability, depression (?), paranoia (?)
Cobalamin (B_{12})	Peripheral neuropathy, subacute combined system degeneration, dementia
Vitamin E	Spinocerebellar degeneration, peripheral axonopathy

Source: Rosenberg and Miller (22).

B_{12}, vitamin C, and riboflavin deficiencies have been associated with decreased memory. Although no changes in the RDAs have been advised, adequate nutrition appears to play a role in neurocognitive function.

I. Vision

Age-related changes include cataract formation and macular degeneration. Both are associated with the increased oxidative effects of ultraviolet exposure and smoking. The protective antioxidant effects of vitamin C, vitamin E, and beta carotene are being explored. No supplemental recommendations above the RDAs are available (23). However, frequently advised increased doses include 1000 mg. of vitamin C, 1000 iu of vitamine E, and 15,000 iu of beta-carotene.

J. Vascular Aging

Atherosclerotic changes are most frequently associated with lipid disorders involving dietary fat and cholesterol. Recent studies correlate premature vascular disease and neurovascular changes with elevated levels of homocysteine (24). The latter is inversely proportional to, and adjusts with changes in, B_{12}, folic acid, and B_6 levels. It would appear that deficiencies in these vitamins have an important effect on the age-related changes of both the neurologic and vascular systems.

IV. SUMMARY

The interrelationship between aging disorders, nutrition, and the gastrointestinal tract has been reviewed. In most cases nutritional adjustments can decrease age-related changes but are not the "fountain of youth." In a few cases, end-organ damages due to specific nutrient deficiencies can be reversed. Age-related GI tract changes alter nutritional absorption to a lesser extent. Fortunately, there is enough reserve and alternative therapy available that GI tract dysfunction is not a significantly limiting factor.

Nutritional intervention can prolong and enhance the quality of life. It is a therapeutic option that should be considered often.

REFERENCES

1. Food and Nutrition Board Committee on Dietary Allowances. Recommended Dietary Allowances. 9th ed. Washington DC: National Academy of Science, 1980.
2. Suter PM, Russel RM. Vitamin requirements of the elderly. Am J Clin Nutr 1987; 45:501–512.
3. Durnin JVGA, Lean MEJ. Nutrition-considerations for the elderly. In: Brocklehurst JC, Tallis RC, Fillit HM, eds. Textbook of Geriatric Medicine and Gerontology. 4th ed. Edinburgh: Churchill Livingstone, 1992:605.
4. McGandy RB, Barrows CH, Spanias A, et al. Nutrient intakes and energy expenditures in men of different ages. J Gerontol 1966; 21:581.
5. Colin SH, Vartsky D, Yasumura S, et al. Compartmental body composition based on total body nitrogen, potassium, and calcium. Am J Physiol 1980; 239:524.
6. Bernstein RS, Thornton JC, Yang MU. Prediction of the resting metabolic rate in obese patients. Am J Clin Nutr 1985; 37:595–602.
7. Rudman D, Feller AG, Nagraj HS, et al. Effects of human growth hormone in men over 60 years old. N Engl J Med 1990; 323(1):1–6.
8. Marton KI, Sox HC, Krupp JR. Involuntary weight loss: diagnostic and prognostic significance. Ann Intern Med 1981; 95:568–574.
9. Cooper C, Melton LJ 3d. Epidemiology of osteoporosis. Trends Endocrinol Metab 199; 3(6):224–229.
10. Riggs BL, Melton LJ 3d. Involutional osteoporosis. N Engl J Med 1986; 314(26):1676–1686.
11. Riggs BL, Melton LJ 3d. The prevention and treatment of osteoporosis. N Engl J Med 1992;327(9):620–627.
12. Parfitt AM, Gallagher JC, Heaney RP, et al. Vitamin D and bone health in the elderly. Am J Clin Nutr 1982; 36:1014–1031.
13. Nordin BEC, Heaney RP. Calcium supplementation of the diet: justified by present evidence. Br Med J 1990; 300:1056–1060.
14. Allen SH. Primary osteoporosis: methods to combat bone loss that accompanies aging. Postgrad Med 1990; 93(8):43–55.
15. Chavance M, Brubacher G, Herberth B, et al. Immunological and nutritional status among the elderly. In: Chandra RK, ed. Nutrition, Immunity and Illness in the Elderly. New York: Pergamon, 1985.
16. Chandra RK. Nutritional regulation of immunity and risk of illness in old age. Immunology 1989; 67:141–146.

17. Diet, Nutrition, and Cancer Prevention: A Guide to Food Choices. Washington: NIH Publ, 1984.
18. Read NW. Dietary fiber and the gut: action in gastrointestinal disorders. In: Sleisenger MH, Fordtran JS, eds. Gastrointestinal Disease. Vol 2, 5th ed. Philadelphia: W.B. Saunders, 1993:2097–2108.
19. Sivrula M, Isokoski M, Vans K, et al. Prevalence of gastritis in a rural population. Scand J Gastroenterol 1968; 3:211–223.
20. Ardeman S, Chanarin I. Intrinsic factor secretion in gastric atrophy. Gut 1966; 7:99–101.
21. Suter PM, Golner BB, Golden BR, et al. Reversal of protein-bound vitamin B_{12} malabsorption with antibiotics in atrophic gastritis. Gastroenterology 1991; 101:1039–1045.
22. Rosenberg IH, Miller JW. Nutritional factors in physical and cognitive function in the elderly. Am J Clin Nutr 1992; 55:1237S–1243S.
23. Jacques PF, Chylack LT Jr. Epidemiological evidence of a role for the antioxidant vitamins and carotenoids in cataract prevention. Am J Clin Nutr 1991; 53:352S–355S.
24. Veland PM, Refsum H. Plasma homocysteine, a risk factor for vascular disease: plasma levels in health, disease, and drug therapy. J Lab Clin Med 1989; 114(5):473–501.

Gastrointestinal Manifestations of Systemic Disorders

Beth Schorr-Lesnick
Albert Einstein College of Medicine, Bronx, and Beth Israel Medical Center, New York, New York

Numerous systemic and extraintestinal disorders have gastrointestinal (GI) manifestations. They exert a significant impact on the health of the elderly. In one study, 18% of all patients in a geriatric clinic had significant GI problems, leading to 27% of all hospital admissions and 20% of all geriatric deaths (1).

Swallowing disorders, constipation, and incontinence are examples of some of the common problems the elderly face when afflicted with the various illnesses to be mentioned in this chapter. Medications commonly used by the elderly are also the cause of GI disturbances. The focus of this chapter will be on the more significant GI manifestations of the frequently encountered systemic diseases of the elderly.

I. NEUROLOGICAL DISORDERS

Several nervous system disorders common in the elderly have important GI manifestations. In general, these disturbances arise from abnormalities in gut motility. Oropharyngeal dysphagia is commonly found in many disorders. There is also altered intestinal and anal motility, causing constipation, impaction, and impaired defecation.

A. Cerebrovascular Accident (CVA)

CVA is a common cause of disability in the elderly, affecting 5% of patients over the age of 65. Conversely, 85% of stroke victims are in that age group

(2). Dysphagia is the most common GI complication of a CVA and occurs in nearly half of patients. Fortunately, most survivors usually regain some swallowing ability after several weeks. Complications arising from dysphagia include tracheal aspiration, nasal regurgitation, and pulmonary infection (3). The diagnosis should be considered in patients with speech impairment and facial weakness. Cine-esophagram is the most accurate and sensitive test to evaluate in these patients.

Management of dysphagia and prevention of aspiration involves intravenous nutrition acutely, and oral feeding after recovery of function. Percutaneous gastrostomy or jejunostomy placement may be necessary for patients with chronic neurologic impairment (3).

Brainstem strokes may be associated with small bowel or colonic pseudo-obstruction, colonic inertia, and esophageal incoordination. Some patients with brainstem strokes are unable to perceive rectal distension and lack the rectoanal inhibitory reflex, resulting in constipation (4).

B. Spinal Cord Lesions Secondary to Tumor

The GI manifestations of spinal cord tumors are diverse and differ according to location of the lesion. A metastatic lesion involving the sacral cord usually disrupts parasympathetic nerve function. This causes an imbalance of extrinsic input to the left colon and rectosigmoid by the sympathetic nerves, leading to increased rectal compliance, flaccid colonic tone, colonic distention, megacolon, megarectum, and fecal impaction (5). In contrast, injury to the lumbar sympathetics causes an increase in parasympathetic input, resulting in increased muscle tone, decreased rectal compliance, and increased frequency of defecation (5).

C. Parkinson's Disease (PD)

While GI symptoms are common in Parkinson's disease, their true frequency and pathophysiology are unclear. Prevalence seems to correlate with duration and severity of disease. Sir James Parkinson, in the original 1918 monograph, graphically described some of the common GI features of the disease (6):

> Food is with difficulty retained in the mouth until masticated; and then as difficultly swallowed . . . the saliva fails of being directed to the back part of the fauces, and hence is continually draining from the mouth . . . the bowels which all also had been torpid, now in most cases, demand stimulating medicines of very considerable power: the expulsion of the feces from the rectum sometimes requiring mechanical aid.

More recently, investigators have identified abnormal salivation, dysphagia, nausea, constipation, and defecatory dysfunction as symptoms common in PD. Additional complications include pulmonary aspiration, sigmoid volvulus, megacolon, and intestinal pseudo-obstruction (7).

Gut dysfunction is multifactorial and may include changes in diet, reduced activity, side effects of anti-PD medications, and the autonomic dysfunction associated with PD itself (7). Abnormal function of the oropharyngeal and upper esophageal sphincter (UES) muscles from PD contributes to dysphagia, excess salivation, and choking. Drooling, once thought to be due to hypersecretion, may be attributed to mechanical difficulties such as dysphagia and decreased frequency of swallowing (6). Defecatory dysfunction may be secondary to an outlet obstruction with abnormal control of the pelvic floor resulting from paradoxical puborectalis contraction. Additionally, the vast majority of patients (80%) exhibit abnormal colonic motility diffusely (6).

Therapeutic interventions should be made on an individual basis. For patients experiencing upper GI symptoms, such as excessive salivation and dysphagia, speech therapy may alleviate symptoms. Patients experiencing defecatory dysfunction from paradoxical muscle contraction seem to benefit from an increase in PD medications (7).

D. Neuropathies

1. Paraneoplastic

Autonomic neuropathy and GI symptoms have been reported in association with small-cell lung cancer or pulmonary carcinoid (2). Clinical manifestations include constipation, gastroparesis, esophageal dysmotilitylike spasm or achalasia, and an autoimmune neuropathy affecting bladder or bowel control (4).

2. Drug Induced

Several of the drugs implicated in the development of autonomic neuropathy are commonly prescribed to elderly patients. Vincristine may cause a paralytic ileus by its effect on the peripheral nervous system, including autonomic nerves. It's presentation may mimic a "surgical abdomen." The ileus will reverse itself with discontinuation of the drug. Vincristine also may have a direct toxic effect on the myenteric plexus. Clonidine, at one time a commonly used antihypertensive, causes reversible constipation and intestinal pseudo-obstruction. It does not result in a chronic neuropathic process, and the precise mechanism is unknown. This side effect of clonidine makes it useful in the treatment of idiopathic diabetic diarrhea (4).

E. Evaluation and Diagnosis

GI motility studies and measurements of transit time may be used to distinguish between neuropathic and myopathic processes, although these tests fail to reliably distinguish between intrinsic (myenteric plexus) and extrinsic neuropathies. Indirect tests of autonomic dysfunction such as tests of pupillary function, orthostatic hypotension, response of heart rate to deep breathing, ECG response to Valsalva maneuvers, sweat tests, and plasma norepinephrine determinations are useful to identify other visceral denervation (4).

II. RENAL DISORDERS

A. Uremia

Uremia has been associated with a host of gastrointestinal manifestations (Table 1). They can be divided into those seen with acute and those seen with chronic renal failure.

1. *Acute Renal Failure (ARF)*

Elderly patients are particularly prone to the development of ARF. This may be due to prerenal causes such as hypovolemia from cardiovascular failure, septic shock, extrarenal obstruction, or exposure to nephrotoxic agents (8).

GI bleeding occurs in over half of patients with ARF and may be due to multiple gastric or duodenal ulcers. Stress-related gastritis is common as well, especially following ARF accompanied by major trauma or surgery. Parenteral H_2 receptor antagonists do not prevent GI bleeding or ulcer development (9). A broad range of gastric acid secretory capacities has been noted in uremic subjects. Patients with hypochlorhydria exhibit hyper-gastrinemia (10).

Table 1 GI Manifestations of Renal Disease

Angiodysplasia
Peptic ulcer
Duodenal polyposis
Bowel obstruction
Bowel perforation
Diarrhea
Uremic enterocolitis
Cecal and rectal ulcers
Stercoral ulcers
"Wasting syndrome"

2. Chronic Renal Failure (CRF)

The annual incidence of chronic renal failure and end-stage renal disease (ESRD) increases with age. As of 1991, 28% of patients with ESRD were over 65 years of age. Since the rate of renal transplants in patients over 50 years of age in the United States is only 1%, this discussion will focus on dialysis patients (11).

A variety of GI symptoms may be associated with CRF including anorexia, hiccups, nausea, vomiting, epigastric pain, heartburn, constipation, and fecal impaction. Thirty-one percent of uremic patients have *H. pylori* in their stomachs. This infection appears to be accompanied by a decrease in stimulated acid production and by gastritis. Histological gastroduodenitis was present in half of all uremic patients whether receiving dialysis or not. The prevalence of peptic ulcer disease and the causes of GI bleeding in dialyzed patients are comparable to a general population. Due to the presence of renal failure as a complicating medical illness, they have a three- to sixfold increased mortality from GI hemorrhage compared to nonuremic patients (10).

The association of renal failure with gastric and intestinal (particularly small bowel) arteriovenous malformations has been noted by several investigators but not confirmed. These malformations have a tendency to bleed. Endoscopic thermal coagulation or an estrogen-progesterone preparation may be used to control bleeding (10). Cryoprecipitate or desmopressin acetate (ddAVP) may improve platelet function in acutely bleeding uremic patients with diffuse gastric bleeding (12).

Constipation and fecal impaction are common problems for uremic patients regardless of dialysis status (10). Contributing factors include aluminum-containing antacids, ion exchange resins, dehydration, and physical inactivity. Nutritional status and digestion are improved in patients undergoing frequent dialysis. Fewer symptoms and enhanced appetite allow patients to ingest more protein to improve their nutritional status. A prolonged orocecal transit time has been reported, as well as abnormalities in local defense mechanisms and in systemic immune function. Ileal bacterial overgrowth may cause abnormal bile acid metabolism and diarrhea in some uremic patients. Patients undergoing hemodialysis are at increased risk for *Salmonella enteritidis* sepsis (9).

It is unusual for patients to die from uremia with the availability of dialysis. Two-thirds of patients who *do* die with renal failure have mild gastrointestinal mucosal abnormalities on autopsy examination. These include edema, congestion, and hemorrhage. The severity of these abnormalities correlates with the prior presence of gastrointestinal symptoms (such as diarrhea or constipation). Bleeding intestinal ulcers are commonly present.

Some are inflammatory, and others may be ischemic. The ileum and colon are the sites of the most severe lesions (10).

Ischemic bowel is a serious, often life-threatening problem for patients with end-stage renal disease. Possible precipitating factors include hypotension, fluid depletion secondary to dialysis, vasoconstrictive medications, and concomitant cardiovascular disease, all of which are common in the elderly. Both hepatitis B and C occur in patients on chronic hemodialysis who receive multiple blood transfusions (13). Since screening for hepatitis C and erythropoietin were not available until recently, elderly patients are at particular risk to have acquired, transfusion-associated hepatitis. Amyloidosis and iron deposition in duodenal and occasionally in gastric mucosa may be seen in patients with renal failure. Amyloid has been associated with intestinal bleeding and bowel infarction. Pancreatitis may complicate chronic renal failure. Otherwise healthy patients with CRF often have an elevated amylase at baseline (up to four times normal), making the diagnosis difficult. Exocrine pancreatic insufficiency improves by pancreatic enzyme replacement, and acalculous cholecystitis has also been noted in hemodialysis patients (10).

III. DERMATOLOGIC DISORDERS

A. Adult Dermatomyositis

Dermatomyositis may sometimes occur in the elderly. "Pneumatosis cystoides intestinalis," characterized by intramural air-filled cysts in the intestine, may be associated. This leads occasionally to abdominal pain, distension, nausea, flatus, constipation, diarrhea, and mucous or bloody rectal discharge. The location of the cysts is the submucosa. Diagnosis may be made by abdominal X-ray, barium enema, CT scan, ultrasound, or unexpectedly on sigmoidoscopy. On abdominal X-ray, one may see linear or curvilinear cystic lucencies in the bowel wall, free air in the peritoneal cavity, and distended, hypomotile loops of bowel. Biopsy is not always diagnostic. Bacterial gas production with breaks in the mucosal integrity may explain most features of the disease. Treatment of pneumatosis cystoides intestinalis is usually conservative and includes nasogastric suction, high flow oxygen, elemental diet, and antibiotics (14).

Some studies indicate an increased risk of visceral malignancy in patients with dermatomyositis (15). Subsequent studies, however, failed to confirm this (9). Nevertheless, since the association of dermatomyositis and cancer may be high in the elderly, a search for cancer is justified (15).

B. Epidermolysis Bullosa (EB)

The GI tract is the commonest extracutaneous site of involvement, affecting primarily the oropharynx and esophagus. Lower GI involvement is also seen. Less commonly, pyloric atresia, complete luminal obstruction, and esophageal spasm are seen (16).

1. Esophageal Involvement

Oral blisters, odynophagia, dysphagia, dental anomalies, microstomia, and pyrosis are common. Eighty-one percent of patients with EB and dysphagia have esophageal pathology, most commonly manifested as esophageal strictures or webs. Although short strictures may be endoscopically dilated, dietary modification (e.g., pureed diet and avoidance of coarse foods) or even total parenteral nutrition may be required. Esophagectomy with colonic interposition may be necessary for severe esophageal stenosis (16). The diagnosis of upper GI involvement is established by barium studies. Given the risk of perforation associated with endoscopy in this condition, the procedure should be avoided (17).

2. Lower GI Involvement

Most patients with lower GI involvement have concomitant upper GI involvement (14). Patients may have anal fissures, strictures, and perianal blisters. Typical symptoms include constipation, hematochezia, and anal pain with defecation. A high-fiber diet and stool softeners may be useful (17).

IV. AMYLOIDOSIS AND THE GI TRACT

Amyloidosis is a systemic disease resulting from extracellular tissue deposition of amyloid protein. Multiple myeloma, chronic infections, and longstanding inflammatory diseases, all seen more commonly in the elderly, are causes (18). All forms involve the GI tract and may affect any segment (9). The rectum is the most frequently involved, and rectal biopsy establishes the diagnosis of amyloidosis in up to 80% of cases. Skin (subcutaneous fat), gingival, and small-bowel biopsies also are positive in more than 75% of patients with systemic amyloidosis (18,19). The chief sites of intestinal amyloid deposition are blood vessel walls (producing ischemia and infarction), muscle layers (causing atrophy and dysmotility), and the muscularis mucosa (impairing absorption). Mucosal infiltration implies massive amyloid deposition (9). Direct pressure damage by amyloid to the myenteric plexus and visceral nerve trunks has been demonstrated as well (4). Despite widespread tissue infiltration, gastrointestinal amyloidosis may be asymptomatic (9) (Table 2).

The liver is involved in about half of patients with systemic amyloidosis. It usually involves the parenchyma and leads to portal hypertension. Hepatosplenomegaly or abnormal transaminases are often present (18,19). Although biopsy is not necessary to confirm liver involvement in patients with known systemic amyloidosis, it is not contraindicated if prothrombin time

Table 2 GI Manifestations of Amyloidosis

Due to direct infiltration	
Bleeding	Mucosal friability
	Ulceration
	Variceal
Obstruction	
Peritonitis	Perforated ulcer
	Hepatic or splenic rupture
	Diverticular perforation
	Ischemia
Macroglossia	
Megacolon, constipation, rectal prolapse, fecal incontinence	
Diverticula	
Related to motility and malabsorption	
Dysphagia	
Intestinal pseudo-obstruction	
Gastric outlet obstruction	Decreased motility
	Mechanical obstruction
Diarrhea	Bacterial overgrowth
	Motility disturbance
Megaloblastic anemia	Decreased intrinsic factor production
Protein-losing enteropathy	Decreased absorption in terminal ileum
Related to hepatobiliary system	
Organomegaly	Hepatomegaly
	Splenomegaly
Jaundice	Intrahepatic, extrahepatic
Ascites	Portal hypertension
	Hypoproteinemia
	Cardiomyopathy
Functional hyposplenism	

and platelet counts are normal and there is no history of a bleeding diathesis (19). The decision to perform liver biopsy should be made on an individual basis.

A. Clinical Features

Fatigue, weight loss, dyspnea on exertion, and edema are the most common symptoms. Macroglossia is pathognomonic for amyloidosis, occurring more often in primary than secondary amyloidosis. In elderly patients with underlying temporomandibular arthritis, drooling and mastication problems may result (9). Esophageal involvement, occuring in two-thirds of patients, weakens the lower esophageal sphincter and disrupts normal esophageal motility. Reflux and dysphagia ensue. Gastric infiltration results in bleeding, gastric outlet obstruction, ulcers, and prominent gastric folds (18). Patients with amyloid deposition in the small intestine may present with diarrhea, obstruction, malabsorption, hemorrhage, infarction, diverticuli, and perforation. Amyloid infiltration of the colon is associated with symptoms mimicking inflammatory bowel disease, such as rectal bleeding, diarrhea, megacolon, fecal incontinence, rectal prolapse, pseudo-obstruction, constipation, and protein-losing enteropathy. Since amyloidosis may complicate Crohn's disease, there may be confusion. Localized amyloid deposition in the bowel may also mimic malignancy. Mesenteric involvement may cause frank bowel obstruction (9). Electrophoretic studies should be performed when the biopsy reveals amyloidosis to establish the relationship to multiple myeloma (18,19).

B. Radiologic Features

There are several modalities that may be helpful in establishing a diagnosis of intestinal amyloidosis. It is important to note that not all patients have radiographic abnormalities. A negative study thus does not exclude the diagnosis. Abdominal ultrasound may reveal thickening of the gastric and colonic walls, primarily in the central echogenic layer (which includes the submucosa). Real-time sonography reveals markedly decreased peristalsis of the small intestine, corresponding to the decreased intestinal motility (20).

On upper GI series, there may be a narrowing from the midportion of the gastric body to the antrum (20). Multiple masses or pyloric obstruction mimic peptic ulcer disease. Diminished or stiff-appearing rugal folds simulating infiltrating submucosal adenocarcinoma may also be seen (9).

Small-intestinal films, however, are often the first to suggest a diagnosis of amyloidosis because small-intestinal involvement is more frequent than stomach or colon. The most common findings are sharply demarcated thickening of the valvulae conniventes, dilatation of the bowel, and the presence of multiple nodular, granular and polypoid lesions. Barium enema may reveal loss of haustration, multiple filling defects, ulceration, or luminal narrowing and rigidity, particularly in the rectum and sigmoid colon (9).

C. Treatment

Therapy aimed at the associated disease may result in regression of amyloid. At present, there is no specific medical therapy for the primary disease.

Total parenteral nutrition has caused resolution of the nodularities and erosions seen on small-intestinal films. Cisapride has been reported to be helpful in the management of amyloid-induced pseudo-obstruction. Intestinal and gastric amyloid seem to portend a particularly grave prognosis (21).

V. CARDIAC DISEASE AND THE GI TRACT

The incidence of cardiac disease increases with increasing age. Thus, GI manifestations are seen frequently in a geriatric population.

A. Arteriovenous Malformation (AVM)

Valvular aortic stenosis (AS) occurs in 4% of elderly people, and is more frequent in males under 80 years of age and in females over 80 (22). One of the complications of AS is the development of AVMs leading to a predisposition for lower GI bleeding (23). Idiopathic hypertrophic subaortic stenosis (IHSS) is also associated with AVMs (24). The presence of bleeding AVMs in association with aortic stenosis is known as Heyde's syndrome (9,18,23,24). Although the relationship between AVMs and aortic valvular disease has recently been called into question (18), the bulk of evidence supports the association (25).

A connective-tissue defect, neurovascular mechanisms, or increased intraluminal pressure with muscle contractions may be responsible for valvular degeneration and colonic vessel dilatation (23). Therapies that increase circulating Von Willebrand factor (VWF) concentrations, such as desmopressin acetate (ddAVP) or cryoprecipitate, successfully correct the hematologic dysfunction seen with AVMs, pointing toward an acquired VWF deficiency as the pathogenesis for AVMs (24).

The location of AVMs is generally in the right colon or cecum although they may be seen anywhere in the GI tract (23,24). Higher intraluminal tension secondary to increased luminal diameter may explain the predominant location. Diagnosis of AVMs is by selective mesenteric angiography (23,24) or by panendoscopy (since AVMs may rarely be found in the stomach or duodenum) (25).

Management of patients should be aimed at controlling the GI bleeding and, if possible, treating the underlying causes of the AVM. Valve replacement with a bioprosthesis (with avoidance of anticoagulation) (23,24) is probably the safest approach to achieving eradication (23,25). Beta blockers diminish outflow obstruction in IHSS and improve perfusion of bowel vessels (24); endoscopic cautery may also be useful. Surgical resection is rarely successful (5% of cases) and recurrence of AVMs and bleeding is common (23).

B.   Congestive Heart Failure (CHF)

CHF occurs frequently in the elderly and may cause a number of GI problems. Congestive hepatopathy has long been recognized as a complication of either acute or chronic congestive right heart failure. Increased hepatic venous pressure leading to central venous and sinusoidal stasis are important factors contributing to hepatic dysfunction. Patients with acute passive liver congestion complain of right upper quadrant discomfort. On physical exam, they may have hepatomegaly, jaundice, peripheral edema, pleural effusion, splenomegaly, malnutrition and protein-losing enteropathy, or ascites (9,19,26). Other signs that may be present include jugular venous distention, hepatojugular reflux, substantial tricuspid valve insufficiency, and a pulsatile liver (19).

Laboratory tests reveal a modest elevation in serum bilirubin, a normal alkaline phosphatase, slight elevations in transaminases, and a prolonged prothrombin time (unresponsive to vitamin K). In general, laboratory abnormalities are more common in patients with acute right-sided CHF than in those with chronic congestion. These abnormalities regress with clinical improvement. Prolonged hepatic congestion can rarely progress to cardiac cirrhosis, not associated with portal hypertension or GI bleeding (18,19).

The diagnosis is primarily clinical. If there is suspicion of additional pathological processes necessitating liver biopsy, it should be postponed until the congestive heart failure has resolved (19). Therapy is aimed at correcting the underlying heart failure.

Acute and chronic left ventricular failure can contribute to a number of GI abnormalities due to decreased perfusion of the liver with decrease in its oxygen supply. "Shock" liver or ischemic hepatitis caused by acute left ventricular failure results in the abrupt onset of centrilobular necrosis. Patients have dramatic elevations of transaminases, an abrupt increase in prothrombin time, and a gradual increase in bilirubin. Passive congestion from preexisting right ventricular failure may predispose to ischemic hepatitis (19). Other manifestations of left heart failure include ischemic colitis, pancreatitis (26), and increased frequency of peptic ulcer disease, sometimes with upper GI bleeding (18).

In addition to the consequences of pump failure itself, drug therapy of cardiac disease may cause GI toxicity (Table 3). Digoxin (especially in excess) may cause anorexia, nausea, and vomiting. Intestinal ischemia due to digitalis-induced constriction of splanchnic vessels may be seen. Quinidine and other antiarrhythmics commonly cause nausea, anorexia, or diarrhea. Diuretics cause constipation or pseudo-obstruction (due to hypokalemia or hypomagnesemia) as well as pancreatitis (e.g., thiazides, furosemide, ethacrynic acid). Potassium supplementation may cause esophagitis, esophageal and intestinal ulcers, and rarely strictures (18).

Table 3 Adverse GI Effects of Cardiac Medications

Drug	Effect
Diuretics	
Furosemide	Constipation, pseudo-obstruction
Hydrochlorthiazide	Constipation, pseudo-obstruction, pancreatitis
Ethacrynic acid	Constipation, pseudo-obstruction, pancreatitis
Potassium supplements	Esophagitis, esophageal and intestinal ulcers, strictures
Antiarrhythmics	
Digoxin	Anorexia, nausea, vomiting, intestinal ischemia
Tocainide	Nausea
Encainide	Nausea
Flecainide	Nausea
Bretylium	Nausea, vomiting
Mexiletine	Nausea, vomiting
Procainamide	Anorexia, nausea
Quinidine	Anorexia, nausea, diarrhea
Calcium channel blockers	Constipation

C. Miscellaneous

Enlargement of the left atrium in patients with mitral valve disease may cause mechanical displacement/compression of the esophagus leading to dysphagia. Chronic cough and long-term bed rest may contribute to reflux esophagitis. Embolization of an atrial or ventricular clot may result in intestinal infarction. Infective emboli from endocarditis may produce distant abscesses (18).

VI. GI MANIFESTATIONS OF EXTRAINTESTINAL MALIGNANCIES

Involvement of the GI tract may occur by direct invasion from nearby organs, by intraperitoneal seeding, hematogenous, or lymphatic spread. Twenty percent of "extraintestinal" neoplasms involve the GI tract in some way. Patterns of spread reflect the location and histologic type of the primary tumor. The most common tumors to metastasize to the GI tract include melanoma, breast, thyroid, and bronchogenic carcinoma. Metastatic tumors may form serosal or mesenteric implants. Local extension from ovarian cancer frequently involves the abdominal viscera. Bladder and prostate cancer sometimes directly infiltrate the bowel wall, lymphatic or neuronal elements causing bleeding, vascular compromise, obstruction, or pseudo-obstruction. Adrenal tumors may cause a Budd-Chiari syndrome by infiltration of the hepatic vein (18). Signs and symptoms include pain, fever, ascites, bleeding, obstruction, and perforation. Intestinal obstruction leads to malnutrition and intestinal infarction, and may cause death. Extramural masses, mucosal ulcerations, "linitus plastica" gastric appearance, or ulcerating masses with a "target" or "bull's eye" appearance may be seen. CT scan is helpful in determining the extent and stage of the primary tumor, and for detection of large serosal implants (9).

Paraneoplastic syndromes often have GI manifestations, such as intestinal stasis or intestinal pseudo-obstruction, as seen with small-cell carcinoma of the lung, or Ogilvie's syndrome. Hypercalcemia secondary to metastatic tumor and multiple endocrine neoplasias (MEN) may also contribute to intestinal dysfunction (9). Nonspecific symptoms such as anorexia, constipation, and diarrhea may occur.

Chemotherapy and radiation therapy usually have GI side effects. Stomatitis, nausea, vomiting, diarrhea, and constipation are common complications of chemotherapy and may contribute to weight loss and generalized wasting. The immunocompromised state that results from systemic chemotherapy predisposes to infection with opportunistic organisms such as *Candida*, herpes, or CMV, causing esophagitis, gastritis, hepatitis, and colitis. Bacteremia with endogenous bowel flora, stercoral ulcers, perianal or perirectal abscesses, pseudomembranous colitis, and necrotizing enterocolitis are also seen (18).

Cancer cachexia (weight loss, anorexia, metabolic disorders) may occur early, but usually occurs with widely disseminated disease (18).

A. Malignant Melanoma

Metastases can occur up to 42 years after the primary melanoma is diagnosed. On occasion, however, metastatic lesions of the GI tract may be the initial manifestation of the disease (27). Frequent sites of metastases include liver, small bowel, stomach, and colon. In the colon, metastases may be mistaken for polyps and must be biopsied (18,27).

Patients with melanoma and GI metastases are usually asymptomatic but may experience nonspecific abdominal pain, anorexia, and GI bleeding. A palpable mass may be present. Bile duct compression may cause jaundice and cholecystitis. Other complications include intussusception, obstruction, bleeding, or perforation (18).

Radiologically, small-bowel metastases appear as multiple mural nodules or ulcerated masses. In the stomach and duodenum they appear as intramural nodules with central ulceration or umbilication ("bull's eye" or "target lesion"). Colonic lesions cause multiple submucosal nodules or, rarely, an infiltrating mass. Regression of GI lesions has been observed in response to chemotherapy (27).

B. Prostate Cancer

Prostate cancer may metastasize to the liver and, rarely, to small bowel, colon, rectum, or stomach. Immunohistochemical stains for prostate-specific antigen (PSA) should be performed on gastric, small-bowel, and rectal biopsies in male patients with adenocarcinoma of unknown origin (28).

Patients with prostate cancer metastatic to stomach are usually asymptomatic or have nonspecific GI complaints such as nausea. They may, however, develop gastric outlet obstruction or hemorrhage with vomiting and/or epigastric pain mimicking peptic ulcer disease (28). Rectosigmoid stricture due to extrinsic rectal masses may simulate colorectal cancer. Rectal involvement occurs in 1.5–11% of cases, and the presentation is usually that of partial or complete bowel obstruction. Spread may be contiguous from the prostate. Rectosigmoid involvement portends a poor prognosis (29).

On sigmoidoscopy, thickened mucosal folds and friable mucosa in the rectosigmoid are most commonly seen, and deep biopsies are necessary to obtain a diagnosis. Routine biopsy of a rectosigmoid stricture is of low yield. An abnormal intravenous urogram, bone scan, and high acid and alkaline phosphatase support a diagnosis of metastatic prostate cancer, as does an elevated PSA in a patient who presents with back pain. With a high annular rectosigmoid stricture and normal-appearing mucosa on sigmoidoscopy, a high index of suspicion of prostate cancer should prevail, even to the point of prostate biopsy (29).

Viral colitis due to cytomegalovirus and herpes simplex virus has also been described in association with advanced prostate cancer. This is probably triggered by the combined immunosuppressive effects of cancer and its therapy (30). Therapy includes withdrawal of the immunosuppressive agent if possible, therapy of the underlying disease, and antiviral medications.

C. Hematologic Neoplastic Disease

Multiple myeloma results from the neoplastic proliferation of monoclonal plasma cells. It usually affects middle-aged and older individuals. When the GI tract is involved, plasmacytomas form and hyperviscosity results. Patients may develop abdominal pain, ulceration, and bleeding, or obstruction, as well as visceral ischemia and thrombosis. Endoscopy or upper GI series is useful to establish the diagnosis and to rule out peptic ulcer disease.

Mesenteric angiography should be avoided if possible, as the contrast dye may precipitate renal failure, particularly in the elderly (18).

Waldenstrom's macroglobulinemia, a malignant proliferation of lymphoplasmacytoid cells that secrete IgM, similarly causes hepatosplenomegaly from infiltration by plasma cells. Diarrhea and steatorrhea due to malabsorption are caused by intestinal IgM deposition (18).

As many as 10% of patients with non-Hodgkin's lymphoma have GI involvement. Prominent clinical features include intestinal obstruction, bleeding, abdominal masses, and perforation. Liver and spleen involvement are common (18).

VII. ENDOCRINE DISORDERS
A. Thyroid Disease (Table 4)
1. Hypothyroidism

Hypothyroidism is common in advanced age, and the diagnosis may be overlooked as the symptoms may be vague and nonspecific in the elderly. It may result from Hashimoto's thyroiditis or therapy of hyperthyroidism. It may be associated with diabetes, or due to primary endocrine failure. Patients have weight gain and anorexia with an accompanying decrease in metabolism (18,31). When Hashimoto's thyroiditis is the cause of hypothyroidism, it may be associated with parietal cell antibodies and atrophic gastritis with hypochlorhydria. Serum gastrin levels are normal unless the atrophy is severe. Myxedematous patients with liver function abnormalities may have other associated autoimmune liver disease as well (31). Rarely, celiac sprue may occur with autoimmune thyroiditis (9).

Lower esophageal sphincter pressure is reduced in hypothyroidism, and there is decreased amplitude and prolonged duration of esophageal contractions. Delayed esophageal emptying and dysphagia, reflux, and esophagitis may persist (31).

Table 4 GI Manifestations of Thyroid Disease

Disease type	Feature
Myxedema	Delayed esophageal transit, gastric hypomotility, megacolon, pseudo-obstruction, fecal impaction, gallbladder hypotonia, ileus, weight gain, hepatic congestion
Thyrotoxicosis	Oropharyngeal dysphagia, abdominal pain, rapid GI transit, vomiting, diarrhea, hepatic dysfunction, weight loss

Hypothyroidism is associated with impaired gut motility, constipation, and abdominal distension. Gastric hypomotility may predispose to phytobezoars (31). When constipation is seen in the elderly, thyroid function tests should be obtained to screen for hypothyroidism. Diarrhea, although rare in hypothyroidism, may occur and may be associated with steatorrhea and malabsorption (9). Intestinal pseudo-obstruction, megacolon, obstipation, obstruction, sigmoid volvulus, rectal prolapse, and fecal impaction have been described (31). Sigmoid stricture mimicking colonic carcinoma but resolving with thyroid hormone replacement may be seen.

Other GI manifestations of hypothyroidism include impaired salivary, gastric, and intestinal secretions and occasionally achlorhydria. Hypotonia of the gallbladder with subsequent gallstones has been described. Ascites and hyponatremia are rare complications of myxedema. Hypothyroidism may be associated with changes in liver architecture suggestive of central congestive fibrosis (31). Routine liver tests are mildly elevated in 50% of hypothyroid patients, especially if congestive heart failure or pericardial effusion is present (9). Thyroid replacement hormone is effective in treating many of the GI symptoms described above (18,31). Surgery should be avoided because of increased morbidity and mortality rates in these patients.

2. Hyperthyroidism

Hyperthyroidism occurs seven times more frequently in persons over 60 than in those under, and should be considered a disease of old age (32). It may affect the stomach, small bowel, and liver (18,32). Gastritis, hypochlorhydria, fasting hypergastrinemia, and increased gastric motility have been described (9,18,32). Coexistent autoimmune gastric disease and antiparietal antibodies are seen in 30% of hyperthyroid patients.

The most common physiologic effect on the GI system is an alteration in intestinal motility resulting in diminished small bowel and colonic transit time (9,18,32). Rapid gastric emptying, mild steatorrhea, increased stool frequency, and (rarely) frank diarrhea may occur. In the elderly, an absence of constipation may be the only clue to the presence of hyperthyroidism. Small-bowel X-rays can show dilation and thickening of the circular folds (31). Symptoms are reversible with therapy (9).

Another GI manifestation of hyperthyroidism is hepatic dysfunction. Increased transaminases, alkaline phosphatase, and bilirubin may occur, as well as decreased cholesterol and albumin (18,33). Although 20–25% of patients in thyroid crisis are jaundiced, it is a relatively rare finding in most hyperthyroid patients, and its presence should prompt a search for infection, underlying liver disease, or heart failure. Hepatic dysfunction portends a poor prognosis (33).

The etiology of liver disease in hyperthyroidism is multifactorial. Centrilobular necrosis due to relative hypoxia of hepatic cells, cholestasis, vascular injury, and portal fibrosis may occur (31,33). Autoimmune thyroid disease (Graves', Hashimoto's thyroiditis) may be associated with autoimmune liver disease as well. Hepatic disease may also be a result of therapy for thyrotoxicosis (18,31).

Patients with hyperthyroidism usually experience hyperphagia with attendant weight loss due to the hypermetabolic state. Paradoxical weight gain may be seen as well (31). Other symptoms seen include anorexia, nausea, and vomiting. Aspiration and subsequent pneumonia may develop in patients with esophageal dysfunction. Occasionally, patients have a change in bowel habits, colicky abdominal pain, or even frank intussusception (9). Apathetic thyrotoxicosis may simulate intraabdominal malignancy.

3. Goiters

Simple goiters are a common occurrence. Most patients are euthyroid and asymptomatic, but if the goiter becomes large enough, it may cause respiratory obstruction and displacement of the esophagus, resulting in dysphagia (18).

B. Diabetes Mellitus

Elderly people appear to be more susceptible to the development of hyperglycemia than younger people. The presence of comorbidity and polypharmacy in elderly diabetics makes treatment more challenging. Seventy-six percent of diabetics seen in the ambulatory setting have complaints affecting virtually any component of the GI tract (Table 5). The majority of symptoms

Table 5   GI Manifestations of Diabetes Mellitus

Organ	Dysfunction	Symptoms
Esophagus	Dysmotility	Dysphagia
	Candida esophagitis	Dysphagia, odynophagia
Stomach	Gastroparesis	Nausea, vomiting, bloating, pain
	Atrophic gastritis	Asymptomatic
Gallbladder	Gallstones and cholecystitis	Abdominal pain
Liver	Steatosis	Asymptomatic, hepatomegaly
	Drug-induced hepatotoxicity (oral sulfonylurea agents)	Occasional jaundice
Small intestine	Diarrhea, steatorrhea	Weight loss
Colon	Dysmotility	Megacolon, constipation
Anal sphincter	Dysmotility	Fecal incontinence

are attributable to abnormal motility (3,34). Blood glucose and electrolyte imbalance, axonal degeneration, and increased susceptibility of diabetics to infection all play a role.

1. Esophagus

Symptoms of esophageal dysfunction are common and include reflux, dysphagia, and odynophagia (3,9,26,35). These abnormalities, likely due to dysmotility, are more commonly seen in the presence of autonomic and peripheral neuropathy. Motility abnormalities are not always associated with delayed transit or even symptoms (35). Promotility agents have been useful in patients with symptoms. Diabetics also have an increased incidence of *Candida* esophagitis which responds well to antifungal therapy. Pill-induced esophagitis also occurs (3,9,34,35).

2. Stomach

Diabetic gastroparesis is seen in up to 50% of all diabetic patients and is often accompanied by autonomic neuropathy, retinopathy, nephropathy, and sometimes poor glucose control. Clinical manifestations include nausea, vomiting, bloating, and epigastric pain. Diminished gastric emptying of liquids and solids leads to formation of obstructive bezoars. These cause erratic absorption of ingested carbohydrates, making control of blood glucose difficult (35). Endoscopy may be used for diagnosis and therapy of bezoars.

The clinical diagnosis of diabetic gastroparesis is made using abdominal X-ray. Gastric emptying studies show prolonged transit time for liquids and solids (3,34,35). Therapy of gastroparesis includes glucose management and antiemetic and promotility agents (3,9,34,35). Abdominal pain with hemorrhagic gastritis often complicates diabetic ketoacidosis (DKA) (9,34). Cholecystitis, appendicitis, pancreatitis, and peritonitis should be considered in the differential diagnosis. Notably, peptic ulcer disease is uncommon in this setting (36). An elevated amylase is often seen in patients with both diabetic ketoacidosis and pancreatitis. Ultrasound, HIDA scan, abdominal X-ray, and upper endoscopy may be required to establish a diagnosis.

Thoracic nerve radiculopathy can cause upper abdominal and lower chest pain and may mimic coronary artery disease, pleurisy, biliary tract disease, or an intraabdominal process. Persistent pain, anorexia, and weight loss suggest intraabdominal malignancy. Diagnosis is confirmed by electromyography. Often the pain subsides spontaneously within 6–12 months (9).

3. Gallbladder

Diabetics have an increased incidence of cholelithiasis. Those with acute cholecystitis classically had significantly increased morbidity and mortality with higher rates of perforation, infection, and emphysematous cholecystitis. Emergency cholecystectomy in diabetics has a 5–10 times greater mortality rate. More recently, morbidity and mortality rates of cholecystectomy or acute cholecystitis have declined in diabetics without comorbid illnesses. Expectant management rather than prophylactic cholecystectomy in patients with silent gallstones appears prudent (3,9,35).

4. Liver

One-third of diabetics have some evidence of liver dysfunction, with elevated triglycerides, increased alkaline phosphatase, and hepatic steatosis. This condition is seen more commonly in type 2, non-insulin-dependent patients and is often asymptomatic (35). Ultrasound reveals an increased hepatic density. Hepatic lesions are usually benign, but progression to cirrhosis can occur (9,35). Therapy includes weight reduction and tight glucose control (9).

Diabetics have enhanced susceptibility to viral hepatitis. In addition, an idiosyncratic reaction secondary to the oral hypoglycemic agents (sulfonylureas) may cause hepatic cholestasis.

5. Small Bowel

Diarrhea occurs in up to 20% of diabetics and is the predominant manifestation of small-bowel involvement. It is usually nocturnal and is more common in males with longstanding, poorly controlled diabetes (3,9,26,35,36). The diarrhea is chronic and is usually unaccompanied by weight loss. Steatorrhea or fecal incontinence of liquid stools may be seen. Impaired regulation of intestinal fluid and electrolyte transport and abnormal sphincter tone have been implicated (9,35,37).

Steatorrhea is commonly seen in diabetics. While it may be idiopathic, pancreatic insufficiency, celiac sprue, and bacterial overgrowth should all be considered as possible causes (35,36). A therapeutic trial with pancreatic enzymes may be valuable as would a trial of antibiotics for bacterial overgrowth. Improvement with pancreatic enzymes should lead the clinician to suspect possible underlying alcohol abuse as a cause of chronic pancreatitis leading to diabetes (3,9,35). Finally, in diabetics the effect of sorbitol (often found in dietetic foods) must be ruled out as a cause of diarrhea (3,9,36). Therapy for diabetics with diarrhea includes psyllium or soluble fiber, kaolin, imodium, clonidine, octreotide, cholestyramine, and biofeedback (35,37).

Acute mesenteric intestinal ischemia, often due to concomitant atherosclerotic disease, is the most serious intraabdominal disease seen in diabetics and may lead to fatal gangrene if not diagnosed (9).

6. Colon

The most common GI complaint of diabetics is constipation, often in patients with autonomic neuropathy. Constipation may cause colonic atony

and dilatation, intestinal pseudo-obstruction, stercoral ulceration, perforation, volvulus, barium impaction with overflow diarrhea, incontinence, and
a blunted gastrocolic response to food. The diagnostic evaluation of constipation is the same in diabetic and nondiabetic patients. Hypothyroidism,
hypercalcemia, and hypomagnesia must be ruled out as well as medications
that cause constipation. Colonoscopy is warranted in patients over 40 years
of age. Therapy is symptomatic. A trial of prokinetic agents may be used
(3,9,35). Colonic ischemia will cause rectal bleeding (9).

VIII. AUTOIMMUNE/RHEUMATIC DISORDERS

A. Scleroderma

Scleroderma is a generalized disorder resulting from deposition of collagen
and other connective-tissue components in the skin, vasculature, and visceral organs (9). Fifty percent of patients have serious GI tract involvement,
with symptoms usually appearing in the fourth to sixth decades of life.

1. Pharynx and Esophagus

Tightening of the perioral skin causes difficulty opening the mouth. Gingivi-
tis and impaired taste sensation may be seen (18). Fifty percent to 80% of
patients have esophageal involvement (18,38). Development of esophageal
disease correlates with duration of scleroderma. Although the presence of
esophageal symptoms almost always indicates the presence of an abnormal
esophagus, up to 20% of asymptomatic patients may have an abnormal
esophagram (38). There is marked acid reflux, dysphagia, and heartburn.
As a result, 60% of patients develop severe reflux esophagitis and esophageal ulcers (9,18). Barrett's metaplasia without an increased incidence of
esophageal adenocarcinoma (9), stricture formation (3.2%) often requiring
dilatation (9), and moniliasis may be seen.

Prokinetic agents increase esophageal tone, correct the clearance defect,
increase lower esophageal pressure, and improve gastric emptying of solids.
H_2 receptor antagonists, omeprazole, and the usual antireflux measures are
all useful in the treatment of reflux esophagitis. Although medical therapy
is preferred in the early stages of scleroderma, antireflux surgery may be
more efficacious after the muscle has undergone fibrosis (39).

2. Stomach

Seventy-five percent of patients have a dilated, flaccid, atonic stomach
with delayed emptying and increased acid secretion. These abnormalities
contribute to esophageal reflux and may respond to promotility and antisecretory agents (9,18,38).

"Watermelon stomach," the presence of antral vascular ectasias, has been described. The lesions may result from repeated trauma to the antral mucosa from prolapse through the pylorus. This entity responds to YAG laser, cautery, and injection sclerotherapy (40).

3. Small Bowel

The incidence of intestinal involvement depends on duration of disease. Small bowel X-rays in asymptomatic patients may reveal early, often occult disease. Ninety percent of patients with small-bowel involvement also have esophageal involvement (41).

Radiographic abnormalities are seen in 42% of patients with scleroderma. Findings include segmentation, flocculation, square-mouthed pseudo-diverticula (9,18,38,41), and "hide-bound" ("wirespring," "accordionlike") small bowel. Finally, "pneumatosis cystoides intestinalis" may also be seen on X-ray (9,38). The diagnosis is made by abdominal X-ray in 58%. The therapy of pneumatosis intestinalis is nasogastric tube suction, hyperbaric oxygen, antibiotics, or surgical bypass of the involved segment. The mortality is related to the underlying disease; in scleroderma, pneumatosis intestinalis usually implies a poor prognosis.

Bacterial overgrowth in the small bowel may cause a "blind loop syndrome" due to stasis. Bacteria may deconjugate bile acids, leading to diminished bile salts, diminished lipid absorption, and steatorrhea (9,18,38,41). Relative pancreatic enzyme deficiency may cause steatorrhea as well (38).

The therapy for malabsorption and intestinal stasis includes antibiotics, promotility agents, or an elemental diet, medium-chain triglyceride supplementation, and total parenteral nutrition (9,41).

Intestinal ischemia and perforation may be seen due to vasculitis and thrombosis (9).

4. Colon and Rectoanal

The colon is involved in approximately 9% of cases (38). The gastrocolic response to eating is uniformly absent. Wide- or square-necked pseudo-diverticula are common (9,18,38). Patients with scleroderma are predisposed to fecaliths with colonic obstruction, pseudo-obstruction, and volvulus (9,18). Most commonly, however, colonic involvement is asymptomatic (38). Patients with scleroderma often suffer from fecal incontinence and rectal prolapse (9,42).

5. Miscellaneous

Calcific pancreatitis and arteritis leading to pancreatic necrosis have been described (9). Telangiectasias throughout the GI tract have been identified as the cause of GI bleeding in scleroderma patients (18). Primary biliary cirrhosis has also been described in patients with limited scleroderma (19).

B. Polyarteritis Nodosa

Vasculitis is a general term referring to a large group of diseases that have
the presence of inflammatory and proliferative changes in the small arteries
and arterioles as their major characteristic. Polyarteritis nodosa (PAN) is
a classic example of this group of diseases. It can occur at all ages but is
most frequent in the fifth and sixth decades (43).

Forty-five percent to 50% of patients with PAN have GI involvement.
Symptoms include nausea, vomiting, bloating, diarrhea, and abdominal
pain. Liver function tests may be abnormal. Obstruction, ulceration, hemorrhage, or intestinal necrosis with perforation may occur. Resection gives
the best chance for survival in patients with perforation. Cholecystitis or
hepatic and pancreatic infarction may be seen as well. The diagnosis may be
suspected clinically in a patient with multisystem involvement. Laboratory
studies are significant for a markedly (often greater than 100 mm/h) elevated
sedimentation rate, microhematuria, casts, elevated serum creatinine, hypertension, high rheumatoid factor, low serum complement, and, in many
cases, abnormal liver function tests. Hypergammaglobulinemia and hepatitis B surface antigenemia may be seen. Angiography may be diagnostic if it
reveals aneurysms in the vasculature of the kidneys and abdominal viscera.
Definitive diagnosis is made by seeing fibrinoid necrosis in the vessel walls
on pathologic exam. Steroids are the primary therapy for this disease
(43,44).

C. Rheumatoid Arthritis

Rheumatoid arthritis (RA) is a disabling multisystem disease with a variety
of GI manifestations and complications (Table 6). Chronic RA may be
associated with temporomandibular arthritis characterized by tenderness,
swelling, crepitus, and difficulty masticating. Patients may exhibit esophageal dysmotility, with low-amplitude persitaltic waves in mid and lower
esophagus, as well as a diminished lower esophageal sphincter pressure.
Heartburn and dysphagia occur infrequently (4,9,26). Gastritis is commonly
found on biopsy, but may be related to the advanced age of the patients
or to the effects of prolonged NSAID or steroid use (3).

Rheumatoid vasculitis may affect 1% of patients with RA. Ten percent
of them have GI involvement. Ischemic bowel ulcers, intestinal strictures
(due to NSAID use), pancolitis, bowel infarction, and hemorrhage may
occur (3,9,26). Rectal biopsy demonstrates a necrotizing arteritis. The prognosis is poor. Response to steroids is fair. Immunosuppressives (such as
azathioprine, cyclosporin, etc.) or plasmapheresis may be promising (9).

Protein-losing enteropathy, secondary amyloidosis, malabsorption, and
Felty's syndrome with intraabdominal abscess are all complications of RA

Table 6 GI Manifestations of Rheumatoid Arthritis

Abnormality	Manifestation
Temporomandibular arthritis	Impaired mastication
Esophageal dysmotility, GI vasculitis	Dysphagia, reflux, abdominal pain, ulceration, acalculous cholecystitis, bowel infarction
Amyloidosis	Pseudo-obstruction, malabsorption, intestinal ulceration and infarction, protein-losing enteropathy, gastric outlet obstruction
Portal hypertension (Felty's syndrome)	Variceal hemorrhage
Gold enterocolitis	Enteritis, diarrhea, fever, eosinophilia, megacolon
Miscellaneous	Gastritis, ischemic colitis, pancreatitis

(3,9). Felty's syndrome may be accompanied by mild hepatomegaly and elevations in transaminases and alkaline phosphatase (19). Pancreatitis and acute cholecystitis have been described in association with RA as well (3).

Gold salts used for the treatment of RA may cause an ulcerative enterocolitis, hepatitis, and jaundice. Withdrawal of the offending drug, supportive measures, sulfasalazine, cromolyn, and bowel rest have all been used with variable success (3,26).

D. Nonsteroidal Antiinflammatory Drugs (NSAIDs)

NSAIDs are the most commonly prescribed drugs worldwide, accounting for 3–9% of all prescriptions. Yet they represent 25% of all reported adverse drug reactions and 31% of the total cost for the treatment of arthritis. In fact, more than 50% of patients with arthritis use NSAIDs. The prevalence of NSAID use increases with age; nearly half of users are older than 60 (45).

Esophageal and intestinal strictures and ulcers are infrequent adverse effects of NSAID use. In the esophagus, there are concurrent disorders of motility, leading to prolonged contact between NSAID and mucosa. Patients should swallow NSAIDs with plenty of fluids and avoid recumbency after ingestion. The small bowel may develop inflammation and increases in permeability (even up to 16 months after discontinuation of the drug) causing hemorrhage and protein loss or perforation. Crohn's disease should be considered in patients with abdominal complaints and a negative upper endoscopy. The small-intestinal inflammation is probably related to an interaction between intestinal bacteria and biliary-excreted NSAIDs and their metabolic products. Diarrhea, proctitis, and an initiation or exacerbation of quiescent ulcerative colitis may be seen with NSAIDs as well (45,46).

Hepatotoxicity occurs rarely and unpredictably. It is prostaglandin-independent. Risk factors include dose, age, concurrent renal insufficiency, alcohol use, polypharmacy, systemic lupus erythematosis, and possibly female gender. Usually asymptomatic, there may be a three- to fivefold increase in transaminases (47). Most NSAIDs follow no consistent pattern, and the mechanism is unclear though it appears to be immunological. Liver function should be monitored 4 weeks after initiating therapy. If hepatotoxicity occurs with one NSAID, one should never rechallenge with the same group of NSAIDs (47) (see Table 4).

The most common and well-known complications of NSAIDs are the effects on the gastroduodenal mucosa (9,46). They occur in 15–35% of patients taking them. NSAID use increases three- to fivefold the risk of gastric ulcers, GI bleeding, GI perforation, GI surgery, and death from GI causes (45). It may also increase the incidence of gastric outflow obstruction (48). Older patients are two to five times more susceptible to serious complications such as ulcer perforation and bleeding. Seventy-five percent of NSAID-induced bleeding and perforation and 90% of NSAID-induced mortality occur in patients over 60 years of age. A significant association has been found between aspirin and uncomplicated gastric ulcer but not uncomplicated duodenal ulcer. Nonaspirin NSAIDs are significantly associated with both uncomplicated gastric and duodenal ulceration (45,48).

NSAID gastropathy is characterized by dyspepsia, nausea, epigastric pain, and heartburn in 50% of patients. Endoscopy may show erythema, diffuse erosions, microscopic bleeding, or frank ulceration. It is the analgesic effect of NSAIDs that is responsible for the poor correlation between symptoms and endoscopically proven gastroduodenal injury (47). This blunting of symptoms may lead to an increase in patients presenting with complications of PUD (e.g., gastric outlet obstruction, hemorrhage, or perforation), as many patients, particularly the elderly, are asymptomatic in early, uncomplicated disease (47–49).

Acute gastropathy begins with erythema leading to diffuse erosions and or microscopic bleeding. Chronic gastropathy is characterized by frank ulceration usually in the antral or pyloric area, which may bleed or perforate without symptoms. Acute and chronic injury seem to arise from different mechanisms, there being no evidence that chronic injury arises from acute injury. They respond differently to drugs and require different management strategies (3,9,49).

The pathogenesis of NSAID-associated mucosal injury is secondary to 1. a direct topical prostaglandin-independent effect, and 2. systemic effects on arachidonic acid metabolism (45). *H. pylori* may potentiate mucosal susceptibility to NSAID-induced damage (49). Half of NSAID-induced ulcers that bleed have type B (antral) gastritis with *H. pylori* infection.

Aspirin, more than the other NSAIDs, has the greatest propensity for producing GI blood loss. This may be due to its irreversible effects on platelet cyclooxygenase. Mucosal ulceration and hemorrhage occur with chronic ASA use, even when buffered and given in low doses (48). Enterically coated aspirin, or prodrugs such as salsalate, cause little or no tissue injury, and their users are relatively free of acute hemorrhagic gastric lesions or superficial erosions (9). Used chronically, however, all can cause focal deep ulcers. Prevention involves avoiding the offending agents, using the smallest dose possible, and substituting acetaminophen for NSAIDs (45,48).

An important consideration in NSAID-induced damage is the phenomenon of "adaptation." Most gastroduodenal erosions and ulcerations occur during the first month of therapy and often disappear in 1 week to 3 months. Adaptation explains the observation that the risk of PUD appears to be highest during the first month of NSAID use. This risk is dose-dependent (45,49).

Certain NSAID users seem to be predisposed to develop complicated peptic ulcer disease (PUD) and may benefit most from ulcer prophylaxis. Risk factors include age greater than 60, dosage and type of NSAID, concomitant steroid use, prior peptic ulcer, and previous NSAID use. Comorbid illness, ethanol use, smoking, stress, increased acid secretion, blood group O, family history of PUD, and *H. pylori* gastritis have also been implicated (45,47,49–51).

The initial approach to patients with GI intolerance from NSAIDs involves stopping or changing the NSAID or decreasing the dose. Taking the medication with food or antacids or adding an H_2 blocker may alleviate symptoms. Tolerance may develop over time, but endoscopy should be performed for persistent symptoms (45).

High-dose or prolonged use of H_2 blockers is quite effective in preventing and treating duodenal ulcers (DU) but is ineffective in preventing gastric ulcer (GU) formation (49,51). Sucralfate prevents and treats DU as well, but is ineffective in the prevention or treatment of NSAID-induced gastric disease. Likewise, omeprazole can prevent DU, but it is unclear if it will prevent GU damage or promote GU healing in patients on NSAIDs. Misoprostol (a prostaglandin E_1 analog) prevents DUs and GUs in patients on NSAIDs and successfully heals NSAID-induced gastroduodenal lesions. Prophylactic therapy may be most beneficial in the first 3 months of NSAID therapy before adaptation occurs (9,46,49,51,52).

Misoprostol may prevent jejunal and ileal ulceration in chronic NSAID users, but the drug's side effects of diarrhea and abdominal cramping may be limiting. Cotreatment with H_2 blockers and misoprostol in patients on

NSAIDs who are a poor surgical risk is reasonable (52). It is unclear whether misoprostol decreases the frequency of PUD or somehow decreases the incidence of life-threatening complications (49,52). Despite misoprostol's beneficial effects on ulcer formation and healing, it does not reduce symptoms (51). Gastric outlet obstruction in elderly patients from NSAID-induced PUD may improve with medical management alone, but the response may be delayed.

REFERENCES

1. McCarthy DM. Acid peptic disease in the elderly. Clin Geriatric Med 1991; 7:231–254.
2. Brust JCM. Stroke. In: Hazzard WR, Bierman EL, Blass JP, Ettinger WH, Halter JB, eds. Principles of Geriatric Medicine and Gerontology. 3rd ed. New York: McGraw-Hill, 1994:1027–1033.
3. Freston JW, Moore JR. Approach to gastrointestinal problems associated with common clinical conditions. In: Yamada T, Alpers DH, Owyang C, Powell DW, Silverstein FE, eds. Textbook of Gastroenterology. Vol 1. Philadelphia: J.B. Lippincott, 1991:928–942.
4. Camilleri M. Disorders of gastrointestinal motility in neurologic diseases. Mayo Clin Proc 1990; 65:825–846.
5. Reynolds JC. Motility disorders of the colon. In: Yamada T, Alpers DH, Owyang C, Powell DW, Silverstein FE, eds. Textbook of Gastroenterology. Vol 2. Philadelphia: J.B. Lippincott, 1991:1715–1733.
6. Edwards LL, Quigley EMM, Pfeiffer RF. Gastrointestinal dysfunction in Parkinson's disease: frequency and pathophysiology. Neurology 1992; 42:726–732.
7. Edwards L, Quigley EMM, Hofman R, Pfeiffer RF. Gastrointestinal symptoms in Parkinson's disease: 18-month follow-up study. Mov Disord 1993; 8:83–86.
8. Anderson S. Nephrology/fluid and electrolyte disorders. In: Cassel CK, Risenberg DE, Sorensen LB, Walsh JR, eds. Geriatric Medicine. 2d ed. New York: Springer-Verlag, 1990:301–311.
9. Sack TL, Sleisenger MH. Effects of systemic and extraintestinal disease on the gut. In: Sleisenger MH, Fordtran JS, eds. Gastrointestinal Disease. Pathophysiology, Diagnosis and Management. 4th ed. Philadelphia: W.B. Saunders, 1989:488–528.
10. Kang JY. The gastrointestinal tract in uremia. Dig Dis Sci 1993; 38:257–268.
11. Cox JR, Macias-Nunez JF, Dowd AB. Renal disease. In: Pathy MSJ, ed. Principles and Practice of Geriatric Medicine. 2d ed. Chichester, England: John Wiley & Sons, 1991:1159–1177.
12. Brenner BM, Lazarus JM. Chronic renal failure. In: Wilson JD, Braunwald E, Isselbacher KJ, et al., eds. Harrison's Principles of Internal Medicine. 12th ed. New York: McGraw-Hill, 1991:1150–1157.
13. Dienstag JL, Wands JR, Isselbacher KJ. Acute Hepatitis. In: Wilson JD, Braunwald E, Isselbacher KJ, et al., eds. Harrison's Principles of Internal Medicine. 12th ed. New York: McGraw-Hill, 1991:1322–1337.

14. Pasquier E, Wattiaux M-J, Peigney N. First case of pneumatosis cystoides intestinalis in adult dermatomyositis. J Rheumatol 1993; 20:499–503.
15. Sorensen LB. Rheumatology: In: Cassel CK, Risenberg DC, Sorensen LB, Walsh JR, eds. Geriatric Medicine. 2d ed. New York: Springer-Verlag, 1990:184–211.
16. Bozymski EM, London JF. Miscellaneous diseases of the esophagus. In: Yamada T, Alpers DH, Owyang C, Powell DW, Silverstein FE, eds. Textbook of Gastroenterology. Vol 1. Philadelphia: J.B. Lippincott, 1991:1178–1197.
17. Gulchin AE, Lin AN, Dannenberg AJ, Carter DM. Gastrointestinal manifestations of epidermolysis bullosa: a study of 101 patients. Medicine 1992; 71:121–127.
18. Neil GA, Weinstock JV. Gastrointestinal manifestations of systemic diseases. In: Yamada T, Alpers DH, Owyang C, Powell DW, Silverstein FE, eds. Textbook Gastroenterology. Vol 2. Philadelphia: J.B. Lippincott, 1991:2135–2157.
19. Cello JP, Grendell JH. The liver in systemic conditions. In: Zakim D, Boyer TD, eds. Hepatology: A Textbook of Liver Disease. 2d ed. Vol 2. Philadelphia: W.B. Saunders, 1990:1411–1437.
20. Shirahama M, Morita S, Koga T, et al. Gastrointestinal amyloidosis associated with multiple myeloma: sonographic features. J Clin Ultrasound 1991; 19:493–497.
21. Fraser AG, Arther JF, Hamilton I. Intestinal pseudoobstruction secondary to amyloidosis responsive to cisapride. Dig Dis Sci 1991; 36:532–535.
22. Williams BO. The cardiovascular system. In: Pathy MSJ, ed. Principles and Practice of Geriatric Medicine. 2d ed. Chichester, England: John Wiley & Sons, 1991:573–623.
23. Schwartz J, Rosenfeld V, Habot B. Cessation of recurrent bleeding from gastrointestinal angiodysplasia, after beta blocker treatment in a patient with hypertrophic subaortic stenosis—a case history. Angiology 1992; 43:244–248.
24. Natowitz L, Defraigne JO, Limet R. Association of aortic stenosis and gastrointestinal bleeding (Heyde's syndrome). Report of two cases. Acta Chir Belg 1993; 93:31–33.
25. Dave PD, Sandberg AR, Weiss RA, Persaud M, Chen WY. Gastrointestinal bleeding after valve replacement (Letter.) J Clin Gastroenterol 1989; 11:238–239.
26. Freston JW, Moore JR. Approach to gastrointestinal problems associated with common clinical conditions. In: Yamada T, Alper DH, Owyang C, Powell DW, Silverstein FE, eds. Atlas of Gastroenterology. Philadelphia: J.B. Lippincott, 1991:92–97.
27. Jubelirer SJ. Multiple colonic polyps as the initial presentation of malignant melanoma. W Va Med J 1992; 8B:279–280.
28. Holderman WH, Jacques JM, Blackstone MO, Brasitus TA. Prostate cancer metastatic to the stomach. J Clin Gastroenterol 1992; 14:251–254.
29. Culkin DJ, Demos TC, Wheeler JS, Castelli M, Canning JR. Separate annular strictures of the rectosigmoid colon secondary to unsuspected prostate cancer. J Surg Oncol 1990; 43:189–192.

30. Hughes J, Kisin MW, Muscat I, Irvin TT, Nuttin BJ, Simpson R. Viral colitis associated with advanced carcinoma of the prostate. J R Soc Med 1989; 82:113–114.
31. Sellin JH, Vassilopoulou-Sellin R, Lester R. The gastrointestinal tract and liver. In: Ingbar SH, Braverman LE, eds. Werner's The Thyroid: A Fundamental and Clinical Text. 5th ed. Philadelphia: J.B. Lippincott, 1986:871–878,1156–1162.
32. Gregerman RI, Katz MS. Thyroid diseases. In: Hazzard WR, Bierman EL, Blass JP, Ettinger WH Jr, Halter JB, eds. Principles of Geriatric Medicine and Gerontology. 3d ed. New York: McGraw-Hill, 1994:807–823.
33. Kimberg DV. Liver. In: Werner SC, Ingbar SH, eds. The Thyroid: A Fundamental and Clinical Text. Hagerstown, Md: Harper and Row, 1971:569–573.
34. Kinsley BT, Gramm HF, Rolla AR. Diabetic gastroparesis. A review. J Diab Complic 1991; 5:207–217.
35. Falchuk KR, Conlin O. The intestinal and liver complications of diabetes mellitus. Adv Intern Med 1993; 38:269–286.
36. Morris JS, Dew MJ, Gelb AM, Clements DG. Age and gastrointestinal disease. In: Pathy MSJ, ed. Principles and Practice of Geriatric Medicine. 2d ed. Chichester, England: John Wiley & Sons, 1991:417–486.
37. Valdovinos MA, Camilleri M. Zimmerman BR. Chronic diarrhea in diabetes mellitus: Mechanisms and an approach to diagnosis and treatment. Mayo Clin Proc 1993; 68:691–702.
38. Poirier TJ, Rankin GB. Gastrointestinal manifestations of progressive systemic scleroderma based on a review of 364 cases. Am J Gastroenterol 1972; 58:30–44.
39. Murphy JR, McNally P, Peller P, Shay SS. Prolonged clearance is the primary abnormal reflux parameter in patients with progressive systemic sclerosis and esophagitis. Dig Dis Sci 1992; 37:833–841.
40. Scolapio JS, Matteson EL. The watermelon stomach in scleroderma. (Letter.) Arth Rheum 1993; 36:724–725.
41. Bluestone R, Macmahon M, Dawson JM. Systemic sclerosis and small bowel involvement. Gut 1969; 10:185–193.
42. Leighton JA, Valdovinos MA, Pemberton JH, Rath DM, Camilleri M. Anorectal dysfunction and rectal prolapse in progressive systemic sclerosis. Dis Colon Rectum 1993; 36:182–185.
43. Kottke BA, Rooke TW. Disorders of the blood vessels. In: Pathy MSJ, ed. Principles and Practice of Geriatric Medicine. 2d ed. Chichester, England: John Wiley & Sons, 1991:625–661.
44. Fauci AS. The vasculitis syndromes. In: Wilson JD. Braunwald E, Isselbacher KJ, et al., eds. Harrison's Principles of Internal Medicine. 12th ed. New York: McGraw-Hill, 1991:1456–1463.
45. Kendall BJ, Peura DA. NSAID-associated gastrointestinal damage and the elderly. Prac Gastro 1993; 17:13,14,17–20,29.
46. Dawes PT, Symmons DPM. Short-term effects of antirheumatic drugs. Bailliere's Clin Rheumatol 1992; 6:117–140.
47. Weinblatt MW. Nonsteroidal anti-inflammatory drug toxicity: increased risk in the elderly. Scand J Rheumatol 1991; 91(suppl):9–17.

48. Bellary SV, Isaacs PET, Lee FI. Upper gastrointestinal lesions in elderly patients presenting for endoscopy: relevance of NSAID usage. Am J Gastroenterol 1991; 86:961–964.
49. McCarthy DM. NSAID-induced gastrointestinal damage. J Clin Gastroenterol 1990; 12(suppl 2):513–520.
50. Taha AS, Angerson W, Nakshabendi I, et al. Gastric and duodenal mucosal blood flow in patients receiving non-steroidal anti-inflammatory drugs—influence of age, smoking, ulceration and *Helicobactor pylori*. Aliment Pharmacol Ther 1993; 7:41–45.
51. Graham DY, White RH, Moreland LW, et al. Duodenal and gastric ulcer prevention with misoprostol in arthritis patients taking NSAIDs. Ann Intern Med 1993; 119:257–262.
52. Ballinger AB, Kumar PJ, Scott DL. Misoprostol in the prevention of gastroduodenal damage in rheumatology. Ann Rheumatol Dis 1992; 51:1089–1093.

16

Surgical Considerations

Howard L. Beaton
New York Downtown Hospital, New York, New York

I. INTRODUCTION

The surgical implications of gastrointestinal disease in the geriatric population are enormous. The proportion of elderly people in the United States population is increasing steadily and represents its most rapidly growing segment. The natural history of gastrointestinal disease must be weighed against this increasing life expectancy, which should not be underestimated, and the risk of surgery in this age group, which is often overestimated.

In the current era of hightened cost-consciousness, the impact of surgical disease in the geriatric population on the utilization and cost of medical services is well recognized. The elderly consume a disporportionately large share of all surgical services, accounting for 40% of all operations, 50% of all surgical emergencies, and 75% of postoperative deaths (1). Whenever possible, the goal of surgical therapy should be the maximization of the patient's lifespan regardless of chronologic age. When advanced or incurable disease is present, surgical treatment can still play an important role in the preservation of function and palliation of pain and suffering.

II. HISTORICAL PERSPECTIVE

The concept of surgery in the elderly is a relatively new and constantly evolving one. A century ago, advanced age alone was generally considered to be a contraindication to elective and emergency surgery. In 1907 a series of 165 patients over the age of 50 undergoing surgery was first reported (2). The most common gastrointestinal disease was acute appendicitis, and the overall mortality rate was 19%. The author stressed, in contrast to the attitude of prevalent at the time, that "because [patients] are old, we must not consider that it is time for them to die. . . . we should endeavor to prolong life, and prolong it in comfort." Progress in the acceptance of this concept, however, was slow. In 1937 a series of surgical patients over 70 was reported and still emphasized the importance of operations performed primarily for the palliation of symptoms (3).

Improvements in surgical technique, anesthesia, and perioperative care occurred rapidly following World War II and the Korean conflict. This permitted operations on steadily older patients with gradually decreasing mortality rates. In 1961 and 1963, two series of patients over the age of 80 undergoing surgical procedures were reported (4,5). Despite this enthusiasm, mortality rate for gastrointestinal surgery in these patients remained high, ranging from 7% for biliary procedures to 39% for gastric surgery (overall 28.7%) (5). Improved survival in this age group was reported in 1979 with a decline in the total death rate to 6.2% for all procedures performed (6).

The results of surgery in 90-year-olds were first published in 1972 (7) and a small series of surgery in centenarians was reported in 1985 (8). Gradually, the concept of an acceptable upper age limit to surgical therapy has faded and major gastrointestinal operations are frequently performed on elderly patients at the current time.

III. DETERMINANTS OF OPERATIVE RISK

As the age barrier to gastrointestinal surgery has been removed, numerous attempts have been made to better determine those factors that effect surgical morbidity and mortality. It is generally accepted that surgical risk increases linearly with advancing age. This seems to be primarily due to decreasing cardiovascular and pulmonary function and coexisting disease. The effects of aging on the immune system remain unclear but are the subject of active investigation.

The first widely accepted, and still currently employed, method of classification of risk was adopted in 1974 by the American Society of Anesthesiology (ASA) (9). This method stratifies patients into five risk groups according to a clinical assessment of their physical status (Table 1). In a prospective analysis of patients over 80, less than 1% of ASA class 2 patients died, (6) whereas 25% of class 4 surgical patients died.

Several attempts to quantitate specific factors responsible for operative risk have led to the use of statistical techniques to simulate clinical judgments. Using linear discrimination analysis, Goldman et al. (10) in 1977 published an important paper describing a "multifactorial index of cardiac risk in noncardiac surgical procedures." Out of a total possible 53 points

Table 1 American Society of Anesthesiologists Physical Status Scale

Class 1	A normally healthy person
Class 2	A patient with mild systemic disease
Class 3	A patient with severe systemic disease that is not incapacitating
Class 4	A patient with incapacitating systemic disease that is a constant threat to life
Class 5	A moribund patient who is not expected to survive 24 hours with or without an operation

in this system, only 5 points were due to age greater than 70 years and 3 points were given for an intraperitoneal operation. The most significant determinates of risk were due to cardiac disease as determined by history, physical examination, or electrocardiographic analysis (Table 2). Using this

Table 2 Computation of the Cardiac Risk Index[10]

Item	Points
History	
Age greater than 70	5
Myocardial infarction within 6 months	10
Physical	
S3 or jugular venous distention	11
Important valvular aortic stenosis	3
Electrocardiogram	
Rhythm other than sinus or the presence of atrial premature contractions on the preoperative ECG	7
More than 5 VPCs per minute at any time prior to surgery	7
Medical status	
Poor general medical status	3
$P_{O_2} < 60$ or $P_{CO_2} > 50$	
$K < 3.0$ or $HCO_3 < 20$ mEq/L	
BUN > 50 or creatinine > 3 mg/dl	
Abnormal SGOT	
Chronic liver disease	
Bedridden due to noncardiac cause	
Operation	
Intraperitoneal, intrathoracic, aortic surgery	3
Emergency surgery	4
Total points	53

Table 3 Risk of Cardiac Complications in
Noncardiac Surgery[13]

Class	Points	Goldman	Zeldin	Detsky
I	0–5	1%	1%	6%
II	6–12	7%	3%	7%
III	13–25	14%	5%	20%
IV	>25	78%	30%	100%

method, patients could preoperatively be divided into four groups, each
with increasing risk for surgery. This has been reevaluated and expanded
by the original author as well as others during the subsequent decade
(Table 3).

The most comprehensive and sophisticated system to date to attempt
to predict hospital mortality in critically ill patients is the APACHE (Acute
Physiology, Age, and Chronic Health Evaluation) method. Its most recent
modification, the APACHE III system proposed in 1991 (14) results from
the addition of three groups of variables (physiology, age, and chronic
health). A cardinal number within a range of 0 to 299 is obtained, of which
only a maximum of 24 points are given for age (Table 4).

Scoring for a wide variety of variables designed to estimate the impact
of physiologic abnormalities, on the other hand, accounts for up to 252
points, or 84%, of the predictive power of this system. Hence, coexisting
disease and not chronologic age is the prime determinant of the risk of
death, even in elderly patients.

In the surgical patient, one must also consider the influence of emergency
and mortality. Numerous studies have emphasized the dramatically in-

Table 4 APACHE III Points for Age

Age, years	Points
≤44	0
45–59	5
60–64	11
65–69	13
70–74	16
75–84	17
≥85	24

creased incidence of death following surgery when performed in the emergency setting. The ASA classification has been modified to include the designation of an "E" to each classification to reflect this difference. In those patients whose ASA classification is I or II, this difference is minimal. However, in ASA Class IV-E or V-E patients, emergency surgery has been found to have a three- to fourfold increase in the complication rate as compared to similar patients undergoing elective surgery (15). The Goldman computation includes 4 points (out of 53 possible points) for emergency operations when calculating the cardiac risk index (10). In the APACHE III risk prediction index, emergency surgery is recognized as a factor increasing the risk of hospital mortality. It is treated as a separate coefficient by which the total score is multiplied (14).

Several retrospective studies have documented this effect of emergency surgery vs. elective surgery on mortality and morbidity rates in separate subgroups of elderly patients and after specific types of surgical procedures. In a large series of patients over 90 years of age the rate of serious perioperative complications was 20.7% and the mortality rate was 17.4% in those undergoing emergency operations. In contrast, in elective patients, the incidence was only 7.5% and 6.8%, respectively (16). In a review of elderly patients requiring surgery for gallstone disease, there was noted to be a 66% morbidity and 19% mortality rate in emergency patients, whereas these declined to 28% and 0.8%, respectively, in elective patients (17).

Unfortunately, there seems to be a tendency for elderly patients to present more frequently than their younger counterparts with conditions requiring emergency surgery. Some of this difference may be due to a difference in the natural history of disease in elderly patients, as in acute appendicitis, which seems to cause perforation more frequently and in less time in the geriatric patient (18). Underestimation of the life expectancy of the elderly may cause inappropriate delay in seeking elective treatment, as in the patient with symptomatic cholelithiasis. In some cases, the aging process may mask the typical presentation of certain conditions, especially when typical signs and symptoms may not occur. Consider the lethargic patient with a mildly distended abdomen; could this be normal or is it an early presentation of intraperitoneal sepsis? Many elderly patients and their families, as well as occasional physicians, still defer diagnostic evaluation or elective surgical intervention out of unfounded fear that such patients are "too old" to undergo surgery. In reality, delay may result in higher mortality as possible elective surgery becomes emergent.

IV. PERIOPERATIVE MONITORING

Cardiac complications, often due to asymptomatic and unrecognized coronary artery disease, are still the most frequent etiology responsible for postoperative death in the geriatric surgical patient. The Goldman index is an important method used to quantitate this risk, relying on readily available static measurement (10). Of importance, 28% of Goldman's 53 points represent potentially treatable and correctible cardiac conditions. In order to evaluate the effect of surgical stress on cardiac reserve, several preoperative methods of assessment have been suggested. Elderly patients who were able to perform a supine bicycle exercise test for 2 minutes and raise their heart rate over 100 were found to have a sixfold decrease in perioperative cardiac complications (19). The most sensitive noninvasive indication of coronary insufficiency currently seems to be the dipyridamole-thallium scan. In patients over 70 years of age undergoing vascular surgery, a positive scan indicated an increase from 3.2% to 30% risk of cardiac complication in the perioperative period (20).

The preoperative evaluation and optimization of cardiac function also requires consultation to treat arrhythmias, congestive heart failure, and hypertension. Chronic medications may require adjustment, and certain short-term pharmacologic measures may be instituted during the perioperative period in order to optimize cardiac reserve in anticipation of the stress induced by the surgical procedure. Preoperative hypovolemia is often present and underappreciated. Chronic diuretic therapy, decreased oral intake, and unrecognized fluid losses may exacerbate this condition. The apparent decreased responsiveness to sympathetic stimuli in elderly patients may further mask the recognition of significant decreases in the intravascular fluid compartment.

Invasive monitoring provides much information about myocardial performance and oxygen delivery. Indwelling arterial catheters and transcutaneous oxygen monitoring provide constant measurements with minimal risk and cost. Central venous pressure monitoring, especially in elderly patients with underlying right ventricular or pulmonary dysfunction, has been found to be inaccurate. Swan-Ganz catheters measure the function of both ventricles and provide the most accurate data to guide perioperative fluid replacement and avoid hemodynamic problems due to hypovolemia. Del Guercio and Cohn used this technique in patients over 65 years of age who had already been "cleared" for surgery (21). Only 13.5% of their patients had normal measured parameters, 63.5% had mild to severe abnormalities, and 23% had functional deficits too severe to permit major surgery. Interestingly, their assessments were in general agreement with ASA classification, but permitted better appreciation of the specific physiologic abnormalities present, as well as providing the data required to optimize function in the intermediate risk groups prior to proceeding with surgery, and guide postoperative ICU management in these patients at increased risk. Most recently, transesophageal Dopplers have been used as a continuous method of assessing cardiac function. Although very sensitive and promising, this technique is currently limited to intraoperative use.

Pulmonary complications are frequent in geriatric gastrointestinal surgery, especially surgery involving incisions in the upper abdomen. It has been estimated that up to 40% of postoperative morbidity and 20% of potentially preventable deaths are due to pulmonary dysfunction (22). Age-related changes in the lung result in decreased compliance and decreased diffusion capacity. Respiratory reserve may be evaluated clinically by a careful functional history, especially related to smoking and any exertional dyspnea or chronic, productive cough. Cessation of smoking preoperatively is universally advocated, although the suggested duration of abstinence has ranged from 2 weeks to 3 months with little scientific supporting data.

Preexisting COPD is an important factor in causing postoperative pulmonary complications. When asymptomatic disease is recognized on chest X-ray, the risk is doubled (23). In severely symptomatic patients, morbidity rates may be increased 20-fold (24). Pulmonary function testing (PFT) may be useful prior to elective surgery, especially in patients who have acceptable results and are thereby found not to be at any increased risk and to require no further testing. A forced expiratory volume (FEV) in 1 second of less that 45% has been shown to be predictive of pulmonary complications (19). Only such patients need to undergo full PFTs with bronchodilation testing and arterial blood gases. In high-risk patients a vigorous pre- and postoperative regimen of chest physiotherapy, bronchodilators, postural drainage, and incentive spirometry may markedly decrease this mobidity. Postoperative monitoring in surgical intensive care units, early use of bronchoscopy when needed, and avoidance of respiratory-depressing narcotics are important in these patients as well.

Renal insufficiency in the geriatric patient is common due to underlying diseases, such as hypertension, diabetes, and generalized atherosclerosis. Routine laboratory data rarely detect the true incidence of this problem, as concurrent loss of muscle mass may keep serum creatinine levels within the normal range. Due to this decreased renal reserve, the kidney in elderly patients is at increased risk from ischemia, hypoperfusion, and the use of nephrotoxic drugs. Likewise, the immune system changes with advancing age. Decreased function of T-cells (as measured by skin test energy), B-cells, and macrophages has been demonstrated (25). Practically, this correlates with increased colonization of the biliary and urinary tracts and increased postoperative infectious morbidity, as well as a decreasing ability to eliminate established infections. The surgeon must be aware of this and employ prophylactic antibiotics frequently in elderly patients. Extra attention should also be given to the nutritional status of elderly patients. Rarely are serum transferrin levels used as an effective early indication of malnutrition. However, a careful history will reveal recent weight loss, and a low serum albumin inflicts longstanding malnutrition, which may predispose to further immunocompromise. In order to be effective, nutritional supplementation must be given preoperatively for at least 10 days to reverse a catabolic state, when possible.

Deep venous thrombosis and pulmonary emoblism can be devastating complications in geriatric gastrointestinal surgery. In a large series of operations in patients over 70 years of age, pulmonary embolism accounted for one-third of all deaths (26). Preoperative inactivity, malignancy, and hemoconcentration may all predispose to increase the incidence of this condition. The long duration of many gastrointestinal surgical procedures further complicates this issue. Prophylactic therapy must be employed in all such elderly patients. Subcutaneous heparin (5,000 units every 12 hours) has been shown to decrease this risk by approximately 50% when started preoperatively (27). Sequential compression devices have been found to have a similar benefit when placed prior to the start of surgery and continued until ambulation has begun.

V. CONDUCT OF THE OPERATION

Surgery is a form of trauma which triggers a predictable cascade of increasingly well understood events at the cellular and hormonal levels. Intraperitoneal surgery is generally considered more "traumatic" than most other forms of surgery, and is given a designation of 3 points alone in the Goldman risk index (10). However, unlike other forms of trauma, the degree of surgical trauma can be minimized by careful surgical technique and well-considered decision making.

The geriatric gastrointestinal surgeon must work closely with the anesthesiologist regarding the selection of anesthetic technique. General anesthetetics exert a depressive effect on most organ function, and the use of such agents must be minimized. Certain simpler gastrointestinal procedures can be performed under monitored local anesthesia or regional technique. Even for major intraperitoneal procedures, the addition of a spinal or epidural anesthtetic may decrease the need for general anesthesia as well as provide effective postoperative pain relief without respiratory depression. The anesthesiologist must be comfortable in the interpretation of physiologic data from invasive monitors and knowledgable in the use of cardioactive drugs.

Although the correct diagnosis is of paramount importance in planning surgery, needless delays for diagnostic procedures must be avoided when the need for emergency laparotomy is clear. Incisions should be planned to minimize interference with postoperative pulmonary function whenever possible. Surgical technique should attempt to be gentle to tissues, yet minimize operating time. Speed can be best influenced by careful intraoperative decision making, especially in selecting less complex procedures, when permitted as in the selection of vagotomy and drainage instead of antrectomy as the preferred operation for bleeding peptic ulcer disease in elderly patients. Incidental procedures have no role in geriatric abdominal surgery. However, other well-considered procedures may minimize postoperative complications. The high-risk pulmonary patient may benefit from a gastrostomy in place of prolonged nasogastric intubation; the malnourished patient may benefit from a feeding jejunostomy instead of intravenous hyperalimentation. The anticipated risk-benefit ratio must be carefully scrutinized for each procedure. Most importantly, the procedure must be carefully tailored to fit the geriatric patient, not vice versa.

No discussion of operative technique today would be complete without mention of laparoscopic surgery. In the initial experience with laparoscopic cholecystectomy, elderly patients were often excluded due to fears arising from the extra duration of the procedure and unknown physiologic effects of prolonged pneumoperitoneum. As techniques have improved, the operating times for laparoscopic and open procedures have become similar, and this is no longer a concern. Increased abdominal pressure, when properly monitored, generally does not significantly compromise venous return to the heart unless combined with extreme patient positioning, and this can easily be monitored and prevented. Pneumoperitoneum using CO_2 for prolonged periods can, however, produce acidosis from CO_2 absorption. (28). The anesthesiologist may have to monitor and compensate for this by adjusting ventilation settings. In elderly patients with severe COPD, laparoscopic surgery may not be feasible. Currently, "gasless" laparoscopy is under investigation, and this technique may be of value in such cases. Successful laparoscopic gastrointestinal surgery may be of perticular benefit in the geriatric patient, as it provides for less postoperative pain, less analgesic use, less respiratory compromise, less paralytic ileus, and greater morbidity. Preliminary investigation seems to indicate that immunologic responsiveness is preserved and, hence, laparoscopic surgery may be "less traumatic" (29).

VI. THE SURGEON'S ROLE

From the above discussion it should be evident that carefully considered, properly timed, and well-executed gastrointestinal surgery is relatively safe in elderly patients. In order to assure maximum benefit and to minimize risk, a coordinated approach including surgeons, anesthesiologists, and medical specialists is required. Additional assistance from geriatric social workers, nurses, and physical therapists may also be needed. Decisions must be made regarding endoscopic or laparoscopic surgery, invasive radiologic procedures, or open laparotomy with a clear knowledge of the risks and benefits of each weighed against the medical condition of the patient and the natural history of the disease to be treated. Education of patients and family members must be undertaken to dispel the myth of patients being "too old" for surgery, as well as knowing the limits of currently available techniques in high-risk or hopeless situations.

Properly, responsibility for this role must be undertaken by the geriatric surgeon, although no recognized subspecialty training or recognition of this field currently exists. No one else is so fully cognizant of all the variables and better qualified to deal with the often difficult decisions that must be made, in concert with all the members of the geriatric team. With such an effort, hopefully, improvement in the outcome for gastrointestinal surgery in the geriatric population will be realized.

REFERENCES

1. Vowles KJD. Surgical problems in the aged. Bristol, England: John Wright & Sons, 1979.
2. Smith O. Med Rec 1907; 72:642–644.
3. Brooks B. Surgery in patients of advanced age. Ann Surg 1937; 105:481–495.
4. Wilder RJ, Fishbein RH. Operative complications and mortality in patients over 80 years of age. Surg Gynecol Obstet 1961; 113:205–211.
5. Marshall WH, Fahey PJ. Operative complications and mortality in patients over 80 years of age. Arch Surg 1964; 88:896–904.
6. Pjokovic TL, Hedley-White J. Prediction of outcome of surgery and anesthesia in patients over 80. JAMA 1979; 242:2301–2306.
7. Denny JL, Denson JS. Risk of surgery in patients over 90. Geriatrics 1972; 27:115–118.
8. Katlic MR. Surgery in centenarians. JAMA 1985; 253(21):3139–3141.
9. Owens WD, Felts JA, Spitznagel EL. ASA physical status classifications: a study of consistency of ratings. Anesthesiology 1978; 49:239–243.
10. Goldman L, Caldera D, Nussbaum S, et al. Multifactorial index of cardiac risk in noncardiac surgical procedures. N Engl J Med 1977; 297;16:845–850.
11. Zeldin R. Assessing cardiac risk on patients who undergo noncardiac surgical procedures. Can J Surg 1984; 27:402.
12. Petsky AS, Abrams H, McLaughlin J, et al. Predicting cardiac complications in patients undergoing noncardiac surgery. J Gen Intern Med 1986; 1:211.
13. Weitz H. Noncardiac surgery in the elderly patient with cardiovascular disease. Clin Geriatr Med 1990; 6(3):511–529.
14. Knaus W, Wagner D, Draper E, et al. The APACHE III diagnostic system: risk prediction of hospital mortality for critically ill hospitalized adults. Chest 1991; 100(6):1619–1636.

15. Tiret L et al. Complications associated with anesthesia: A prospective study in France. Can Anaesth Soc J 1986; 33:336–344.

16. Hosking MP et al. Outcome of surgery on patients 90 years old and older. JAMA 1989; 261:1909–1915.

17. Houghton PW, Jenkinson LR, Donaldson LA. Cholecystectomy in the elderly: a prospective study. Br J Surg 1985; 72:220–222.

18. Lau WY, Fan ST, Yiu TF, et al. Acute appendicitis in the elderly. Surg Gynecol Obstet 1985; 161:157–161.

19. Gerson MD, Hurst JM, Hertzberg VS, et al. Prediction of cardiac and pulmonary complications related to elective abdominal and noncardiac thoracic surgery is geriatric patients. Am J Med 1990; 88:101–107.

20. Boucher CA, Brewster DC, Darling C, et al. Determination of cardiac risk by dipyridamole-thallium imaging before peripheral vascular surgery. N Engl J Med 1985; 312(7):389–394.

21. DelGuercio L, Cohen JD. Monitoring operative risk in the elderly. JAMA 1980; 243(13):1350–1355.

22. Seymour DG, Pringle R. Post-operative complications in the elderly surgical patient. Gerontology 1983; 29:262.

23. Boghosian SG. Usefulness of routine preoperative chest roentgenograms in elderly patients. J Am Geriatr Soc 1987; 35:142.

24. Stein M, Koota GM, Simon M, et al. Pulmonary evaluation of surgical patients. JAMA 1962; 181:765.

25. Powers DC et al. In: Katlic MR, ed. Geriatric Surgery. Baltimore, MD: Urban & Schwartzenberg, 1990:173–181.

26. Palmberg S, Hirsjarvi E. Mortality in geriatric surgery. Gerontology 1979; 25:103.

27. Collins RC, Scrimgeour A, Yusuf S, et al. Reduction in fatal pulmonary embolism and venous thrombosis by perioperative administration of subcutaneous heparin. N Engl J Med 1988; 318:1162.

28. Wittgen CM et al. Analysis of the hemodynamic and ventilatory effects of laparoscopic cholecystectomy. Arch Surg 1991; 126:997–1000.

29. Trokel M. Personal communication.

17

Geriatric Gastroenterology in the Nursing Home

Carole A. Michelsen and Mark Chu
Beth Israel Medical Center, New York, New York

I. IN THE NURSING HOME

The nursing home is a challenging environment in which to provide medical care. The large and diverse population of nursing home residents has grown and currently consists of over 1.6 million people. While approximately only 5% of those over age 65 reside in a nursing home, one-quarter of all those over age 85 will at some time require nursing home care. As the "baby boomers" bound into old age and current socioeconomic trends (i.e., the two-income family) continue, it is anticipated that this population will also grow.

The nursing home is the most highly regulated healthcare setting, by both the individual states and federal regulation. OBRA, or the 1987 Omnibus Budget Reconciliation Act, is a law enacted to improve the standards of nursing home care. It linked compliance with regulation and reimbursement, and addressed many issues related both to quality of care and quality of life.

The purpose of this chapter is to highlight commonly encountered gastrointestinal problems in nursing home patients, and suggest practical treatment options.

II. MEDICATION USE

Medication use in the elderly is more complicated than in younger populations for a variety of reasons. The older person rarely has only one disease process to account for symptoms or which requires treatment. Polypharmacy is frequently encountered and often results in adverse drug effects and hospitalization.

There are significant federal regulations regarding the use of drugs in long-term-care facilities. These include the adequate dosing of drugs, surveillance for the use of duplicate therapy, time periods for the use of a specific drug, and the use of guidelines for monitoring purposes.

Inappropriate medication use is common in nursing homes. All too often orders are written at the time of admission and periodically renewed but less frequently assessed for efficacy, necessity, and ongoing need. It is essential to regularly determine the appropriateness of each resident's drug regimen. Common examples are the following:

1. NSAIDs are commonly used for extended periods without obtaining a hemoglobin level.
2. NSAID use in the presence of positive stool occult blood without explanation.
3. Vitamin B_{12} use in the absence of documented B_{12} deficiency or a diagnosis of pernicious anemia.
4. H_2 receptor antagonists used for greater than 3 months without an attempt to decrease the dose (except in cases of Zollinger Ellison syndrome or gastroesophageal reflux disease).

All of the above are easily avoided by carefully reviewing the medication regimen of the resident, and in cooperation with the interdisciplinary team including nurses, pharmacists, and other clinicians.

III. GASTROENTERITIS

Outbreaks of gastroenteritis occur in nursing home facilities from time to time. It is extremely important to quickly identify cases that may be related in order to develop strategies to investigate and contain an outbreak, and to minimize the risks for residents and staff.

An outbreak should be suspected whenever there is documentation of three or more cases in a single nursing unit, or when 30% or more of a facility's population develop symptoms, generally diarrhea and vomiting, with onset during a 7-day period. The diarrhea typically is three or more loose stools per day or an unexplained increase in the frequency of formed stools. Symptoms range in severity and may be associated with fever, anorexia, lethargy, nausea, and decline in functional status. Staff must also be assessed, though symptoms may vary from the residents affected.

The etiological agents responsible for outbreaks include *Shigella*, *Salmonella*, *Staphylococcus*, *E. coli*, and *Listeria* as well as viral agents, including hepatitis A. Management is generally symptomatic, and if a particular pathogen is identified, tailored to treat that organism. As soon as an outbreak is suspected, interim control measures are instituted, including the following:

1. Staff education on infection control technique
2. Emphasis on the importance of handwashing
3. Inspection of the kitchen area and any other areas possibly related to the outbreak
4. Enteric precautions when appropriate

In addition, the following might need to be considered, based upon the etiologic agent, severity of symptoms, number of residents and staff affected and other facility specific characteristics:

1. Restriction of new admissions to affected units or the facility
2. Limitation of off-unit activities
3. Restriction of visitors

Antiperistaltic agents should be avoided. Fluid balance should be assessed and maintained for all residents. In some cases, intravenous therapy will be needed, and in severe cases, hospitalization.

As soon as an initial assessment of the outbreak is made, the local area health department should be notified. The health department will often have information available regarding other facility and area outbreaks, and can be of great assistance in identifying the causative agent and providing helpful information to manage these situations. Of course the residents and families need to be informed of the facility's efforts, and education must be provided to reassure all involved.

IV. CONSTIPATION

Constipation cannot be described as a disease but as a symptom due to other causes. The complaints of decreased frequency of bowel movements and straining on defecation in the elderly population are labeled constipation. Some have characterized constipation as the inability to pass stool despite the urge to do so. Others may complain that their stools are too small or too hard and that defecation is painful or associated with abdominal distension and cramping with flatulation. There is general agreement that constipation is no more than two bowel movements per week and/or difficulty with defecation as described above. These are the wide ranges of subjective interpretations by the patients that vary with a physician's criteria for constipation.

A. Complications

In the nursing home, constipation, real or imagined, is a very common complaint. It is often disregarded as a minor symptom but is a major cause of abdominal discomfort and could lead to severe complications such as megacolon, volvulus, and fecal impaction. The most serious complication is fecal impaction, which can lead to fecal incontinence with frequent diarrhea, intestinal obstruction, stercoral ulcerations, and ischemic bowel. Hemodynamic compromise from increased intrathoracic pressure during straining can cause decreased flow to coronary, cerebral, and peripheral circulation.

B. Normal Physiology—Defecation

The stimulus for initiating defecation is from distension of the rectum by fecal mass. This occurs when stool is delivered from the sigmoid colon via movement due to peristalsis. There is involuntary relaxation of the puborectalis muscle and internal anal sphincter, as well as contraction of the external sphincter, which is under voluntary control. The individual can therefore push the bolus past the external sphincter.

C. Causes of Constipation

Colonic motility in healthy, elderly subjects shows no decline with aging. However, there is marked increase in colonic transit times in patients with constipation, especially in the area of the left colon and rectum, resulting in decreased fecal bulk from water reabsorption and harder stools. This could be due to decreased intrinsic innervation of the myenteric plexus and or increase in beta-endorphin concentrations in the plasma, which bind to opiate receptors in the gut. In the rectum, there are two observed changes in patients with constipation. First, there is increased rectal tone with decreased rectal compliance. Second, there is reduced tone with an impaired rectal threshold that requires a larger amount of stool in the rectal ampulla to initiate reflex relaxation of the internal anal sphincter.

Constipation in the elderly can be attributed to underlying medical illnesses, medications, dietary fiber, and fluids. It is believed that immobility and bed rest contribute to decreased colonic motility. This is because the gastrocolic reflex needs physical activity to move fecal bolus through the gastrointestinal tract. Patients with poor dietary intake of fiber have been correlated with chronic constipation. Paradoxically, in patients with chronic constipation, fiber can increase the large amount of feces already present and exacerbate the symptoms. Dehydration can cause reabsorption of water from the fecal bolus and resultant decrease in fecal bulk and hard stools. Medications with strong anticholinergic properties affect the contractility of the smooth muscle of the gut by an antimuscarinic action at acetylcholine receptor sites.

Drugs commonly used in the nursing home can cause constipation (Table 1). Psychiatric illness does not predispose a patient to become constipated, but associated factors such as immobility, psychotropic medications, and poor diet are risk factors for constipation.

Diseases that affect the autonomic and peripheral nervous systems such as Parkinson's disease and diabetes cause constipation through bowel dysmotility, muscular weakness, and incoordination. Electrolyte abnormalities such as hypokalemia decrease acetylcholine effect on gut smooth muscle. Hypercalcemia causes delayed innervation of the gastrointestinal tract. The underlying metabolic and/or endocrinologic pathologies are possibly correctable with specific therapy and must be investigated.

Table 1 Causes of Constipation

Incorrect subjective view	Drugs	Metabolic
Low-fiber diet	Antacids (calcium,	Hypercalcemia
Dehydration	aluminum)	Hypokalemia
Immobility	Opiates	Hypomagnesemia
Fecal impaction	Anticholinergics	Obstruction
Depression	Anticonvulsants	Tumors
Dementia	Antidepressants	Adhesions
Stroke	Antipsychotics	Chronic volvulus
Parkinson's disease	Antianxiety	Hernias
Multiple sclerosis	Antiparkinsons	Ischemic colitis
Paraplegia	Antiemetics	Radiation
Aganglionosis	Calcium channel	Diverticular disease
Hirschsprung's disease	blockers	Irritable bowel
Chagas' disease	Iron	syndrome
Laxative induced	Diuretics	Anorectal disease
(irritants)	Calcium	Hemorrhoids
	Endocrine	Rectal prolapse
	Hypothyroidism	Fissures
	Hyperthyroidism	Fistulas
	Diabetes	Perirectal abscess
	Hyperparathyroidism	
	Hypopituitarism	

Obstructive colonic pathologies are more prevalent in the geriatric population and if symptoms are of recent onset, one should suspect the presence of tumor.

Laxative use and abuse are common in our elderly population due to poor patient education and belief that if daily stools do not occur, they are constipated. Chronic habitual use of laxatives may result in the cathartic colon. This is due to the degeneration of the myenteric plexus as a result of overstimulation.

D. H & P

Evaluation of constipation requires a detailed bowel history of the patient including frequency of bowel movements, necessity to strain during defecation, and character of stools. The presence of incontinence of urine and feces, pain on defecation, and history of laxative use are indicators in diagnosing clinical constipation. Recent dietary changes and medication use should be noted. An accurate medical history is required to rule out treatable organic causes along with the physical examination that includes a digital rectal exam. This exam will identify hemorrhoids, rectal impaction, sphincter tone, and painful anorectal conditions. Stool is checked for occult blood and if present, workup to locate the source with barium enema and/ or endoscopy is indicated. When the history and physical do not point to a possible cause of constipation, serum electrolytes and thyroid function studies should be reviewed.

E. Radiologic Studies

Diagnostic imaging studies should start with the plain abdominal film. The plain film can demonstrate fecal impaction, fecoliths, obstructions, megacolon, and perforations. Barium enemas are indicated for any patient with a long history of constipation. Disease states that can be identified easily are diverticulosis, Hirshsprung's disease, hernias, chronic sigmoid volvulus, radiation changes, and carcinomas.

Intestinal transit study gives a good estimate of bowel motility and can localize segments of small intestine or colon with abnormal peristalsis. Patients are asked to swallow radiopaque markers, and successive abdominal radiographs are taken. Locations of the markers are documented over the next 5 days, with a normal study showing 50–80% of marker being eliminated. If greater than half the markers are present, the abnormal segment of bowel can be identified.

The observed physiologic changes in the elderly constipated patient are mainly in the area of the left colon and rectum. Since the 1960s, cineradiographic studies have been utilized to study anorectal physiology and evacuation. The procedures involved in defecography are easy to perform and to interpret. The indications for defecography include abnormal intestinal transit study with localization in the rectosigmoid, incomplete evacuation, pain, constant urge to defecate with difficulty in emptying the rectum, and fecal incontinence. Defecography is also used to identify prolapse of perineal structures and changes that occur with straining.

F. Treatment of Constipation

The initial approach to constipation is to identify underlying treatable causes and employ appropriate therapy. If none, the fluid status of the patient must be assessed. Dehydration should be corrected by encouraging fluid intake unless contraindicated by a medical condition. Fiber should only be used in a mobile patient since it can cause exacerbation of constipation. The recommended treatment can be with 6–15 g of bran daily or psyllium 10 g twice daily. The patient must take advantage of the gastrocolic reflex that occurs after meals by toileting themselves. Ambulating after a mean is encouraged since this will increase colonic motility. Irritant laxatives should be avoided such as senna, phenolphthalein, bisacodyl, and caster oil. Saline laxatives such as milk of magnesia have a rapid onset of action by stimulating cholecytokinins and causing osmotic movement into the intestinal lumen.

Lactulose and sorbitol act as osmotic agents and shorten transit time but are nonabsorbable, and long-term safety has been shown in the elderly (with lactulose). Stool softeners such as docusate have not been shown to cause a laxative effect but aid in evacuating bulkier stool. Enemas with phosphate and soap can cause mucosal damage; a safer alternative is tap water. Lubrication with glycerine suppositories and mineral oil are also effective as well as safe.

V. *CLOSTRIDIUM DIFFICILE* IN THE NURSING HOME

Clostridium difficile is the Gram-positive obligate anaerobic bacterium responsible for pseudomembranous colitis, and a major cause of nosocomial diarrhea. It is often suspect in the nursing home when there is an outbreak of diarrhea, especially after antibiotic therapy. The prevalence of this bacterium in the nursing home has an adverse effect on the morbidity and mortality of the patient population in that facility.

A. Pathophysiology

The pathogenesis of the diarrhea observed in *C. difficile* colitis is due to two exotoxins, A and B. Toxin A is an enterotoxin and primarily responsible for the symptoms caused by mucosal damage, intestinal inflammation, and secretion of fluids into the intestinal lumen. Toxin B is a cytotoxin which disrupts the actin-cytoskeleton of a cell and causes rounding of a culture cell. There is a laboratory method by which infection with *C. difficile* can be identified. The toxins bind to a receptor on an enterocyte and enters a cell that causes an inflammatory reaction with neutrophil chemotaxis and release of cytokines from macrophages. The pseudomembranous changes seen during endoscopy are due to exudate consisting of fibrin, mucin, leucocytes, and debris that cover an ulceration and necrosis of the mucosa. The presentations of these lesions vary with the severity of the symptoms from diffuse to none.

The elderly have been shown to be more susceptible to colonization with *C. difficile* and are often asymptomatic. The older patient has physiologic age-related immunodeficiencies such as the decreased ability to phagocytize *C. difficile* organisms by polymorphonuclear leucocytes. Also, it was found that serum of elderly patients who are infected with *C. difficile* have decreased toxin-neutralizing antibodies. Other factors that predispose a nursing home patient to infection are frequent use of antibiotics, contamination of an area with *C. difficile* spores, presence of nasogastric and/or gastrostomy tubes, fecal incontinence, and any medications that can change the environment of the bowel such as laxatives and stool softeners. Antibiotic use is clearly a precipitating factor due to destruction of normal flora and overgrowth with resistant *C. difficile*. The most common antibiotics implicated are the cephalosporins, penicillins, and clindamycin. The least likely antibiotics are aminoglycosides, metronidazole, and vancomycin. The role of the healthcare worker in preventing transmission of the infection is crucial. Handwashing with a disinfectant, chlorohexidine soap, use of disposable gloves, and disposable single-use thermometer may help reduce outbreaks but can still occur.

B. Presentation

Patients with *C. difficile* infection can present in many ways including an asymptomatic carrier state, antibiotic-related colitis without pseudomembranes, pseudomembranous colitis, and fulminant colitis. The asymptomatic carrier plays a major role in outbreaks of *C. difficile* in a medical environment. They are reservoirs of the organism that contaminates an area and perpetuate the chain of infection. Treatment of asymptomatic carriers with metronidazole or vancomycin has shown no effect in reducing the rate of outbreaks and is not recommended. In fact, treatment can prolong the carrier state and cause symptoms by supressing normal flora.

The presentation of *C. difficile* infection is with diarrhea, diffuse crampy abdominal pain, chills, fever, dehydration, and peripheral leucocytosis.

Symptoms usually present during or slightly after antibiotics treatment but can appear later, in 4–6 weeks. In antibiotic-related colitis without pseudomembranes, the symptoms are usually mild and subside when the antibiotics are stopped. Medications that cause decreased motility must be avoided since prolonged colonic exposure to toxins can result in toxic megacolon. Pseudomembranous colitis presents with the above symptoms, and sigmoidoscopy reveals the characteristic yellow-white raised plaques (2–10 mm in diameter) over large areas of mucosa. This can progress to fulminant colitis if not treated and can result in toxic megacolon, perforation, peritonitis, and death. This condition requires immediate treatment with metroindazole or vancomycin.

C. Diagnosis

The diagnosis of *C. difficile* is made by stool-cytotoxin studies by observing the action of toxin B on culture cells. This is the gold standard due to high sensitivity and specificity. However, overnight incubation of samples is necessary and the test is expensive. There is a rapid latex agglutination test that is designed to detect toxin A but has cross-reactivity with strain of nonpathogenic clostridia. The enzyme immunoassay test detect either toxin A or B and has better sensitivity and specificity than the latex agglutination and can provide results in a few hours.

D. Treatment

The initial treatment of *C. difficile* infection is oral metronidazole 250 mg four times daily. Another option is oral vancomycin 125 mg four times daily is very effective and is not absorbed by the intestines. Rapid improvements in symptoms should appear within 2–3 days, with return to normal bowel movements in 7–10 days. Despite the fact that metronidazole-resistant *C. difficile* exists, it is preferred initially over vancomycin due to cost. Metronidazole can be used in situations where oral medication is contraindicated such as surgery. It is given parenterally and has excretion into the bile and exudation through the inflamed colonic mucosa to achieve high concentrations in the lumen. Bacitracin has good activity against *C. difficile* and, like vancomycin, is poorly absorbed from the gut. The cost of therapy is very expensive, and recurrence is great. Anion exchange resins such as cholestyramine bind to toxin and can be used in some cases of relapse, but this should not be a first-line drug of choice.

Relapse of symptoms occur in 10–25% of patients when antibiotic therapy is withdrawn. This usually occurs 1–3 weeks after therapy has ended. If symptoms are mild, therapy may be withheld. If diarrhea persists or is severe, patient may be retreated with metronidazole. Various attempts to restore normal flora have been tried such as bacteriotherapy with fecal enema prepared from healthy people and ingestion of lactobacilli cultures.

VI. FECAL INCONTINENCE

The term fecal incontinence has been defined as involuntary excretion or leakage of stool at inappropriate times. Fecal incontinence is a common problem in the elderly and the nursing home patient. It is also associated with functional impairment such as dementia, and family members have a difficult time caring for the person. This is a common reason for referral to a skilled nursing facility for management. It is estimated that about 50% of nursing home patients suffer from this distressing and embarrassing condition.

A. Physiology of Continence

The maintenance of continence is through the sphincteric mechanisms, ability to sense rectal filling, and compliance of the colon and rectum to store feces. The internal sphincter, under involuntary control, is in a state of contraction at rest, and the external sphincter can remain voluntarily contracted for only a few minutes. As stool enters the distal rectum, the internal sphincter relaxes and the external sphincter reflexively contracts simultaneously. The puborectalis muscles act as a sling to keep the anorectal angle acute and to control passage of stools. This muscle acts in accordance with the external anal sphincter. After the rectum is filled with stool (approximately 150–200 ml), the internal sphincter will relax completely. When convenient, the external sphincter and puborectalis muscle can relax and stool is passed, but, if inconvenient, the internal sphincter contracts again.

B. Causes of Fecal Incontinence

In the institutionalized, elderly patient with fecal incontinence, the problem is usually due to fecal impaction and leakage of liquid stool around the obstruction. In a majority of patients with fecal impaction, the abnormality found was impairment in rectal sensation that required larger volumes of stool to cause feelings of fullness and desire to defecate. These patients did not have reflexive relaxation of the internal anal sphincter, and therefore the external anal sphincter, along with the puborectalis muscle, did not contract to prevent leakage of stool. With impaction, there is also increased and prolonged straining at stool. This causes stretching and compression of nerves with degeneration and secondary loss of muscle tone. These degenerative changes are also seen in patients with rectal prolapse and perineal descent (Table 2).

Neurologic disorders such as peripheral neuropathy due to diabetes cause fecal incontinence through a number of reasons. In the colon, neuropathy can cause decreased motility and constipation resulting in impaction. Diabetic involvement of the small intestine is usually characterized by diarrhea. The pathophysiology of the diarrhea is unclear, but speculations range from malabsorption of bile salts to bacterial overgrowth due to decreased motility. There is also weakened sphincteric function, especially in patients with longstanding diabetic neuropathy. However, it is unclear whether the dysfunction is secondary to defective peripheral or autonomic nervous regulation.

Functional impairment due to dementia and immobility are common causes of fecal soiling. Patients with moderate to severe dementia are unable to inhibit intrinsic rectal contractions that result from distension and usually pass formed stools occurring after meals in accordance with the gastrocolic reflex. Immobility causes chronic constipation, impaction, and overflow diarrhea.

Conditions that cause decreased rectal capacity are surgery, radiation, tumors, and fibroelastic changes seen with normal aging. The rectum has higher pressures with a smaller amount of stool which increases urgency and inhibits sphincter tone. Also, there are decreased strength of the external anal sphincter and decreased resting tone of the internal anal sphincter.

C. Evaluation

Evaluation of the patient begins with a history and physical exam. The information gathered in the history should describe urgency and frequency

Table 2 Causes of Fecal Incontinence

Fecal impaction	Decreased rectal compliance
Functional impairment	Radiation
Dementia	Tumor
Confusion	Surgery
Immobility	Aging
Weakness	Ischemia
Neurologic conditions	Anorectal injury from trauma
Diabetes with neuropathy	Rectal prolapse
Spinal chord lesion (low lesion)	Diarrhea
Multiple sclerosis	Infectious diarrhea
Strokes	Inflammatory bowel disease
Perineal descent with neuropathy	Laxative abuse

versus true incontinence. History of trauma, surgery, anorectal disease, and irradiation should be sought. Also, underlying medical conditions and medications may be exacerbating the symptoms and must be addressed. Once the diagnosis of true incontinence is decided, the severity of the condition needs to be assessed. This can be determined through questions on necessity of diapers and passage of liquid or formed stools. A good physical examination of the anus, rectum, and perineum during rest and straining must be done. A digital rectal exam will allow palpation of external sphincter and puborectalis muscle tone at rest and during voluntary contraction. At the same time, one must check for presence of hard stools and occult blood. The next step would be confirmation of the diagnosis through physiologic testing. Anal manometry measures the pressure generated by sphincter both at rest and during contraction. This exam also evaluate sensation and rectal compliance. Cinedefecography shows actual defecation of a barium paste that assesses rectal capacity, anorectal angle, and presence of rectoceles, enteroceles, or prolapse. Electromyography can demonstrate the integrity of sphincter innervation. Sigmoidoscopy will allow visualization of tumors, strictures, and inflammation.

D. Treatment

Treatment of fecal incontinence should begin with identification of an underlying cause and give specific treatment if possible. Fecal impaction should be removed using enemas daily or twice daily until the colon is empty. Manual disimpaction may be necessary in severe cases. After the colon is cleansed, the immobile, demented patient must be placed on a restricted fiber diet to prevent increased fecal mass. Enemas should be used on a weekly basis to prevent reaccumulation of stools.

In the intact elderly patient, biofeedback programs and bowel training show good results. Biofeedback training consists of insertion of an anorectal manometer and visual display to self-regulate anal sphincter responses. Biofeedback is successful in all types of patients, but certain criteria must be met to start the program. Patients must have some evidence of rectal sensation and motivation and be free of neurologic diseases that would impair ability to follow instructions. Bowel habit training consists of using the gastrocolic reflex with regular toileting. If there is no defecation after 2–3 days, an enema or suppository can be used to stimulate a bowel movement.

Chronic loose stools and incontinence due to decreased rectal compliance can be treated with low dietary fiber and planned toileting; if all else fails, loperamide can be administered. If prolapse is the cause of soiling, surgery is the best option. Multiple surgical procedures are available to repair prolapse from rectopexy to rectosigmoidectomy. Long-term, controlled studies are needed to compare the efficacy of surgical repair to conservative techniques.

E. Weight Loss

One frequently encountered problem in the long-term care setting is weight loss. This finding must always be addressed promptly, as it impacts on the resident's quality of life, risk for illness, and, ultimately, survival. Many reversible causes can be identified and treated, resulting in stabilization of the resident's condition.

All residents should be weighed regularly and, at the least, monthly. For residents who are new to a facility, experience an illness, become hospitalized, or show a functional decline, weekly weight will be of benefit to quickly identify and any negative trend. Prompt identification evaluation and treatment are crucial for both planning and avoidance of complications.

One of the most common causes of weight loss is depression. Medication use and medication adjustment including psychotropic drug reduction are also major causes of weight loss. Dementia and swallowing disorders are both common and result in chronic progressive weight loss. Medical conditions including COPD, CHF, cancer, infections, and dehydration also contribute to this common problem.

The investigation of weight loss should include a careful review of the time of onset, relation to medication use or changes, and the medical condition. Physical examination might be helpful, and evaluation of the mental status and screening for depression are helpful. Laboratory investigations can complete a review after an adequate history and physical examination.

F. Ethical Issues

Ethical dilemmas regarding therapies that sustain life are frequently encountered in the long-term care setting. One particularly difficult situation is the resident with advancing dementia or cognitive loss where a decision regarding feeding tube insertion must be made. As many nursing homes now provide care to increasing numbers of younger people with AIDS, this is no longer an ethical dilemma of the elderly.

Despite the enactment of the Patient Self Determination Act, most nursing residents do not have health-care proxies, nor have they ever discussed advanced directives or care preferences before admission. Meaningful decisions are not possible by the time a resident is admitted. In other cases, though information might be provided, more can be done to assess and document care preferences to help clinicians and family in decision making when the resident loses capacity.

Studies regarding limitations of treatment document that many healthy nursing home residents would reject life-sustaining tube feedings. Many physicians also support the limitations of tube feedings, particularly if the care preferences of residents are known. Sometimes there is discordance between resident and family; education can benefit family members and aid in the decision making processing.

It is known that terminal phase of dementia can be prolonged in the nursing home by tube feedings. It is, however, also known that the terminal phase of dementia cannot be reversed and that tube feeding is a temporizing measure at best, and eventual death is inevitable.

Individual cases are often complicated by the lack of a meaningful doctor-patient-family relationship, physicians' biases toward care options, and the variability of both state regulation and legal precedent. Each situation must be addressed as it arises, promptly and thoroughly; often persons distanced from the case may be of assistance.

The roles of institutional ethics committees are evolving and their expertise should be sought to facilitate decision making. Perhaps the area where physicians can be of greatest assistance is in encouraging the use of advanced directives for their patients and discussing issues that occur at the end of life when patients are able to reflect and consider choices. These discussions are both accepted by and not distressing for patients. In properly explaining the choices, the physician can ease the burden of those making the ethical decisions.

REFERENCES

1. Barrett JA. Colorectal disorders in elderly people. Br Med J 1992; 305:774–776.
2. Beers MH, Ouslander JG, Fingold SF, et al. Inappropriate medication prescribing in skilled-nursing facilities. Ann Intern Med 1992;117:684–689.
3. Elon R, Pawlson LG. The impact of OBRA on medical practice within nursing facilities. J Am Geriatr Soc 40:958–963.
4. Ench P. Biofeedback training in disordered defecation, a critical review. Dig Dis Sci 1993; 38(11).
5. Harari D, Gurwitz JH, Minaker KL. Constipation in the elderly. J Am Geriatr Soc 1993; 41:1130–1140.
6. Hold PR. Diarrhea and malabsorption in the elderly. Gastroenterol Clin North Am 1990; 19(2).
7. Kane RL, Kane RA. A nursing home in your future? N Engl J Med 1991; 324(9):627.
8. Kelly CP, Pothoulakis C, LaMont JT. *Clostridium difficile* colitis. N Engl J Med 1994; 330:257–262.

9. Kemper P, Murtaugh CM, Lifetime use of nursing home care. N Engl J Med 1991; 324(9):595.
10. Levenson SA. Medical Direction in Long-Term Care, A Guidebook for the Future, Second Edition. Carolina Academic Press, 1993.
11. Libow LS, Starer P. Care of the nursing home patient. Med Intelligence 321(2):93–96.
12. Madoff RD, Williams JG, Causbal PF. Fecal incontinence. N Engl J Med 1993;326(15):1002–1007.
13. Morley JE, Kraenzle D. Causes of weight loss in a community nursing home. J Am Geriatr Soc 1994;42:583–585.
14. Murray FE, Bliss CM. Geriatric constipation: brief update on a common problem. Geriatrics 1991; 46:64–68.
15. Ogbonnaya KI, Arem R. Diabetic diarrhea, pathophysiology, diagnosis, and management. Arch Intern Med 1990; 150.
16. Ouslander JG, Tymchuk AJ, Krynski MD. Decisions about enteral tube feeding among the elderly. J Am Geriatr Soc 1993; 41:70–77.
17. Ouslander JG, Osterweil D, Morley J. Medical Care in the Nursing Home. New York: McGraw-Hill, 1991.
18. Peck A, Cohen CE, Mulvihill MN. Long-term enteral feeding of aged demented nursing home patients. J Am Geriatr Soc 1990; 38:1195–1198.
19. Simor AE, Yake SL, Tsimidis K. Infection due to *Clostridium difficile* among elderly residents of a long-term care facility. Clin Infect Dis 1993; 17:672–678.
20. Thomas DR, Bennett RG, et al. Postantibiotic colonization with *Clostridium difficile* in nursing home patients. J Am Geriatr Soc 1990; 38:415–420.
21. Wald A. Constipation and fecal incontinence in the elderly. Gastroenterol Clin North Am 1990; 19(2).
22. Walker KJ, Gililand SS, et al. *Clostridium difficile* colonization in residents of long-term care facilities: prevalence and risk factors. J Am Geriatr Soc 1993; 41:940–946.
23. Von Preyss–Friedman SM, Uhlmann RF, Cain KC. Physicians' attitudes toward tube feeding chronically ill nursing home patients. J Gen Intern Med J 1992; 46–51.

Index